Genitourinary Ultrasound

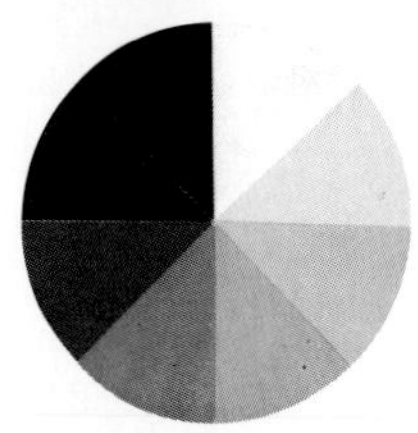

CLINICS IN DIAGNOSTIC ULTRASOUND
VOLUME 18

EDITORIAL BOARD

Volumes Already Published

Vol. **1** Diagnostic Ultrasound in Gastrointestinal Disease, Kenneth J.W. Taylor, Guest Editor

Vol. **2** Genitourinary Ultrasonography, Arthur T. Rosenfield, Guest Editor

Vol. **3** Diagnostic Ultrasound in Obstetrics, John C. Hobbins, Guest Editor

Vol. **4** Two-dimensional Echocardiography, Joseph A. Kisslo, Guest Editor

Vol. **5** New Techniques and Instrumentation, P.N.T. Wells and Marvin C. Ziskin, Guest Editors

Vol. **6** Ultrasound in Cancer, Barry B. Goldberg, Guest Editor

Vol. **7** Ultrasound in Emergency Medicine, Kenneth J.W. Taylor and Gregory N. Viscomi, Guest Editors

Vol. **8** Diagnostic Ultrasound in Pediatrics, Jack O. Haller and Arnold Shkolnik, Guest Editors

Vol. **9** Case Studies in Ultrasound, Harris J. Finberg, Guest Editor

Forthcoming Volumes in the Series

Genitourinary Ultrasound

Edited by

Hedvig Hricak, M.D.

Associate Professor of Radiology and Urology
Department of Radiology
University of California, San Francisco
School of Medicine
San Francisco, California

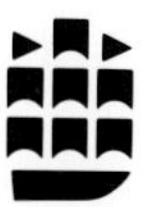

CHURCHILL LIVINGSTONE
NEW YORK, EDINBURGH, LONDON, MELBOURNE
1986

Acquisitions Editor: Robert Hurley
Copy Editor: Michael Kelley
Production Designer: Charlie Lebeda
Production Supervisor: Sharon Tuder
Compositor: Kingsport Press
Printer/Binder: Halliday Lithograph

Accurate indications, adverse reactions, and dosage schedules for drugs are provided in this book, but it is possible that they may change. The reader is urged to review the package information data of the manufacturers of the medications mentioned.

Distributed in the United Kingdom by Churchill Livingstone, Robert Stevenson House, 1–3 Baxter's Place, Leith Walk, Edinburgh EH1 3AF and by associated companies, branches and representatives throughout the world.

First published 1986

Printed in USA

ISBN 0–443–08409–2

7 6 5 4 3 2 1

Library of Congress Cataloging-in-Publication Data
Main entry under title:

Genitourinary ultrasound.

   (Clinics in diagnostic ultrasound; v. 18)
   Includes bibliographies and index.
   1. Genito-urinary organs—Diseases—Diagnosis.
2. Diagnosis, Ultrasonic. I. Hricak, Hedvig.
II. Series. [DNLM: 1. Genital Diseases, Male—
diagnosis. 2. Urologic Diseases—diagnosis.
3. Ultrasonic Diagnosis. W1 CL831BC v.18 / WJ 141
G3315]
RC874.G46 1986   616.6'07543   85–24273
ISBN 0–443–08409–2

Manufactured in the United States of America

Contributors

Sharon L. Abrams, M.D.
Assistant Clinical Professor of Radiology, University of California, San Francisco, School of Medicine, San Francisco, California

Peter Burns, Ph.D.
Research Associate, Department of Diagnostic Radiology, Yale University School of Medicine, New Haven, Connecticut

Barbara A. Carroll, M.D.
Associate Professor of Radiology, Duke University Medical Center, Durham, North Carolina

Roy A. Filly, M.D.
Professor of Radiology, Obstetrics and Gynecology, and Reproductive Medicine, Chief, Section of Diagnostic Ultrasound, Department of Radiology, University of California, San Francisco, School of Medicine, San Francisco, California

Gerald W. Friedland, M.D.
Professor of Radiology, Stanford University School of Medicine, Stanford, California; Staff Radiologist, Palo Alto Veterans Administration Medical Center, Palo Alto, California

Debora Green, M.D.
Fellow in Ultrasound, Department of Radiology, Stanford University School of Medicine, Stanford, California

William K. Hoddick, M.D.
Clinical Instructor, Department of Radiology, University of California, San Francisco, School of Medicine, San Francisco, California

Hedvig Hricak, M.D.
Associate Professor of Radiology and Urology, Department of Radiology, University of California, San Francisco, School of Medicine, San Francisco, California

R. Brooke Jeffrey, Jr., M.D.
Assistant Professor of Radiology, University of California, San Francisco, School of Medicine, San Francisco, California

Neal Joseph, M.D.
Director of Cardiovascular and Interventional Radiology, Department of Radiology, The Western Pennsylvania Hospital, Pittsburgh, Pennsylvania

Ewa Kuligowska, M.D.
Associate Professor of Radiology, Boston University School of Medicine; Chief of Ultrasound Section, Boston City and University Hospitals, Boston, Massachusetts

Alfred B. Kurtz, M.D.
Professor of Radiology, Obstetrics and Gynecology, Department of Radiology, Jefferson Medical College of Thomas Jefferson University; Staff Radiologist, Thomas Jefferson University Hospital, Philadelphia, Pennsylvania

Tom F. Lue, M.D.
Assistant Professor of Urology, University of California, San Francisco, School of Medicine, San Francisco, California

Barry S. Mahony, M.D.
Assistant Professor of Radiology, Duke University Medical Center, Durham, North Carolina

Kenneth Marich
Product Manager, Peripheral, Vascular/Operative, Diasonics, Inc., San Francisco, California

Harvey L. Neiman, M.D.
Clinical Professor of Radiology, University of Pittsburgh School of Medicine; Chairman, Department of Radiology, The Western Pennsylvania Hospital, Pittsburgh, Pennsylvania

Inder Perkash, M.D., F.R.C.S.
The Paralyzed Veterans of America, Professor of Spinal Cord Injury Medicine, Professor of Surgery, Stanford University School of Medicine, Stanford, California; Chief, The Spinal Cord Injury Center, Veterans Administration Medical Center, Palo Alto, California

Matthew D. Rifkin, M.D.
Professor of Radiology, Jefferson Medical College of Thomas Jefferson University; Staff Radiologist, Thomas Jefferson University Hospital, Philadelphia, Pennsylvania

Thomas L. Slovis, M.D.
Clinical Professor of Radiology, Wayne State University School of Medicine, Detroit, Michigan

Kenneth J.W. Taylor, M.D., Ph.D., F.A.C.P.
Professor of Diagnostic Radiology, Yale University School of Medicine, New Haven, Connecticut

Robert L. Vogelzang, M.D.
Assistant Professor of Radiology, Northwestern University Medical School; Associate Attending Medical Staff, Northwestern Memorial Hospital, Chicago, Illinois

Contents

CASE STUDIES

Sharon L. Abrams

Preface

Ultrasonography has emerged in the last decade as one of the most frequently applied and useful diagnostic modalities. The broad scope in which this method is applied to the diagnosis and evaluation of abnormalities of the urogenital tract is effectively demonstrated in the chapters of this book.

Hardly any pathologic condition of the kidneys, urinary bladder, prostate, testicles, or uterus escapes scrutiny by this most versatile approach. Ultrasonography has so many advantages in this area, that it has, in most of the world, become the primary diagnostic modality. It is relatively inexpensive, has excellent spatial and temporal resolution, and has no harmful genetic or other biologic effects. It can be applied at the bedside and can provide images in any desired plane. Its disadvantages of low signal to noise ratio, lack of contrast media, and operator-dependence are relatively minor in view of its overwhelming usefulness.

The applications of ultrasound in the genitourinary tract are still expanding, as is clearly shown in the many new points brought out in the following chapters. It can be said truthfully that uroradiology has been re-born with the introduction of ultrasonography. With the new generations of radiology residents obtaining excellent training in this modality, its importance will only be enhanced and its use expanded.

Hedvig Hricak, M.D.

1 The Genitourinary System in Utero

BARRY S. MAHONY
ROY A. FILLY

GENERAL CONSIDERATIONS

Antenatal sonography readily demonstrates normal and abnormal fetal anatomy.[1] The use of ultrasound in the antepartum period provides an effective diagnostic tool with which to examine fetal organs in detail and to evaluate a variety of congenital malformations.[2-5] The fetal urinary tract, for example, can be delineated sonographically by the fifteenth menstrual week.[6] Since cystic or obstructive genitourinary lesions constitute the majority of causes for neonatal abdominal masses, since sonography accurately depicts fluid-filled pathological lesions, and since standards for assessment of normal fetal renal growth and echotexture exist, careful evaluation of the fetal abdomen will reliably detect many fetal genitourinary abnormalities.[7,8] Most renal anomalies are incidental findings, however, and are not detected unless a complete sonographic examination is performed.

Following detection of a fetal genitourinary anomaly, thorough evaluation of each of the components of the genitourinary system will frequently enable an accurate antenatal diagnosis. Knowledge of the normal sonographic appearance of the fetal genitourinary system and of the expected ultrasound features of the different anomalies assists in this task. The information supplied by antenatal sonography regarding fetal genitourinary anomalies assists the obstetrician and perinatalogist in prompt postnatal management. Furthermore, on the basis of information provided by anatenatal sonography, fetuses can be identified who may benefit from in utero therapy, since recent advances in urological management now permit diversion of significant obstructive urinary tract lesions.[9-11]

THE NORMAL FETAL GENITOURINARY SYSTEM

In the last half of gestation, most of the amniotic fluid arises from fetal urination.[12] An assessment of the quantity of amniotic fluid, therefore, constitutes the initial step in the evaluation of the fetal genitourinary system. A normal amount of amniotic fluid implies the presence of at least one functioning kidney.

Although the extreme variability of fetal positioning and the lack of subject contrast between kidney and the surrounding tissues do not permit consistent identification of both fetal kidneys, normal fetal kidneys may be identified in their paraspinous location as early as 15 menstrual weeks. In longitudinal section they appear as bilateral elliptical structures, and in transverse section they have a circular appearance adjacent to the lumbar spinal ossification centers bilaterally. Later in pregnancy echogenic retroperitoneal fat, which surrounds the kidneys, assists in their sonographic visualization. The echopenic fetal renal pyramids are arranged in anterior and posterior rows in a configuration corresponding to the calices (Fig. 1.1). The echotexture of the normal fetal renal cortex, which usually approximates or may even be slightly greater than that of the surrounding tissues, often highlights the relatively echopenic pyramids. Identification of the characteristic configuration of the pyramids in anterior and posterior rows avoids any potential confusion between renal pyramids and parenchymal cysts. Within the pelvocalyceal system a small amount of fluid may reside in the absence of obstruction.[13] We recently studied 100 consecutive fetal kidneys and observed a small amount of fluid in the intrarenal collecting system of 59 (Fig. 1.2).[14]

The fetal kidneys grow throughout gestation. Standards for renal length, width, thickness, volume, and circumference have been established as a function of menstrual age and correspond with measurements of renal size obtained on stillborn fetuses postnatally.[6-8] Throughout pregnancy the ratio of kidney circumference to abdominal circumference remains constant at 0.27 to 0.30. In the absence of another process, such as ascites, which will increase the abdominal circumference, significant deviation from this pattern permits antenatal detection of renal enlargement. Diminution in renal size is more difficult to detect because the exact renal border may be partially obscured and because of the wide standard deviation in renal size.

The normal fetal ureter cannot be routinely identified. However, as early as 15 menstrual weeks the normal fetal urinary bladder can be identified. Since the fetus normally fills and empties the urinary bladder every 30 to 45 minutes, the bladder will frequently be seen to increase in size and to empty during the course of a sonographic examination. At 32 weeks of gestation the maximum fetal bladder volume measures 10 cc.[15] By term, the normal fetal bladder volume quadruples. Similarly, fetal urine production, as calculated by determination of change in bladder volume with time, increases from 9.6 ml/hr at 30 weeks to 27.3 ml/hr at 40 weeks menstrual age.[16] Filling and emptying of the fetal urinary bladder confirms that the fetus produces urine but does not indicate the quality of urine produced. The normal fetal urinary bladder, the wall of

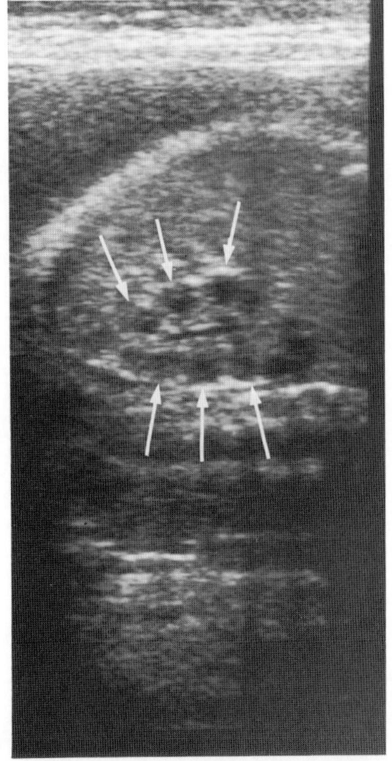

FIG. 1.1. High-resolution real-time sonogram of the fetal kidney at 35 menstrual weeks clearly demonstrates the echopenic renal pyramids (arrows) arranged in anterior and posterior rows.

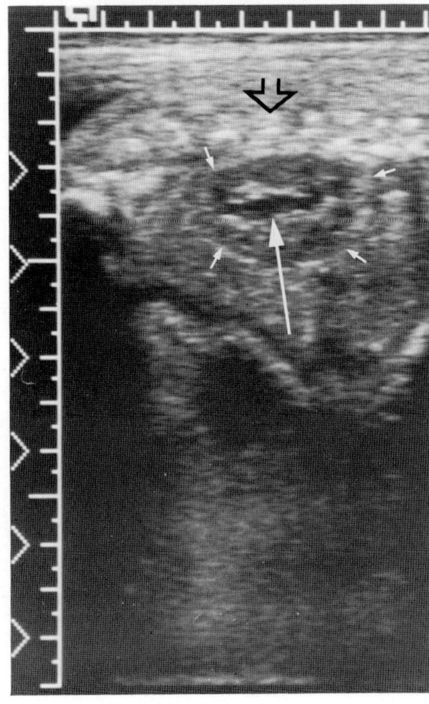

FIG. 1.2. A small amount of fluid (long arrow) resides within the renal pelvis of this fetal kidney (small arrows) at 31 menstrual weeks. Open arrow = fetal spine.

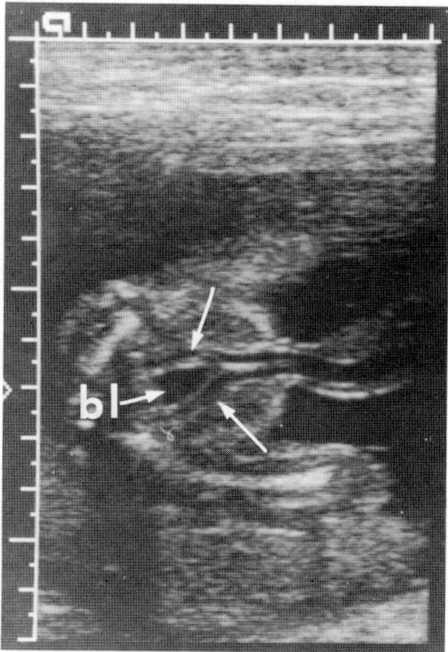

FIG. 1.3. The wall of the normal fetal urinary bladder is very thin or virtually invisible. In this 22-menstrual-week fetus, the iliac arteries (arrows) which course lateral to the urinary bladder (bl) delineate the bladder wall. This appearance should not be mistaken for bladder wall thickening.

which is very thin or virtually invisible, occupies a midline position within the fetal pelvis (Fig. 1.3). When distended, the urinary bladder becomes spherical or elliptical in configuration. Changes in volume of the urinary bladder with time differentiate it from other cystic pelvic structures. The normal fetal urethra may be identified as an echogenic line extending the length of an erect penis. In females and in males imaged at a time when the penis is flaccid, the normal urethra is more difficult to identify.

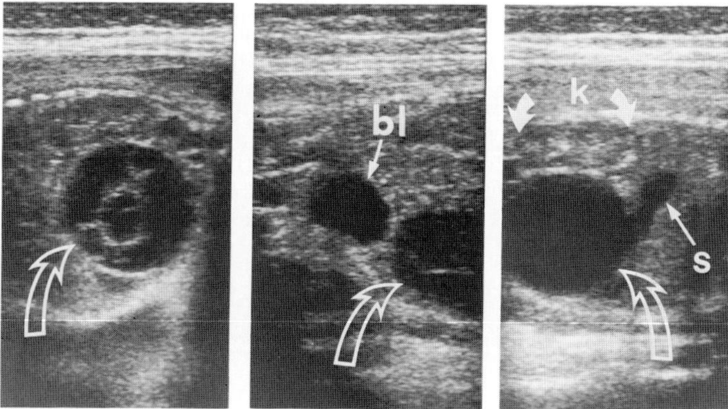

FIG. 1.4. A complex left pelvic cystic mass (open arrows) was noted on this antenatal sonogram at 32 menstrual weeks. Based upon the identification of the normal fetal urinary bladder (bl), kidneys (k), and stomach (s) which were separate from the mass, the antenatal diagnosis of a left ovarian cyst was made.

Previous reports regarding the fetal genital system have centered primarily upon determination of fetal sex.[17-19] Sex determination in the second trimester of pregnancy among fetuses at risk for severe X-linked disorders is of critical importance since unequivocal identification of a female fetus excludes the possibility of the fetus being affected with the disorder. Based upon visualization of the fetal penis, scrotum, or labia, Birnholtz reported a 99 percent accuracy of sex determination among fetuses of 15 or more weeks' gestational age.[17] However, in 31 percent of his 855 subjects, the external genitalia could not be visualized. Testicular descent into the scrotum occurs between 28 and 30 menstrual weeks in 62 percent of male fetuses and in 93 percent of male fetuses of greater than 32 menstrual weeks. Visualization of the ovaries, uterus, and vagina occurs less frequently unless these organs are enlarged and produce a pelvic mass such as occurs with a large ovarian cyst or with hydrocolpos (Fig. 1.4).

FETAL GENITOURINARY ANOMALIES

Renal Agenesis or Severe Hypoplasia

Absence of renal function, almost always secondary to bilateral renal agenesis or severe bilateral renal hypoplasia, represents a severe and lethal form of renal disease. Early identification of these lethal anomalies allows elective termination. Bilateral renal agenesis occurs in 1 of 4,000 births, more commonly in males than in females.[20,21] This entity is caused by embryological disturbance of the mesonephric duct which causes failure of the metanephric blastema to differentiate and leads to failure of the kidney and ureter to form. The absence of urine production causes severe oligohydramnios which results in pulmonary hypoplasia, the reason these infants die.

Sonographic observations which enable a confident diagnosis of absence of renal function to be made prior to the twentieth menstrual week include: (1) identification of severe oligohydramnios and (2) absence of urine within the fetal urinary bladder (Fig. 1.5). Unfortunately, the profound oligohydramnios and absence of fluid within the stomach and urinary bladder increase the difficulty in imaging these fetuses. In such circumstances, nonvisualization of the urinary bladder is more significant than apparent visualization of the kidneys because the fetal adrenal glands or bowel may simulate kidneys. This may lead to a false impression of the presence of kidneys. The most reliable feature which discriminates a kidney from either bowel or adrenal gland in the renal fossa is identification of medullary pyramids. Neither bowel nor adrenals are capable of simulating this appearance. In bilateral renal hypoplasia, the hypoplastic kidneys may be identified but the sonographic and clinical appearance is otherwise identical to that of bilateral renal agenesis.

If the fetal urinary bladder cannot be visualized over a period of approximately 2 hours, intravenous infusion of furosemide into the mother may be performed. The furosemide normally induces fetal diuresis approximately 15

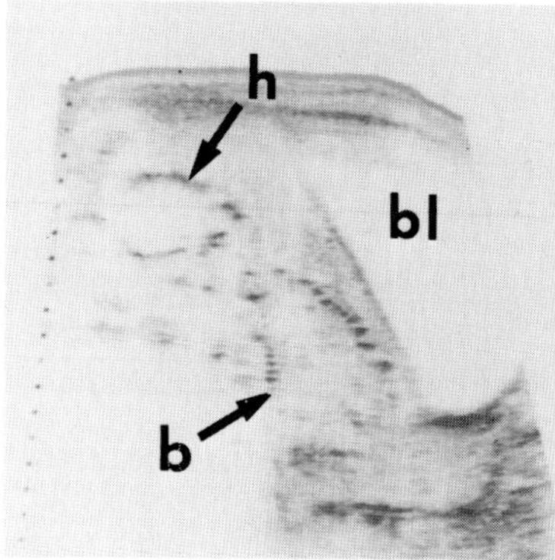

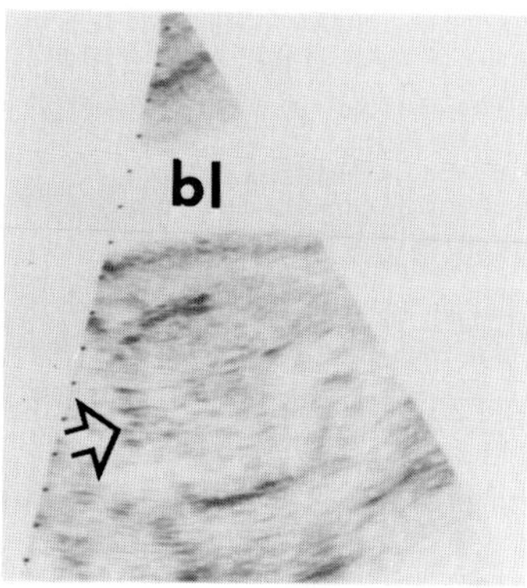

FIG. 1.5. Representative static sonograms of the gravid uterus at 18 menstrual weeks demonstrate profound oligohydramnios. No urine was present within the fetal urinary bladder. This fetus had bilateral renal agenesis. Although no fetal kidneys were seen adjacent to the fetal spine (open arrow), this is an unreliable sign of renal agenesis. h = Fetal head; b = fetal body; bl = maternal urinary bladder.

to 45 minutes following maternal administration.[22] Absence of urine in the fetal urinary bladder following maternal administration of furosemide provides evidence of fetal anuria, a condition incompatible with extrauterine life. Of note, however, is a recent case reported by Rosenberg and Bowie[23] of severe oligohydramnios and absence of urinary bladder filling following maternal furosemide infusion in a fetus with intrauterine growth retardation but normal postnatal renal function. Growth retardation is unlikely to be the cause of a false-positive furosemide test in fetuses examined in the second trimester. The furosemide test, however, only provides evidence which is highly suggestive of decreased fetal renal function; confirmation of renal agenesis or hypoplasia requires postmortem examination.

Infantile Polycystic Kidney Disease

Although some renal malformations do not produce a specific sonographic appearance, if the sonogram is performed because of a risk for a specific congenital renal disorder, an unequivocal renal abnormality indicates recurrence of the disease. Infantile polycystic kidney disease, for example, which is inherited in an autosomal recessive manner, exhibits variable expression dependent upon the degree of renal involvement.[24] Several reports confirm the diagnosis of infantile polycystic kidney disease as early as 17 menstrual weeks on the basis of renal abnormalities seen on the antenatal sonogram.[3,4,7,25-28] Medullary ectasia producing numerous- 1 to 2-mm cysts of nonobstructed renal collecting tubules in bilaterally enlarged kidneys characterizes the disorder.[29] Sonographic descriptions of infantile polycystic kidney disease in the fetus and neonate include bilaterally enlarged fetal kidneys which maintain their reniform shape but exhibit increased renal echogenicity.[3,27,30] Early in pregnancy the renal cor-

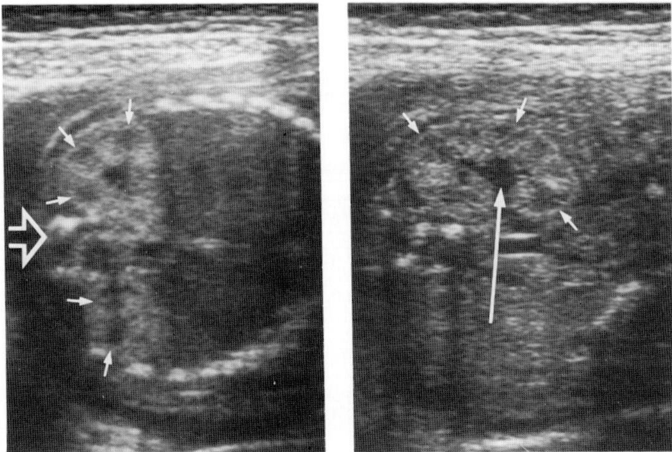

FIG. 1.6. Real-time sonograms at 21 menstrual weeks of a fetus with infantile polycystic kidney disease demonstrate kidneys which have an echogenic cortex and echopenic pyramids (small arrows). A small amount of fluid is present within the renal pelvis (long arrow). Open arrow = fetal spine.

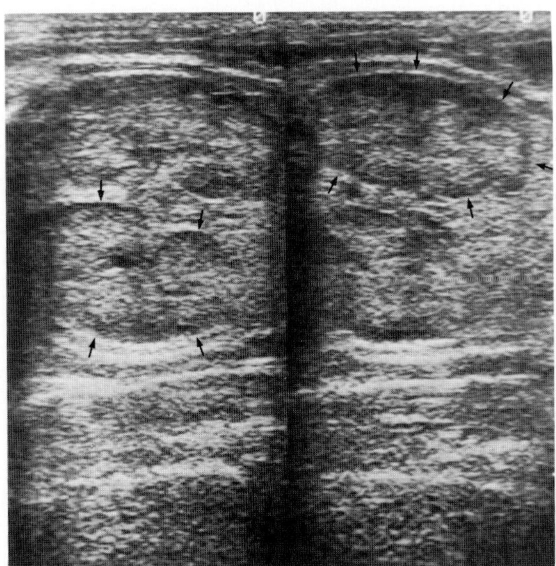

FIG. 1.7. Scans of a fetus with infantile polycystic kidney disease at 33 menstrual weeks display enlarged kidneys (arrows) with echogenic medullae surrounded by a rim of echopenic renal cortex. Oligohydramnios is present.

tex may appear echogenic, whereas the medullae appear echopenic (Fig. 1.6). Later in pregnancy, however, the pattern reverses; a peripheral rim of hypoechoic renal cortex surrounds the echogenic medullae (Fig. 1.7).[5] Although the numerous tiny cysts are usually smaller than the limit of sonographic resolution, the multiple interfaces produced by these cysts result in the characteristic diffusely increased renal echogenicity. Sonographic visualization of fetal renal cysts suggests cystic dysplasia rather than infantile polycystic kidney disease, although a few macroscopic cysts may be seen in this disorder, particularly late in pregnancy. Diminished renal function usually produces nondilated renal pelves, ureters, and bladder with a decreased amount of amniotic fluid.

When bilaterally enlarged kidneys occur in a fetus at risk for infantile polycystic kidney disease, the diagnosis of the syndrome should be made. On the other hand, a normal fetal sonogram early in gestation of a fetus at risk for infantile polycystic kidney disease does not assure absence of this genetic disease. We recently encountered a case of infantile polycystic disease in which the fetal urinary tract appeared sonographically normal at 19 to 20 menstrual weeks, but ultrasound at 24 to 25 menstrual weeks demonstrated unequivocally enlarged, echogenic kidneys.[31] The reasons for this finding remain unclear but imply that, at least in some cases, the pathological abnormality in infantile polycystic kidney disease expresses itself only following completion of nephron induction.

In the absence of a genetic risk for infantile polycystic kidney disease, sonographic visualization of enlarged, fetal kidneys raises the possibility of either bilateral mesoblastic nephromas or congenital metabolic diseases, such as glycogen storage disease or tyrosinosis. To our knowledge these entities have not yet been detected by an antenatal sonogram but might be difficult to distinguish from infantile polycystic disease. In such instances however, oligohydramnios and absence of urine within the urinary bladder would favor infantile polycystic kidney disease over the other entities.

Hydronephrosis

Hydronephrosis is the most common cause of an abdominal mass in the neonate. Antenatal sonography readily detects fetal hydronephrosis ranging from minimal pyelectasis to severe hydronephrosis with virtual complete loss of renal parenchyma. Careful assessment of the sonographic features of fetal hydronephrosis usually permits localization of the level of urinary tract obstruction. This information is essential when in utero diversion of the obstruction is contemplated.

Minimal Pyelectasis

Not infrequently, minimal dilatation of the fetal renal pelvis is demonstrated on routine obstetrical sonographic examinations.[13,14] Among 100 fetal kidneys prospectively examined, 18 demonstrated minimal pyelectasis (maximum diameter of the fetal renal pelvis equal 3 to 11 mm). Furthermore, within the pelvis of 41 additional fetal kidneys, small amounts of sonographically detectable fluid (1 to 2 mm) were seen. To assess the relationship of this finding with states of maternal hydration, we examined 17 fetal kidneys following maternal hydration and again following maternal dehydration. Among the 17 fetal kidneys with mild pyelectasis following maternal oral hydration, only 4 kidneys (23 percent) showed complete or almost complete resolution of the pyelectasis following maternal abstention of oral intake for 12 hours. The remaining 13 kidneys demonstrated little or no change in the degree of pyelectasis following maternal dehydration. This suggests that maternal oral hydration is not a major cause of minimal fetal renal pyelectasis. Experimental evidence with sheep, which shows no change in fetal urine output after maternal volume expansion with 1,000 cc of saline administered over 1 hour, supports this finding.[32]

An alternative explanation for the common occurrence of minimal fetal renal pyelectasis, other than the current state of maternal oral hydration, would include the major physiological changes which accompany pregnancy. Increases in maternal blood volume begin in the first trimester of pregnancy and, at term, the maternal plasma volume is increased by 40 percent.[33,34] Concomitant increases in maternal renal plasma flow and glomerular filtration rate occur. Maternal hydronephrosis is a well-known accompaniment of pregnancy. Hormonal influence on the urinary tract is a strong contender as the etiology of this finding in the mother. Since the fetus is subject to similar endocrinological stimuli, these factors may lead to minimal fetal pyelectasis. Although the etiology of this finding remains uncertain, its impressive frequency suggests that it is unlikely to be of clinical significance. The frequency of detection of minimal fetal pyelectasis renders it impractical to observe all cases sequentially for progression.

Moderate-to-Severe Hydronephrosis

When moderate dilatation of the infundibula and calices occurs, sonography visualizes uniformly sized, branching, fluid-filled structures radiating from the central portion of the kidney toward the margin of the renal sinus (Fig. 1.8). In less severe cases, the thickness of the renal parenchyma remains normal. Worsening hydronephrosis leads to progressive dilatation of the renal calices, and the renal parenchyma thins to the point that, in the most severe cases, only a large paraspinous cystic structure is seen. Because the normal morphology of the kidney is lost in severe cases of hydronephrosis, distinction between other abdominal masses may be difficult. However, documentation that the mass touches the fetal spine assists in localization of the mass to the genitourinary system (Fig. 1.9). Since renal anomalies constitute the vast majority of fetal retroperitoneal masses, we observe the general rule that a fetal flank mass touching the spine is genitourinary in origin. In cases of severe hydronephrosis the urinary tract may rupture and produce a perinephric urinoma which may decompress the urinary tract. A perinephric urinoma appears as a large unilocular cystic flank mass which touches the fetal spine (Fig. 1.10).

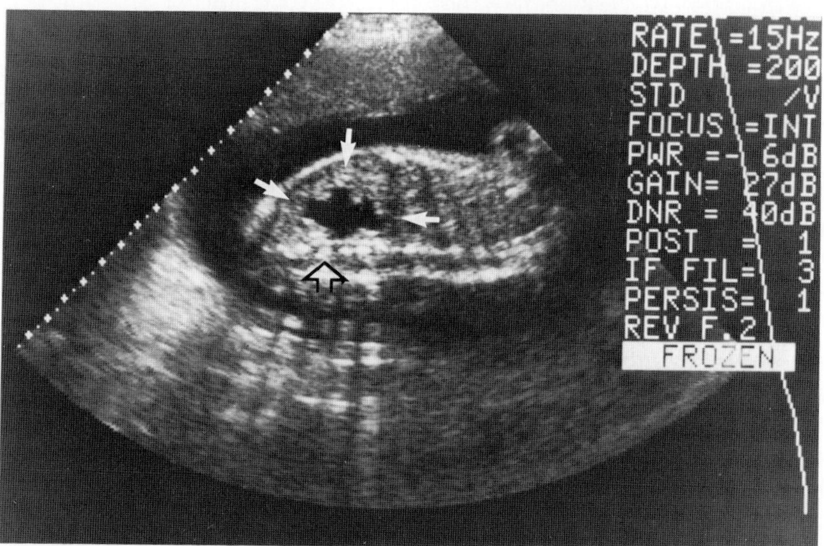

FIG. 1.8. Longitudinal scan of the abdomen of a fetus with unilateral ureteropelvic junction obstruction shows moderate dilatation of the infundibulae and calices (white arrows). A normal amount of amniotic fluid is present. Open arrow = fetal spine.

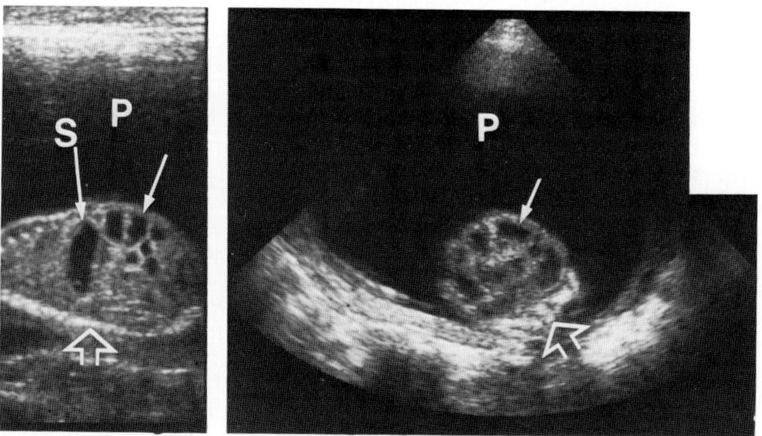

FIG. 1.9. Longitudinal (left) and transverse (right) sonograms of a fetus with small bowel obstruction demonstrate numerous fluid-filled structures of the fetal abdomen (arrows). The presence of polyhydramnios (p) in conjunction with the demonstration that none of the fluid-filled structures are paraspinous imply the presence of bowel obstruction rather than urinary tract obstruction. s = Fetal stomach; open arrows = fetal spine.

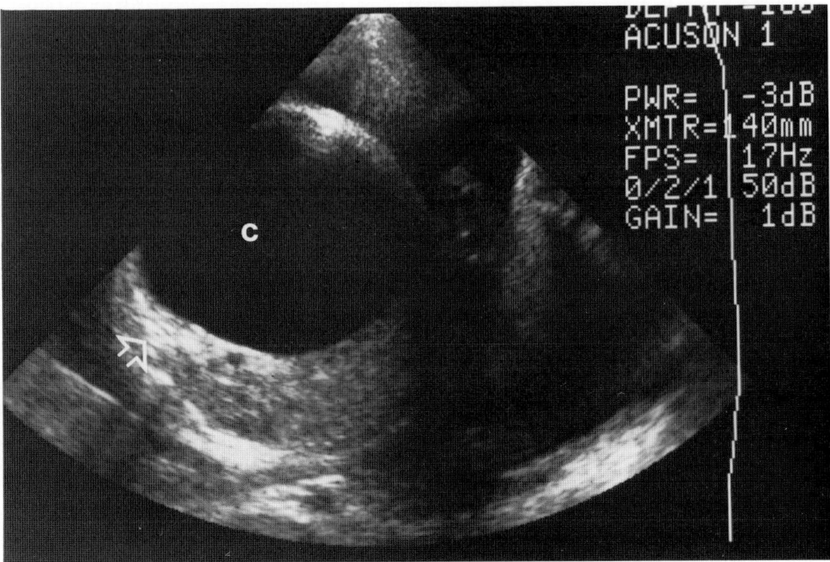

FIG. 1.10.   A large unilocular cystic left flank mass (c) touches the fetal spine (open arrow) of this 37-menstrual-week fetus who had a left ureteropelvic junction obstruction. The unilocular cystic flank mass represented a perinephric urinoma which had resulted from rupture of the urinary tract.

Severe Hydronephrosis Versus Multicystic Dysplastic Kidney

Although sonographic distinction between a hydronephrotic fetal kidney that demonstrates predominant infundibular and calyceal dilatation and a multicystic dysplastic kidney may be more difficult, a variety of observations permit distinction between these two entities.[5] When prominent dilatation of the minor infundibula and calices occurs, these rounded fluid-filled structures may resemble numerous renal cysts. In cases of hydronephrosis, however, the reniform contour is maintained, the dilated calices and infundibula are of uniform size, communicate with each other, and are arranged in anterior and posterior rows; renal parenchyma is seen at the periphery of the hydronephrotic structures. In multicystic dysplasia, on the other hand, the reniform contour is lost, the cysts are of variable size without identifiable communication or anatomical arrangement, and any tissue which may resemble possible renal parenchyma is interspersed between these cysts (Fig. 1.11). The pathological appearance of a multicystic dysplastic kidney correlates with the sonographic appearance described above. The renal pelvis and ureter are usually atretic and not visualized sonographically. Occasionally, however, the distal ureter may be dilated in proximal ureteral atresia, and the renal pelvis may be dilated in distal ureteral atresia.[35] Contralateral renal disease occurs in approximately one-third of patients with multicystic dysplastic kidney. Even when the contralateral kidney cannot be adequately visualized, a normal amount of amniotic fluid and normal

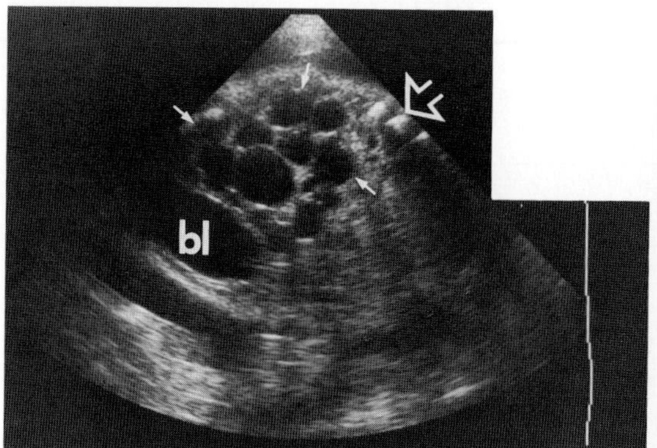
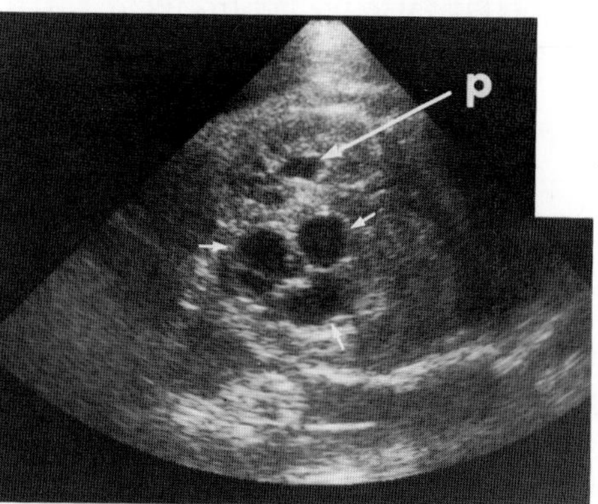

FIG. 1.11.   A paraspinous mass (small arrows) containing numerous cysts of variable size without identifiable communication or anatomical arrangement is present in this 34-menstrual-week fetus with a unilateral multicystic dysplastic kidney. The contralateral kidney has minimal pyelectasis (p) but is otherwise unremarkable. bl = Fetal urinary bladder; open arrow = fetal ribs.

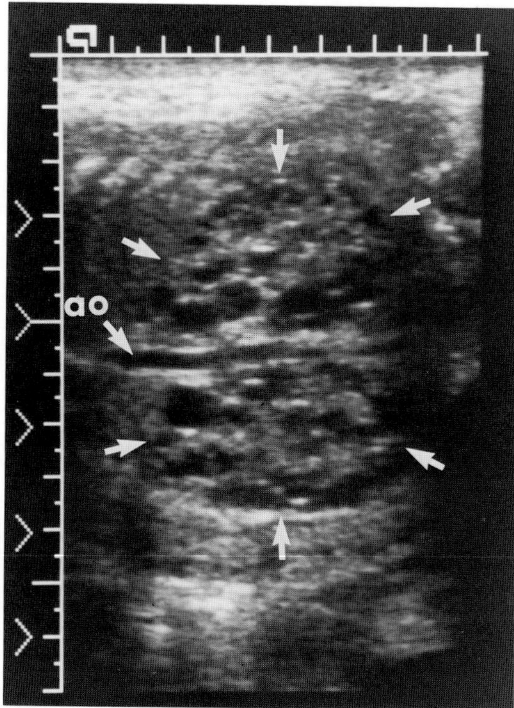

FIG. 1.12.   Coronal sonogram of a fetus at 29 menstrual weeks shows bilateral flank masses (arrows) with numerous variably sized cysts without anatomical arrangement or identifiable communication. Profound oligohydramnios is present. This appearance is typical of bilateral multicystic dysplastic kidney. ao = Fetal aorta.

emptying and filling of the fetal urinary bladder suggest normal contralateral renal function. Approximately 10 percent of patients with a multicystic dysplastic kidney have contralateral hydronephrosis, usually from obstruction at the ureteropelvic junction. In such cases, the degree of obstruction determines the amount of amniotic fluid, since the obstructed kidney is the only potentially functional one. Profound oligohydramnios and absence of fetal urinary bladder filling, on the other hand, suggest bilateral multicystic dysplasia which occurs in approximately 20 percent of cases or contralateral renal agenesis which occurs rarely in conjunction with multicystic dysplasia. With bilateral multicystic dysplasia, typical flank masses are evident (Fig. 1.12). When only a unilateral multicystic dysplastic kidney is seen in the setting of profound oligohydramnios and absence of bladder filling, the diagnosis of contralateral renal agenesis can be made. The absence of functioning renal tissue renders both entities uniformly lethal.

Level of Obstruction

The guidelines outlined above enable reliable distinction between a multicystic dysplastic kidney and obstructive uropathy and between unilateral and bilateral disease. When obstruction is present, characteristic sonographic features permit determination of the site of obstruction.[5] Knowledge of the level of the obstructive lesion is necessary if antenatal or prompt postnatal surgical management is contemplated. Even when early surgical management is not deemed necessary, antenatal identification of urinary tract obstruction permits increased surveillance so that the patient does not return later in childhood with loss of renal function from unobserved progression of an obstructive lesion which had been clinically silent.

The most common cause of neonatal hydronephrosis is obstruction at the ureteropelvic junction.[36] In unilateral ureteropelvic junction obstruction the renal pelvis, infundibula, and calices may be dilated (Fig. 1.13). In severe cases only a single fluid-filled structure with a thin rim of surrounding parenchyma is present. The ureters are not dilated and are not visible sonographically. Since the contralateral kidney is normal, the amount of amniotic fluid is normal, and the urinary bladder fills and empties normally, even if the degree of obstruction is severe enough to cause renal damage on the ipsilateral side.

We have encountered several cases in which unequivocal unilateral fetal hydronephrosis without hydroureter compatible with ureteropelvic junction obstruction has been detected, but a sonogram obtained on the first day following birth showed no evidence of hydronephrosis. This was presumably secondary to relative neonatal dehydration because scans obtained several days later again confirmed the presence of unilateral hydronephrosis. A normal renal sonogram in a neonate who had unequivocal hydronephrosis in utero, therefore, should not alter the diagnosis of urinary tract obstruction.

Bilateral ureteropelvic junction obstruction occurs in approximately 30 percent of cases (Fig. 1.13).[37] Involvement is usually asymmetric and, fortunately, severe bilateral ureteropelvic junction obstruction is rare. In cases with severe

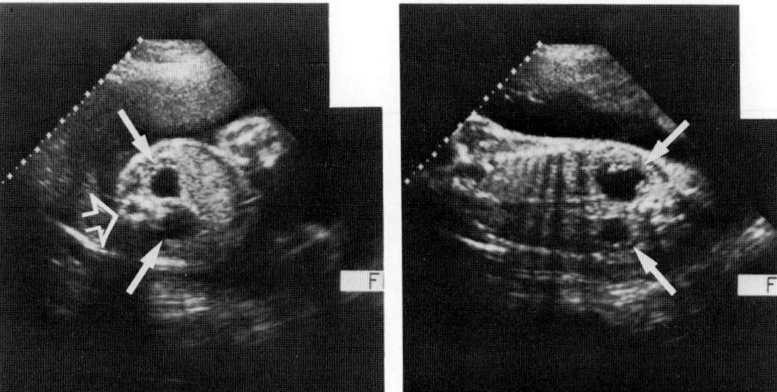

FIG. 1.13.   Bilateral dilatation of the renal pelves and infundibulae (closed arrows) are identified in this fetus with bilateral ureteropelvic junction obstruction. A normal amount of amniotic fluid is present. Open arrow = fetal spine.

bilateral ureteropelvic junction obstruction oligohydramnios is present, and the urinary bladder may be empty. As mentioned above, unilateral ureteropelvic junction may be associated with contralateral multicystic dysplastic kidney or renal agenesis, both of which will produce profound oligohydramnios if the ureteropelvic junction obstruction is severe.

Fetal obstruction at the ureterovesical junction is rare. In most cases it is caused by an ectopic ureterocele associated with ureteric duplication and obstruction of the upper pole moiety. Sonography visualizes dilatation of the obstructed ureter leading to a hydronephrotic upper pole. Occasionally, a redundant, dilated ureter may mimic fluid-filled bowel. Documentation that the serpentine fluid-filled structure touches the fetal spine and originates from the renal pelvis distinguishes hydroureter from fluid-filled bowel. In ureterovesical junction obstruction secondary to ectopic ureterocele, the hydronephrotic upper pole moiety may displace the unobstructed lower pole inferiorly. The urinary bladder is normally distended and of normal wall thickness. Ectopic ureterocele occurs bilaterally in approximately 15 percent of cases.[36] Unless the obstruction is severe bilaterally, the amount of amniotic fluid in cases with ectopic ureterocele is normal. The ureteroceles may rarely be seen as cystic structures within or adjacent to the collapsed urinary bladder.[4] Occasionally, other cystic structures in the fetal pelvis, such as an ovarian cyst, hydrocolpos, or an anterior meningocele, may mimic the urinary bladder. Documentation that a midline pelvic fluid collection changes in volume with time distinguishes the urinary bladder from other cystic pelvic masses.

Posterior urethral valves commonly cause obstruction of the urinary bladder and obstructive uropathy in the male fetus. Although severely affected male fetuses demonstrate a broad spectrum of findings, a dilated posterior urethra and massively dilated, thick-walled urinary bladder represent convincing evidence of posterior urethral valvular obstruction (Fig. 1.14). In posterior urethral

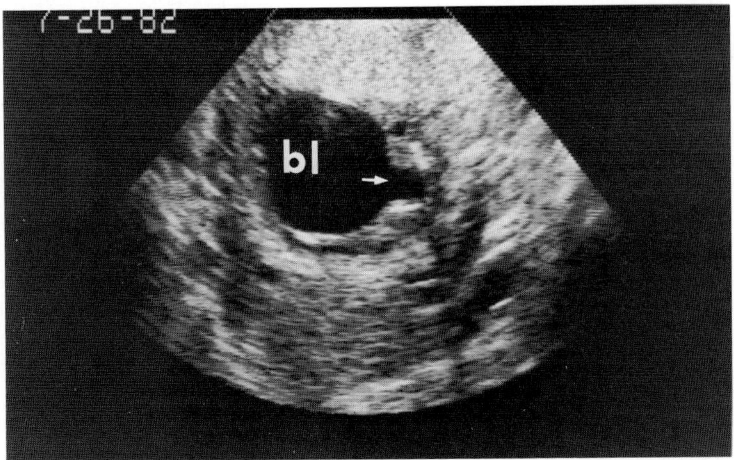

FIG. 1.14.   Real-time sonogram of the fetal pelvis discloses a dilated urinary bladder (bl) and posterior urethra (arrow). Oligohydramnios is present. This fetus had posterior urethral valvular obstruction.

valvular obstruction hydroureter is usually more pronounced than is hydronephrosis.[5] Urine ascites or uriniferous perirenal pseudocysts (urinomas) from spontaneous decompression of the urinary tract may occur as early as the beginning of the second trimester of pregnancy.

When the diagnosis of posterior urethral valvular obstruction is considered, careful scanning of the fetal perineum should be performed to document the presence of male genitalia. If male genitalia cannot be documented in cases with massive distension of the fetal urinary bladder, the diagnosis of the caudal regression anomaly should be considered. This entity, although less common than posterior urethral valvular obstruction, can occur in a fetus of either gender.

The association between spinal dysraphism and hydronephrosis secondary to poor bladder emptying has been well documented.[38-40] Ten to forty-seven percent of neonates and children with myelomeningocele have hydronephrosis.[41] We have been concerned, therefore, that in a male fetus with megacystis, hydroureter, and hydronephrosis the leading differential diagnostic possibilities would include posterior urethral valves and spinal dysraphism. In a recent review of 14 fetuses with spinal dysraphism, however, hydronephrosis was present in only 1 fetus.[41] Conversely, only 1 of 27 fetuses with hydronephrosis had associated spinal dysraphism. Spinal dysraphism, therefore, is uncommonly associated with dilatation of the fetal urinary tract.

In severe fetal urethral-level obstruction the bladder may dilate to the point that it distends the fetal abdomen and elevates the fetal hemidiaphragms. Urine ascites may further distend the abdominal wall and lead to lax abdominal musculature characteristic of the "prune belly syndrome."[42] Of more prognostic significance however, is the presence of oligohydramnios which causes pulmonary hypoplasia, the reason neonates with severe obstructive uropathy frequently die. When oligohydramnios occurs in the setting of urinary tract obstruction, it is usually secondary to severe and persistent obstruction which does not permit egress of fluid from the fetal urinary tract. Alternatively, however, it may also result from diminished renal function in the absence of persistent obstruction. Interventive procedures such as aspiration of fetal urine and catheter measurement of fetal urine production provide detailed information regarding whether the predominant feature is lack of egress of fluid from the urinary tract or from diminished renal function.[7,8] However, increased fetal risk accompanies these procedures. Furthermore, these methods do not provide information regarding reversibility of renal damage.

Renal Dysplasia

In light of the recent urological capabilities which permit diversion of significant fetal obstructive urinary tract lesions, our recent efforts in cases of fetal obstructive uropathy have been directed toward determining whether the fetus has poor renal function and, in cases with poor renal function, whether the potential for reversibility of renal function exists.[9-11,43] Accurate prediction of irreversible renal damage is necessary since any salutary effect of decompression of fetal urinary tract obstruction presupposes that the fetus has not already suffered extensive irreversible renal damage. Renal dysplasia, defined as abnormal parenchymal development from anomalous differentiation of metanephric tissue, implies irreversible renal damage.[44-47] The functional capacity of an affected kidney depends upon the extent and severity of the dysplasia. A dysplastic kidney is characterized pathologically by disorganized epithelial structures surrounded by abundant fibrous tissue. Cortical cysts are often but not necessarily present.

Studies on the morphogenesis and incidence of renal dysplasia indicate that approximately 90 percent of dysplastic kidneys are associated with urinary tract obstruction during nephrogenesis and that the severity of obstruction as well as patterns of dysplasia correspond with the site of obstruction.[47-49] On this basis Bernstein[44] classifies renal dysplasia into four major headings: (1) multicystic dysplasia, invariably associated with ureteropelvic occlusion; (2) focal and segmental cystic dysplasia, usually caused by obstruction related to ectopic ureterocele with ureteral duplication; (3) cystic dysplasia associated with lower urinary tract obstruction, most commonly from posterior urethral valves; and (4) heredofamilial cystic dysplasia. Only the latter category, a smaller group of dysplastic uropathy, results from nonobstructive causes.

In an attempt to determine if a reliable prediction of irreversible renal damage (dysplasia) can be made solely on the basis of antenatal renal sonographic features, we recently reviewed sonograms on 49 fetal kidneys with obstructive uropathy who had renal pathological follow-up (Fig. 1.15).[43] Among the 49 kidneys histologically evaluated, 34 kidneys had dysplasia, and 15 had no evidence of dysplasia. In each case we recorded the presence or absence of

FIG.   1.15. Representative antenatal real-time sonograms demonstrate typical features of posterior urethral valvular obstruction with bilateral renal cystic dysplasia. The urinary bladder (bl) is distended and thick-walled with trabeculations. Dilatation of the posterior urethra (pu) and of the ureters (u) are evident. Within the echogenic kidneys (curved arrows) are numerous small cortical cysts (small arrows). Open arrows = fetal spine.

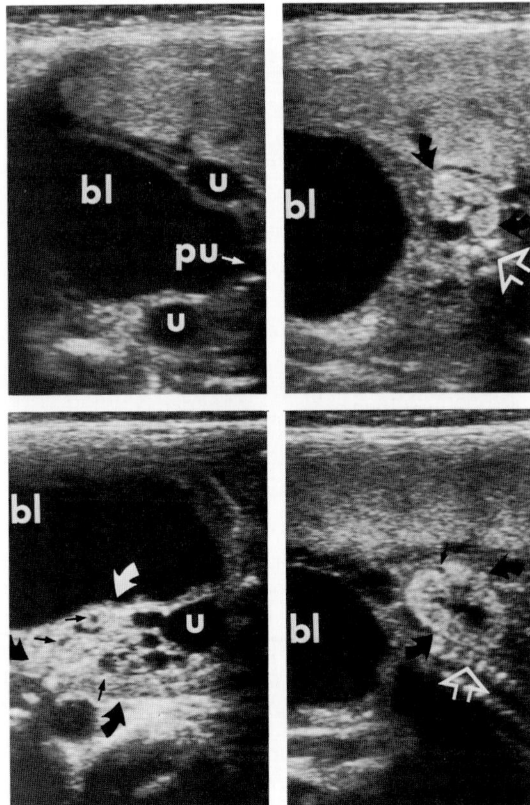

renal cortical cysts and the degree of renal echogenicity and of hydronephrosis. Only when cortical cysts were unequivocally visualized and could be reliably distinguished from ectatic calices were they recorded as being present. Only those kidneys which were easily discriminated as being significantly more echogenic than the surrounding tissues were recorded as being echogenic. Similarly, we assessed unequivocal hydronephrosis only when calyceal blunting and/or parenchymal thinning was evident. We subsequently correlated the fetal renal sonographic data with the pathological follow-up.

Among the 49 fetal kidneys with obstructive uropathy, sonographic demonstration of renal cysts invariably signified the presence of dysplasia, and in no cases without dysplasia were renal cysts sonographically visible. In these fetuses with known obstructive uropathy, therefore, sonographic demonstration of renal cysts effectively indicated the presence of dysplasia and irreversible renal damage which would not respond to urinary tract diversion. The identification of sonographically visible renal cysts in fetal obstructive uropathy also correlated with the severity of involvement. Of the 15 kidneys with visible cysts, 13 were evaluated either at autopsy or following nephrectomy.

When renal cysts were not sonographically visible, however, we could not accurately exclude the presence of dysplasia. We visualized cysts in only 44 percent of dysplastic fetal kidneys, and only 44 percent of kidneys without demonstrable cysts were free of dysplastic changes. Several reasons account for the inability of antenatal sonography to detect cysts in dysplastic fetal kidneys. First, not all dysplastic kidneys have cysts and, when cysts are present, they may be smaller than sonographic resolution capabilities.[47] Second, fetal position and degree of oligohydramnios may prohibit adequate renal visualization. Although ultrasound is ideally suited for the detection of fluid-filled pathological lesions, small cysts may not be seen in the "down-side" kidney since it often resides in the far field of the sonographic beam where resolution decreases or may be effectively shadowed by the fetal spine. Oligohydramnios minimizes the opportunity for the fetus to alter its position such that either of these deficiences would be rectified.

Assessment of fetal renal echogenicity provided a less accurate prediction of renal dysplasia than did visualization of renal cortical cysts. In our study, assessment of renal echogenicity yielded a specificity of only 80 percent and an accuracy of a positive prediction of 89 percent. Importantly, not all fetal kidneys that are of greatly increased echogenicity were dysplastic. A spectrum of fetal renal echogenicity exists, even in the normal state, and normal fetal kidneys may demonstrate slightly increased echogenicity relative to surrounding tissues. Problems inherent in an operator-dependent modality such as ultrasound further diminished the assessment value of fetal renal echogenicity. Assessment of fetal renal echogenicity is more difficult when: (1) severe hydronephrosis compresses the renal parenchyma, (2) urine ascites increases sound transmission, or (3) the fetal kidney resides in the sonographic near field where parenchymal visualization may be impaired. For all these reasons, assessment of fetal renal echogenicity offered only limited predictive value of dysplasia in obstructive uropathy.

Similarly, the degree of pelvocalyceal dilatation was not necessarily predictive of the presence of dysplasia in fetuses with obstructive uropathy. Only 14 of 34 (41 percent) kidneys which were dysplastic secondary to urinary tract obstruction had significant hydronephrosis at the time of sonographic evaluation. Numerous observations explain this apparent discrepancy between urinary tract obstruction and lack of hydronephrosis. First, dilatation of the urinary tract secondary to posterior urethral valvular obstruction is often most pronounced in the bladder and ureters, whereas the kidney may demonstrate only minimal pelvocalcyceal dilatation.[50,51] Second, some fetuses may decompress the urinary tract by rupturing the bladder or by developing urinomas in response to urinary tract obstruction.[52] Third, a decrease in urine production and in dilatation of the urinary tract may occur following the development of dysplastic changes.[50] Fourth, in multicystic dysplasia caused by pelviureteric atresia, no opportunity exists to visualize dilatation, even though the obstruction is at its most extreme.[50] And fifth, urethral obstruction in the first half of gestation in fetal lambs produces dysplasia whereas obstruction which originates during the second half of gestation causes only hydronephrosis and atrophy without evidence of dysplasia.[54,55]

In summary, careful evaluation of the fetal abdomen and amount of amniotic fluid will frequently enable an accurate antenatal diagnosis when a genitourinary abnormality is detected. In cases with obstructive uropathy, the site of obstruction may be delineated. Sonographic visualization of renal cortical cysts accurately predicts the presence of severe dysplasia.

OBSTETRICAL AND UROLOGICAL MANAGEMENT

The ability of antenatal sonography to detect and define fetal renal anomalies has dramatically changed obstetrical management. In cases with distension of the fetal abdomen from urine ascites or from a massively distended urinary bladder, prenatal fetal paracentesis or bladder drainage may prevent dystocia. Alternatively, elective cesarean section may be considered to optimize perinatal care. Early detection of lethal disorders such as bilateral multicystic dysplastic kidney, renal agenesis, or infantile polycystic kidney disease may provide the parents with the option of elective termination. Detection of unilateral renal disease or bilateral disease without evidence of severe irreversible renal damage suggests that the anomaly may be amenable to early postnatal or prenatal therapy.

A careful sonographic examination of the fetal abdomen may detect a hydronephrotic kidney which might not otherwise be clinically detected following birth. Relief of urinary tract obstruction in the young infant minimizes the risk of ongoing damage. Similarly, when urinary tract obstruction is detected in a fetus who has not yet suffered irreversible renal damage, in utero diversion of the obstruction may prevent ongoing renal damage. Early urological decompression of an obstructed fetal urinary tract may prevent oligohydramnios, thereby avoiding the risk of pulmonary hypoplasia. Antenatal sonographic delineation of the site of obstruction and assessment of potential reversibility of renal damage assist the urologist in choice and timing of surgical procedures and in patient selection.

REFERENCES

1. Johnson ML, Rees GK, Hattan RA: Normal fetal anatomy. p. 410. In Callen PW (ed). Ultrasonography in Obstetrics and Gynecology. Saunders, Philadelphia, 1983
2. Rumack CM, Johnson ML, Zunkel D: Antenatal diagnosis. Clin Diag Ultrasound 8:210, 1981
3. Hobbins JC, Grannum PAT, Berkowitz RL et al.: Ultrasound in the diagnosis of congenital anomalies. Am J Obstet Gynecol 134:331, 1979
4. Hadlock FP, Deter RL, Carpenter R et al.: Sonography of fetal urinary tract anomalies. AJR 137:261, 1981
5. Chinn DH, Filly RA: Ultrasound diagnosis of fetal genitourinary tract anomalies. Urol Radiol 4:115, 1982
6. Lawson TL, Foley WD, Berland LL et al.: Ultrasonographic evaluation of the kidneys. Analysis of normal size and frequency of visualization as related to stage of pregnancy. Radiology 138:153, 1981
7. Grannum P, Bracken M, Silverman R et al.: Assessment of fetal kidney size in normal gestation by comparison of ratio of kidney circumference to abdominal circumference. Am J Obstet Gynecol 136:249, 1980

8. Jeanty P, Dramaix-Wilmet M, Elkhazen N et al.: Measurement of fetal kidney growth on ultrasound. Radiology 144:159, 1982

9. Harrison MR, Filly RA, Parer JT et al.: Management of the fetus with a urinary tract malformation. JAMA 246:635, 1981

10. Golbus MS, Harrison MR, Filly RA et al.: In utero treatment of urinary tract obstruction. Am J Obstet Gynecol 142:383, 1982

11. Harrison MR, Golbus MS, Filly RA et al.: Fetal surgery for congenital hydronephrosis. N Engl J Med 306:591, 1982

12. Abramovich DR: The volume of amniotic fluid and its regulating factors. p. 31. In Fairweather D, Eskes T (eds). Amniotic Fluid-Research and Clinical Application. 2nd Revised Ed., Elsevier/North Holland Biomedical Press, (Amsterdam), 1978

13. Scheible W, Talner LB: Grey-scale ultrasound and the genitourinary tract. A review of clinical applications. Radiol Clin North Am 17:281, 1979

14. Hoddick WK, Filly RA, Mahony BS et al.: Minimal fetal renal pyelectasis. J Ultrasound Med, 4:85, 1985

15. Campbell S, Wladimiroff JW, Dewhurst CJ: The antenatal measurement of fetal urine production. J Obstet Gynaecol Br Commonn 80:680, 1973

16. Wladimiroff JW, Campbell S: Fetal urine production rates in normal and complicated pregnancy. Lancet 1:151, 1974

17. Birnholtz JC: Determination of fetal sex. N Engl J Med 309:942, 1983

18. Dunne MG, Cunat JS: Sonographic determination of fetal gender before 25 weeks gestation. AJR 140:741, 1983

19. Scholly TA, Sutphen JH, Hitchcock DA et al.: Sonographic determination of fetal gender. AJR 135:1161, 1980

20. Potter EL: Bilateral absence of ureters and kidneys. Obstet Gynecol 25:3, 1965

21. Dubbins PA, Kurt AB, Wapner RJ et al.: Renal agenesis: Spectrum of in utero findings. J Clin Urol 9:189, 1981

22. Wladimiroff JW: Effect of furosemide on fetal urine production. Br J Obstet Gynecol 82:221, 1975

23. Rosenberg ER, Bowie JD: Failure of furosemide to induce diuresis in a growth retarded fetus. AJR 142:485, 1984

24. Madewell JE, Hartman DS, Lichtenstein JE: Radiologic-pathologic correlations in cystic disease of the kidney. Radiol Clin North Am 17:261, 1979

25. Garrett WJ, Grunwald G, Robinson DE: Prenatal diagnosis of fetal polycystic kidney by ultrasound. Aust NZ J Obstet Gynecol 10:7, 1970

26. Reilly KB, Rubin SP, Blanke BG et al.: Infantile polycystic kidney disease: A difficult antenatal diagnosis. Am J Obstet Gynecol 133:580, 1979

27. Habif DV, Berndon WE, Yeah M-N: Infantile polycystic kidney disease: In utero sonographic diagnosis. Radiology 142:475, 1982

28. Shenker L, Anderson C: Intrauterine diagnosis and management of fetal polycystic kidney disease. Obstet Gynecol 59:385, 1982

29. Potter EL: Normal and Abnormal Development of the Kidney. Year Book Medical Publishers, Chicago, 1972, p. 141

30. Boal DK, Teele RL: Sonography of infantile polycystic kidney disease. AJR 135:575, 1980

31. Mahony BS, Callen PW, Filly RA et al.: Progression of infantile polycystic kidney disease in early pregnancy. J Ultrasound Med, 3:277, 1984

32. Hurley JK, Kirkpatrick SE, Pitlick PT et al.: Renal responses of the fetal lamb to fetal or maternal volume expansion. Circ Res 40:557, 1977

33. Pritchard JA: Changes in blood volume during pregnancy and delivery. Anesthesiology 26:393, 1965

34. Ueland K: Maternal cardiovascular dynamics. VII. Intrapartum blood volume changes. Am J Obstet Gynecol 126:671, 1976

35. DeKlerk DP, Marshall FF, Jeffs RD: Multicystic dysplastic kidney. J Urol 118:306, 1977

36. Lebowitz RL, Griscomb NT: Neonatal hydronephrosis—146 cases. Radiol Clin North Am 15:49, 1971

37. Johnston JH, Evans JP, Glassberg KI et al.: Pelvic hydronephrosis in children. A review of 219 personal cases. J Urol 117:97, 1971

38. Harlowe SE, Merrill RE, Lee EM et al.: A clinical evaluation of the urinary tract in patients with meningomyelocele. J Urol 93:411, 1965

39. Wilcock AR, Emery JL: Deformities of the renal tract in children with meningomyelocele and hydrocephalus, compared with those of children showing no such central nervous system deformities. Br J Urol 42:152, 1970

40. Miller JH, Reid BS, Kemberling CR: Utilization of ultrasound in the evaluation of spinal dysraphism in children. Radiology 143:737, 1982

41. Lirette M, Filly RA: Relationship of fetal hydronephrosis to spinal dysraphism. J Ultrasound Med 2:495, 1983

42. Pramanik AK, Altshuler G, Light IJ et al.: Prune-belly syndrome associated with Potter (renal non-function) syndrome. Am J Dis Child 131:672, 1977

43. Mahony BS, Filly RA, Callen PW et al.: Fetal Renal Dysplasia: Sonographic Evaluation. Radiology 152:143, 1984

44. Bernstein J: A classification of renal cysts. p. 7. In Gardner KD (ed). Cystic Diseases of the Kidney. John Wiley, New York, 1976

45. Risdon RA: Renal dysplasia. J Clin Pathol 24:57, 1971

46. Kissani JM: The morphology of renal cystic disease. p. 31. In Gardner KD (ed). Cystic Diseases of the Kidney. John Wiley, New York, 1976

47. Bernstein J: The morphogenesis of renal parenchymal maldevelopment (renal dysplasia). Pediatr Clin North Am 18:395, 1971

48. Rubenstein M, Meyer R, Bernstein J: Congenital abnormalities of the urinary system. I. A postmortem study of developmental anomalies and aquired congenital lesions in a children's hospital. J Pediatr 58:356, 1961

49. Mackie GG, Stephens FD: Duplex kidneys: A correlation of renal dysplasia with position of the ureteral orifice. J Urol 114:274, 1975

50. Glazer GM, Filly RA, Callen PW: The varied sonographic appearance of the urinary tract in the fetus and newborn with urethral obstruction. Radiology 144:563, 1982

51. Rattner WH, Meyer R, Bernstein J: Congenital abnormalities of the urinary system. IV. Valvular obstruction of the posterior urethra. J Pediatr 63:84, 1963

52. Parker RM: Neonatal urinary ascites: A potentially favorable sign in bladder outlet obstruction. Urology 111:589, 1974

53. Bernstein J: Renal hypoplasia and dysplasia. p. 547. In Edelmann CM (ed): Pediatric Kidney Disease. Vol. 2. Little Brown, Boston, 1978

54. Beck AD: The effect of intrauterine urinary obstruction upon the development of the fetal kidney. J Urol 105:784, 1971

55. Glick PL, Harrison MR, Noall RA et al.: Correction of congenital hydronephrosis in utero. III. Early mid trimester ureteral obstruction produces renal dysplasia. J Pediatr Surg 18(6):681, 1983

2 Ultrasound of the Urinary Tract in Pediatrics

THOMAS L. SLOVIS

The speed, accuracy, and noninvasive aspects of ultrasound evaluation have made this modality the first imaging procedure (after plain films) in examining the pediatric urinary system.[1-4] We can, however, be seduced into a false sense of security if the ultrasound examination is not meticulously performed and if we are not aware of its limitations. Rather than repeat the instances where ultrasound is universally accepted as the indicated procedure, this chapter will discuss the newer and more controversial clinical indications. The emphasis is on those instances in which sonography can stand alone and those situations in which sonography should be combined with a second imaging modality for optimal diagnostic accuracy. Although the answers to each issue will not necessarily be given, a perspective and a philosophy will hopefully emerge. Since technical considerations and anatomical differences between the pediatric patient and the adult are important for comprehension of the clinical controversies, these sections will begin the chapter.

TECHNICAL CONSIDERATION

Ultrasound is a tomographic discipline; as more sections are obtained, more of the anatomy will be seen, and the chances of showing an abnormality are improved (Fig. 2.1).

To examine the urinary tract, we advocate the use of a real-time unit and images recorded on the hard copy and a video tape. The examination is performed in a prescribed manner by the sonographers and/or the physicians with longitudinal and transverse transabdominal sections of the kidneys obtained with the patient supine. Coronal sections are produced by making transverse and longitudinal scans through the patient's side (Fig. 2.2). The inferior vena cava and aorta are recorded in all of these planes whereas the other viscera (liver, gallbladder, pancreas, and spleen) are given a cursory evalu-

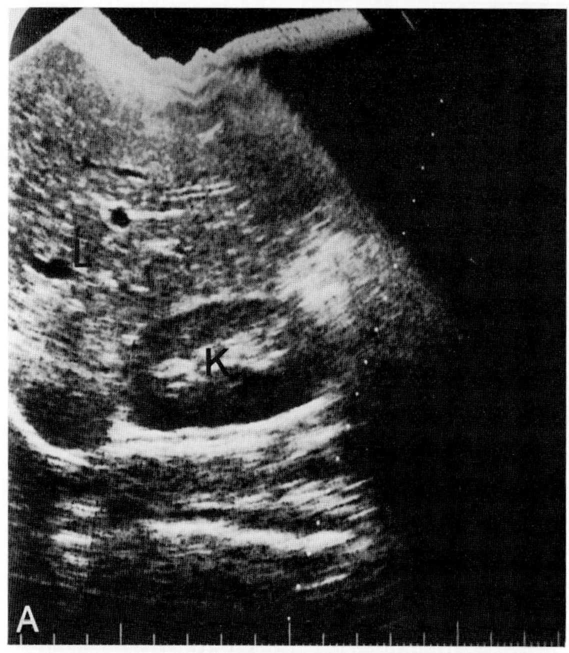

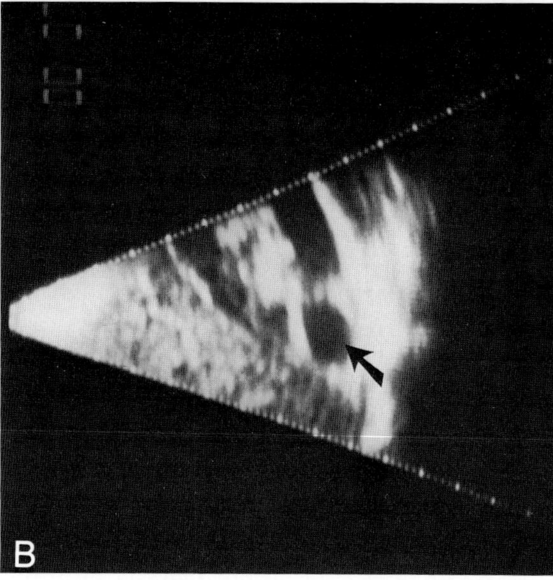

FIG. 2.1. Ultrasound is a tomography discipline. Detection of an obstructed duplication in the upper pole. (A) Supine static scan on an 8-year-old girl with urinary tract infection reveals an apparently normal right kidney. L = liver; K = kidney. (B) Real-time scan on the same patient shows a lucency (arrow) in the extreme upper pole not visualized by the static scan (Figure continues).

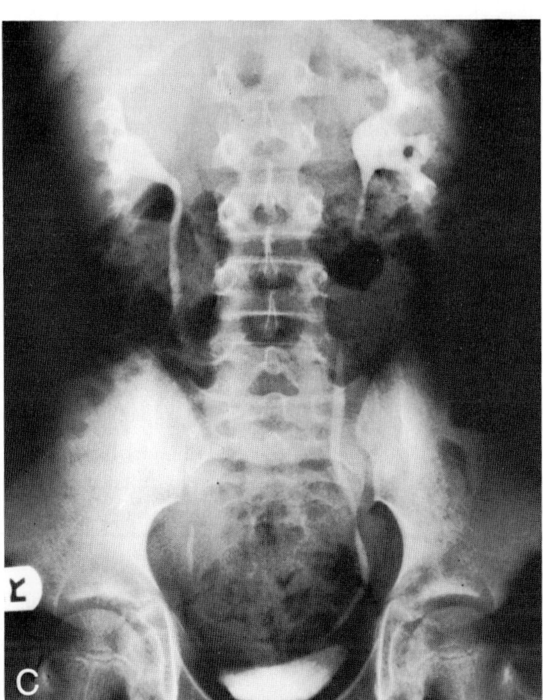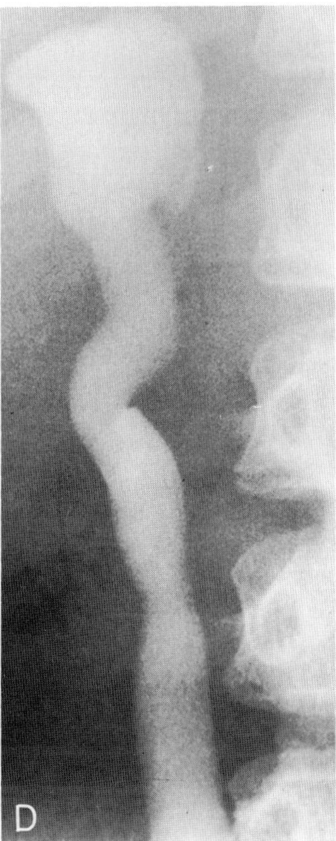

FIG. 2.1 (Continued). (C) Intravenous pyelogram shows the depression of the lower segment of the right kidney and lateral position of the visualized calyces relative to the spine. The right ureter is deviated laterally from the spine. (D) Retrograde urethrogram of the right kidney reveals the fluid-filled upper pole of the duplicated system and the enlarged tortuous ureter. The ureteral dilation explains the position of the lower pole ureter.

ation. Hard-copy images of the kidneys are obtained in the most definitive of the four planes. If an abnormality or variant is detected, multiple oblique planes are studied. In all renal examinations, the bladder is evaluated as well as the pelvic genital organs. The converse is also true; that is, in genital abnormalities the kidneys are evaluated because of the high incidence of associated renal anomalies. Patients examined for the first time are then studied in the prone position with the static scanner and additional hard-copy images are generated.

In order to accomplish these multiple views, it is manditory that the young infant be relatively still. Rather than sedation, we prefer the liberal use of tape for immobilization (Fig. 2.3).

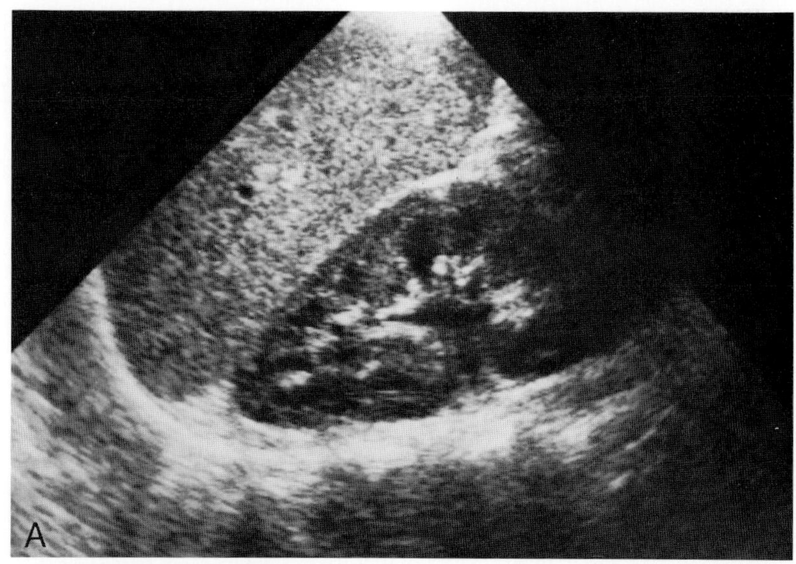

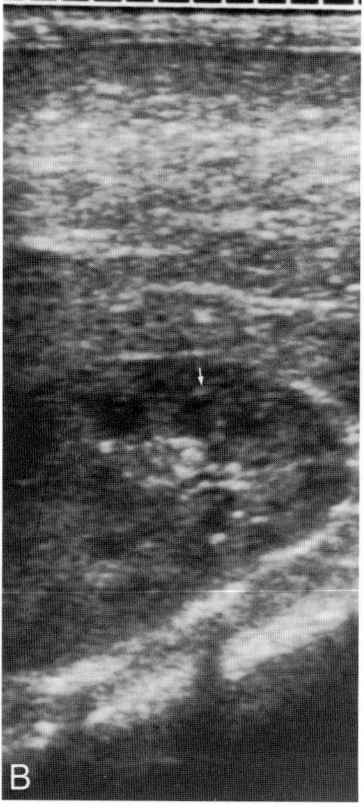

FIG. 2.2. The normal kidney in the older child. (A) Longitudinal scan produced through the patients side (coronal section) shows the echogenic sinus (mostly fat) and the medullary pyramids. The cortex is less echogenic than the liver. The collecting system is easily seen in the midst of the central sinus fat because of an extremely full bladder. (B) Linear scan shows the arcurate artery (arrow) and medullary pyramid in this 4-year-old. The renal outline is easily seen, and the cortical echoes are present though less echogenic than the liver.

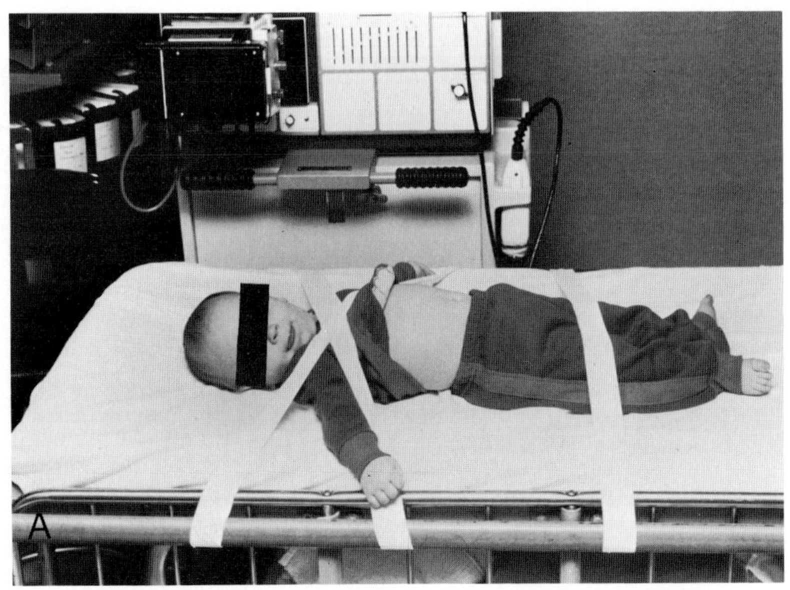

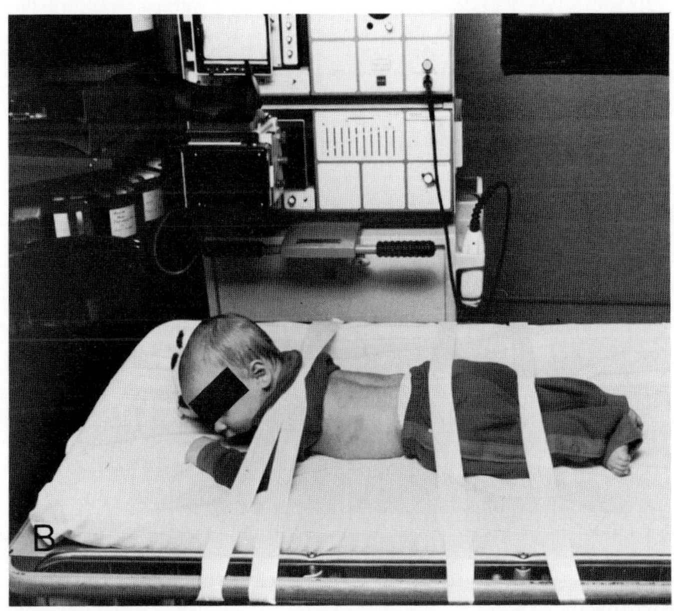

FIG. 2.3. Immobilization of the infant. (A) With the patient supine, tape is placed over the knees and in an "X" configuration above and below the arms. The hands are free so the patient can suck his thumb or play with small objects while the abdominal scan is being done. When necessary, diapers or towels are used to mummify the patient prior to the taping. (B) Prone scan showing the tape passing over the popliteal fossa, tape over the buttocks and over the shoulders.

ANATOMY

The ultrasound appearance of the kidney of the older child and adult is different from that of the neonate (Figs. 2.2 and 2.4).[5-7] The neonatal kidney has large sonolucent medullary pyramids which are arranged in an elliptical pattern midway between the outer edge of the cortex and the central collecting system. The medullary pyramids are larger with regard to the cortex (1:1 ratio) during this period than at any other time (adult 3:1 cortex-medulla). In addition, the cortex may be quite echogenic, equaling the echogenicity of the liver. This finding is explained by the presence of the maximum number of glomeruli—nephrogenesis ceases at 36 weeks' gestation—crowded together in a smaller volume of cortex.[8] The neonatal glomeruli are also histologically different from mature glomeruli, with prominent epithelial cells on the glomerular tuft. There is conspicuous absence of the bright echoes in the renal pelvis (the central sinus region) as there is little fatty tissue.

As the kidney matures, the cortex increases in thickness as a result of tubular growth with resultant separation of the glomeruli. Since the tubules are not

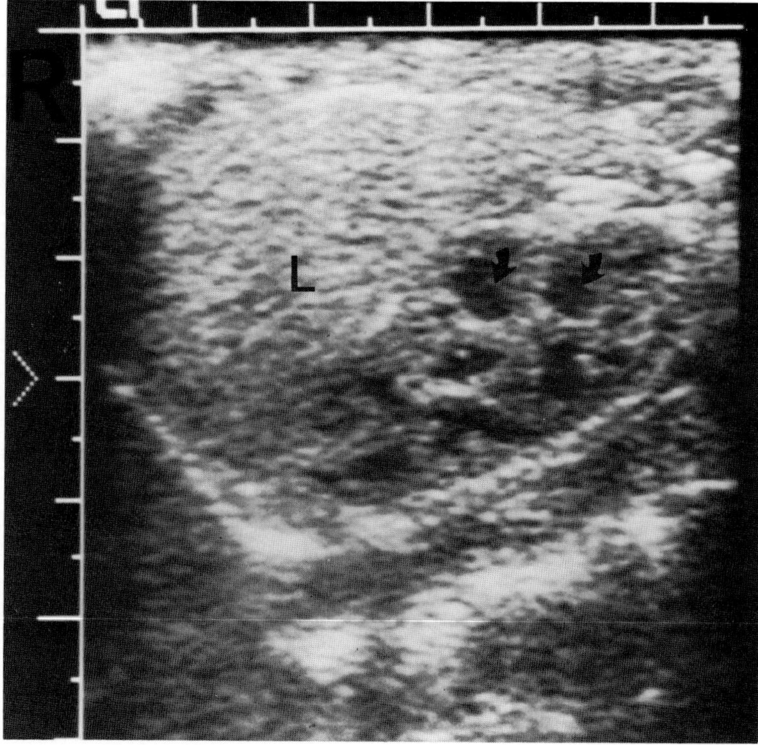

FIG. 2.4. Neonatal kidney of a 20-day-old. Longitudinal scan showing the cortical parenchyma in relationship to the liver. The cortical echoes are of similar intensity to the liver. The medullary pyramids are easily seen (arrows). L = liver.

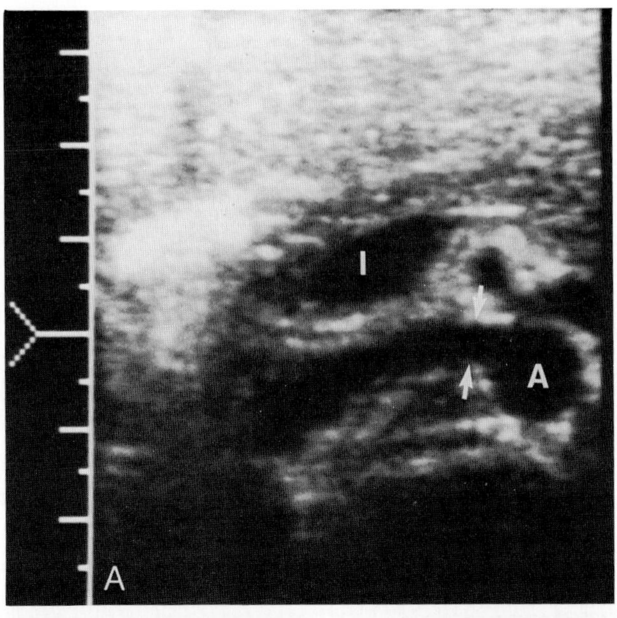

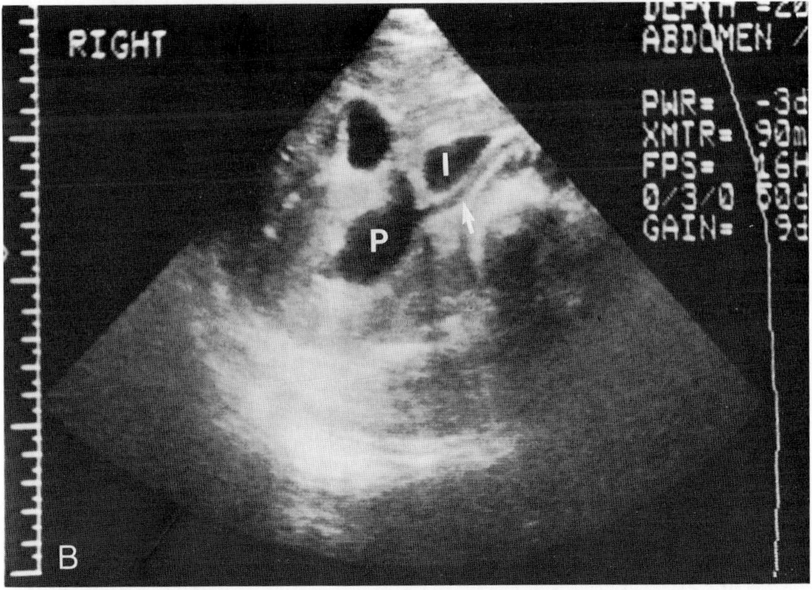

FIG. 2.5.   Renal vascular anatomy. (A) Cone-down transverse section shows the aorta (A) and the origin of the right renal artery (arrow). The inferior vena cava (I) is easily seen. (B) Transverse section to the right of the spine shows the course of the renal artery (arrow), the inferior vena cava (I), and a rather bulbous renal pelvis (P). The gallbladder is seen above the kidney (Figure continues).

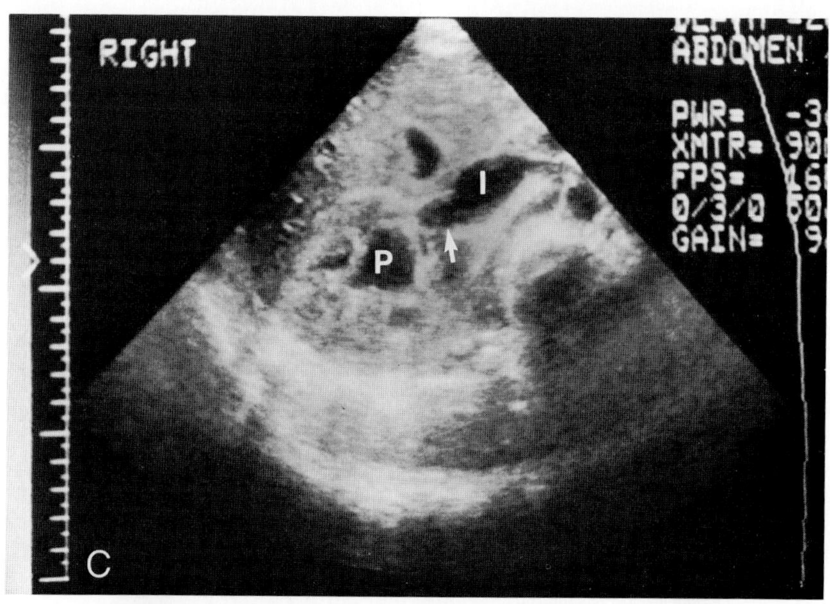
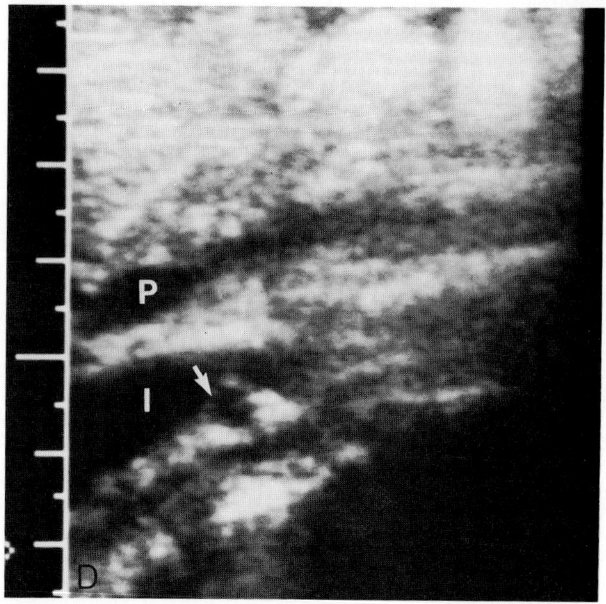

FIG. 2.5 (Continued). (C) Transverse section to the right of the spine reveals the inferior vena cava (I) and the left renal vein. The left renal vein runs above the aorta and below the superior mesenteric artery. The right renal vein is enlarged (arrow). Again note the large renal pelvis (P). (D) Longitudinal scan of the inferior vena cava (I) at the level of the portal vein (P) reveals the right renal artery in cross section (arrow).

echogenic, the cortical echogenicity diminishes. The renal sinus accumulates fat and increases in echogenicity.

In the older child, the cortex is less echogenic than the liver, the medullary pyramids are smaller but always seen, and the arcuate arteries are frequently visualized. The transverse scans (either on transabdominal or coronal) reveal the renal artery, renal vein, and ureter at the hilum. The course of both the renal vein and artery is demonstrated (Fig. 2.5).

CLINICAL INDICATIONS, LIMITATIONS, AND CONTROVERSIES

The general indications of urinary sonography are given in Table 2.1. In almost all of these instances, ultrasound provides the diagnosis or reveals positive findings and directs the workup. It is important to consider the questions,

TABLE 2.1 Accepted indications for ultrasound of the urinary system in pediatrics

1. Abdominal masses in children[9,10]
   a. Defines nature of mass (cystic vs. solid)
   b. Defines viscus of origin
   c. Shows intravascular invasion (IVC)
   d. Directs the workup
2. The oliguric-anuric patient[11,12]
   a. Reveals the dilated collecting system
   b. May show architectural changes of advanced medical renal disease (i.e., increased cortical echogenicity)
   c. Aids in the diagnosis of renal vein thrombosis
   d. Reveals renal agenesis
3. Follow up of known disease(s)[13]
   a. Posturological surgery
   b. Posttumor treatment (surgical or medical)
   c. The patient with a myelomeningocele
   d. The patient with a neurogenic bladder
   e. Urinary tract infection (follow-up)
4. Specific syndromes which may have renal changes[14,15]
   a. Tuberous sclerosis
   b. Aniridia, hemihypertrophy (nephroblastomatosis, etc.)
5. Renal infiltration as in leukemia[16]
6. Renal and perirenal abscess[17]
7. Evaluation of acute transplant rejection[18]
8. Evaluation of residual bladder volume[2]
9. Screening for congenital anomalies[13]
10. Detection of nephrocalcinosis[19]
11. Contraindication to intravenous contrast agent (i.e., sensitivity)

TABLE 2.2 Controversial topics

1. "First" urinary tract infection
   a. Renal evaluation
   b. Sonographic cystogram
2. Histological diagnosis by ultrasound architecture
   a. The echogenic kidney
      1. The neonate
      2. The older child
   b. Separation of recessive from dominant polycystic disease
   c. Tumors
   d. Renal duplication vs. cyst
3. Renal trauma
   a. Functional impairment
   b. Extent of injury
   c. Follow-up
4. Renal calculi

Does the sonogram provide all of the information of the test it replaces? If it does not, should we be doing the sonogram? Radiation should be avoided if it is excessive or repetitive, but radiological tests may provide the only means of acquiring important information. Table 2.2 lists those conditions which will be analyzed from these perspectives.

"First" Urinary Tract Infection

The evaluation of renal size has been the province of the intravenous urogram.[20] The strength of the urogram lies in the ability to depict the whole kidney in *one* picture. It lets you see the *normal* ureter and any ureteral deviation. Precise evaluation of renal size and cortical outline is easily obtained. Since ultrasound and computed tomography (CT) are tomographic modalities, the broad overview of size and cortical outlines is not easily obtained. In fact, renal length is even difficult to evaluate, not so much by absolute measurement but relative to the individual as there is a great deal of variation within each age range.[21] The old urographic rule of 4 to 4½ vertebral bodies is still a good standard, and there is no sonographic counterpart. The best "eyeball" estimate compares the renal length with that of liver. Similiarly, renal volume is useful as an internal comparison. The volume and areas measurements are time consuming but will be advocated by some.[22]

Those concepts of cortical margins and size are particularly useful to remember when evaluating a child with a first urinary tract infection. An important finding is that of a focal scar. These scars denote previous upper tract damage (be it by reflux or pyelonephritis) and change the present diagnosis to recurrent urinary tract infection with a different treatment plan (Fig. 2.6). Sonography

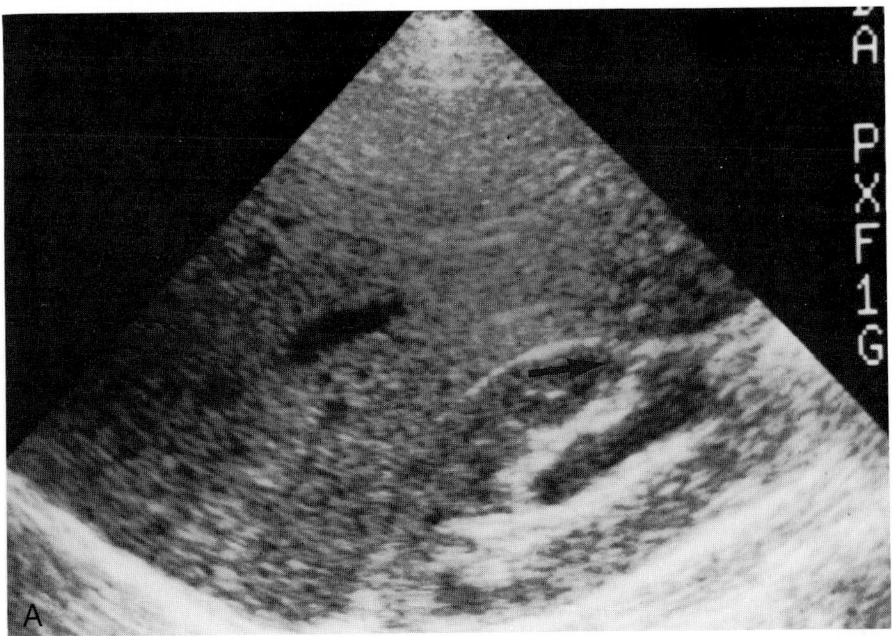

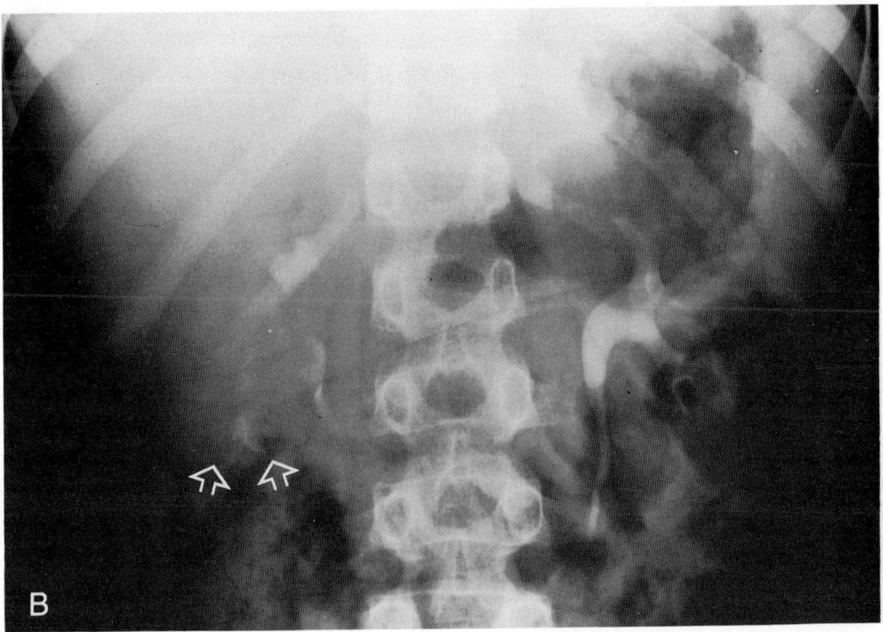

FIG. 2.6. Renal scarring. Sonographic detection of a moderately severe lesion. (A) Longitudinal scan of the right kidney shows the central sinus fat adjacent to the lower pole cortical margin (arrow). (B) Intravenous pyelogram shows decreased (arrow) parenchyma of the lower pole compared with the rest of the kidney. This was a 9-year-old girl with documented reflux.

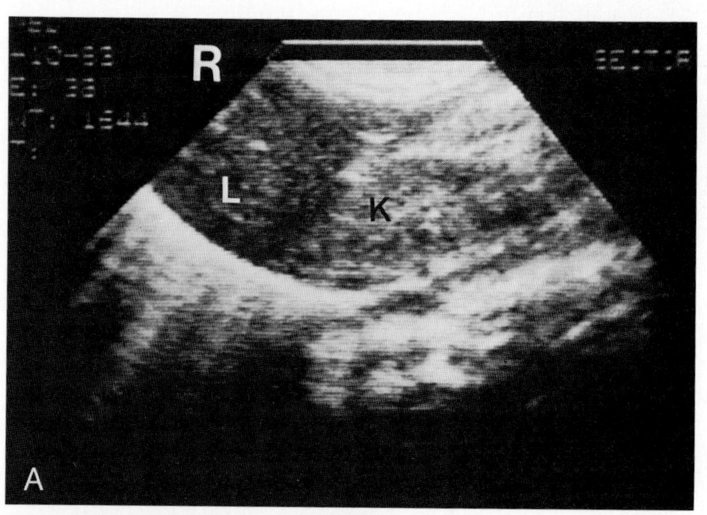

A

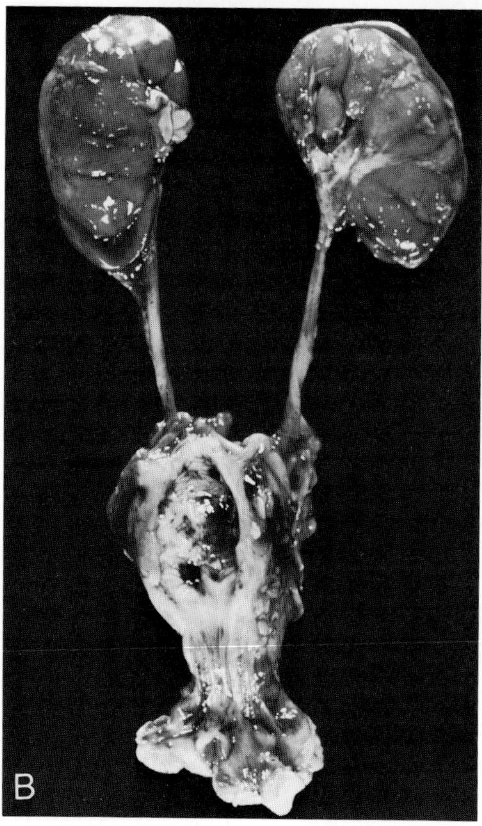

B

FIG. 2.7. The neonatal echogenic kidney. (A) This 1,644-g male had multiple abnormalities including severe intracranial hemorrhage at birth. He was anuric. Longitudinal ultrasound of the right kidney revealed this echogenic kidney with abnormal architecture. The kidney was much more echogenic than the liver, and the medullary pyramids were not seen. A left kidney was difficult to see because of the abundant gas. L = liver; K = kidney; R = right. (B) At autopsy, this infant had two normal kidneys on both gross and microscopic examination. (C) This full-term infant had ischemia at birth. Longitudinal ultrasound of the left kidney (K) reveals the normal size, shape, and architecture. (D) Evaluation of the right kidney in longitudinal view reveals lack of the normal medullary pyramids and architecture and increased echogenicity relative to the liver. L = liver; R = right. (E) At autopsy, the left kidney was of normal size but ischemic from renal artery thrombosis. The right kidney was found to be swollen and mildly congested but otherwise unremarkable.

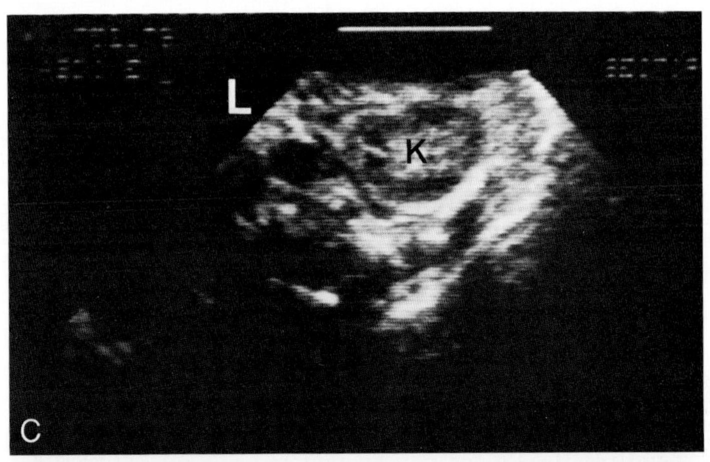

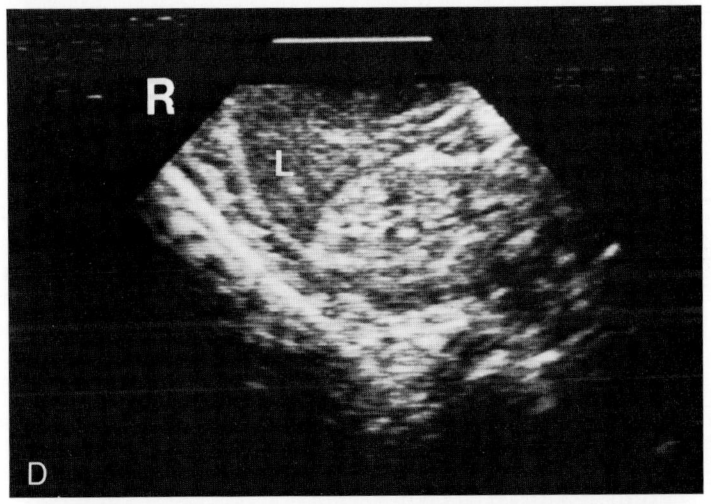

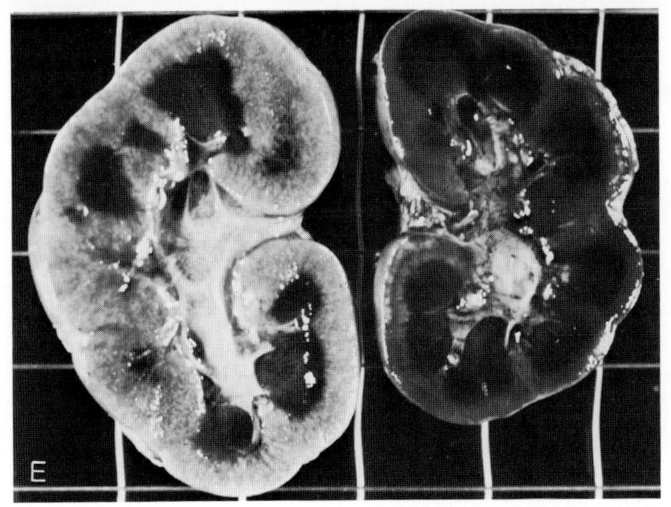

is being touted as *the* imaging procedure for the first infection.[23-26] However, these studies indicate that focal scars can be missed but congenital anomalies and obstructive disease should be detected. Sonography does not make the definitive diagnosis of chronic renal insult, and therefore does not provide all the information the urogram does. The sonogram does eliminate the possibility of contrast reaction and radiation. How much radiation does a child receive? This varies with the number of films obtained and the patient's age and sex. In a four-film urogram, the skin entrance dose ranges from 200 to 750 mR and the gonadal dose from 44 to 140 mR in a female and 4 to 22 mR in a male.[27] The battle lines are clear, the answer is not.

The complete workup for a child with a first urinary tract infection should include evaluation of both the upper and lower urinary system. The urethra, bladder, and perhaps ureteral orifices are evaluated with a voiding cystography. Preliminary work on the sonographic cystogram has suggested that the injection of air bubbles into the sterile fluid can be detected as the bubbles ascend up the ureter to the renal pelvis.[28] Even the most enthusiastic advocate of this technique admits that vesicoureteral reflux into the distal ureter (grade I) will go undetected. However, it is uncertain how important the detection of grade 1 reflux is. The major clinical effect of finding this type of reflux is the duration of antibiotic therapy and how closely the patient is followed. Reflux into the proximal ureter and kidney also can be missed but with less frequency (sensitivity of 87 percent). Here the failure to detect reflux may change a surgical treatment to a medical one. Does cystographic sonography meet our proposed criterion?

Histological Diagnosis by Sonographic Architecture-Tissue Signature

Histological diagnosis in a noninvasive manner is the ultimate goal of sonography. How far are we from attaining this goal? A good example is the echogenic kidney (Fig. 2.7).[19,29] In the neonate, the abnormal echogenic kidney is one that is much more echogenic than the liver. It is found in neonates with severe hypoxic injury (presumably renal cortical and tubular necrosis), dehydrated neonates (prerenal azotemia), in severe dysplastic kidneys, in congenital medical renal disease such as nephrotic syndrome, and in the polycystic disease of both recessive and dominant types (see below).[30,31] It may be associated with large-, normal-, or small-sized kidneys; it may be transient. The findings of an echogenic kidney in a neonate suggests a differential diagnosis but is not prognostic. The reasons for the increased echogenicity, of course, depends on the etiology, but the simplest common denominator is an increased number of acoustical interfaces, be it microcysts or edema.

In the older child, an echogenic kidney also should suggest a differential diagnosis. In this age group, the normal kidney is far less echogenic than the liver. The differential diagnosis includes the infiltrated kidney (i.e., leukemia), the severely dysplastic kidney, the severely diseased kidney (advanced medical

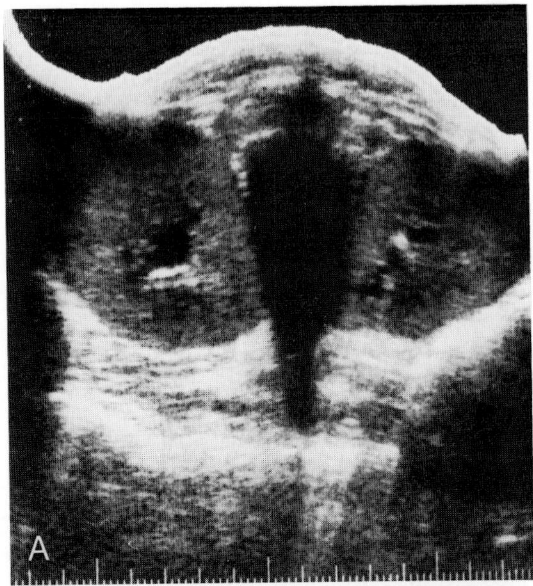

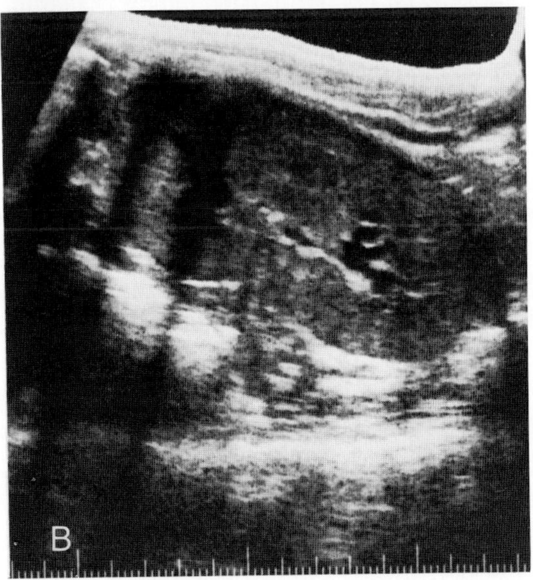

FIG. 2.8.   The echogenic kidney in an older child with leukemia. (A) Prone transverse scan reveals the kidneys to be quite devoid of normal architecture with mild central sinus dilatation. (B) Longitudinal prone scan reveals the central sinus fat but increased echogenicity of the entire kidney. This child had leukemia and was treated with chemotherapy (Figure continues).

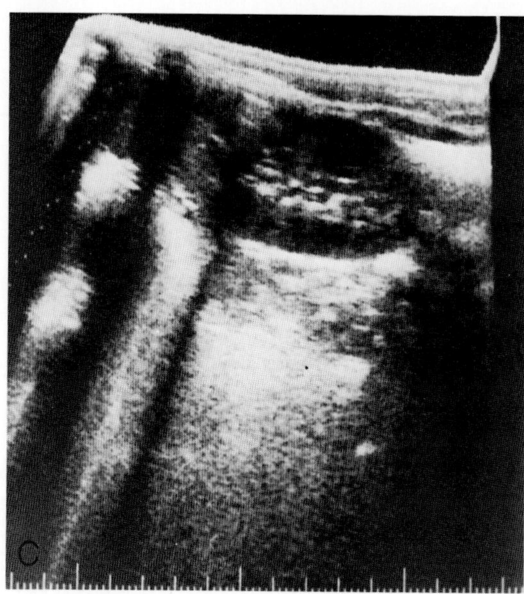

FIG. 2.8 (Continued). (C) Prone scan done several months after initiation of therapy shows the normal size and architecture of the kidney.

renal disease of any type), and the severely impaired chronic shrunken kidney (Fig. 2.8). It is apparent that this sonographic change is *not* necessarily an early sign of disease in the older child and, except for some of the reversible infiltrative diseases, is a poor prognostic sign.

Another important area of controversy is the ability of the sonogram to separate the types of polycystic kidney disease in the neonate and young infant.[30,31] The hallmark of the *recessive* type of polycystic disease is dilatation of collecting ducts and collecting tubules. This type of polycystic disease may be so severe that the neonate is born with massive kidneys, markedly impaired renal function, and dies within the first days. The urogram shows the classic spoke-wheel appearance, with the collecting ducts containing contrast. The sonogram reveals large echogenic kidneys and many small cortical cysts are *now* seen. At the other end of the spectrum in recessive polycystic disease is the neonate with mildly enlarged kidneys and minimal renal impairment. On the sonogram the kidney is echogenic with small cysts, but the collecting system is visualized. The infant has minimal renal impairment. Urography reveals contrast-filled collecting ducts and tubules (tubular cystic ectasia), as well as contrast in the renal pelvis (Fig. 2.9). Although the hallmark is elongated ductal cysts, the size of the cysts is not diagnostic, and larger cysts may be present (Fig. 2.9).

In the *dominant* form of this disease, the kidneys can also be large and echogenic (Fig. 2.10). There may or may not be larger cysts present in the neonatal period. On architecture alone, these two entities may not be truly separable. The urogram, however, is very helpful, and the presence of contrast-filled tubules separates the two forms.[32,33] Occasionally in the neonate and certainly

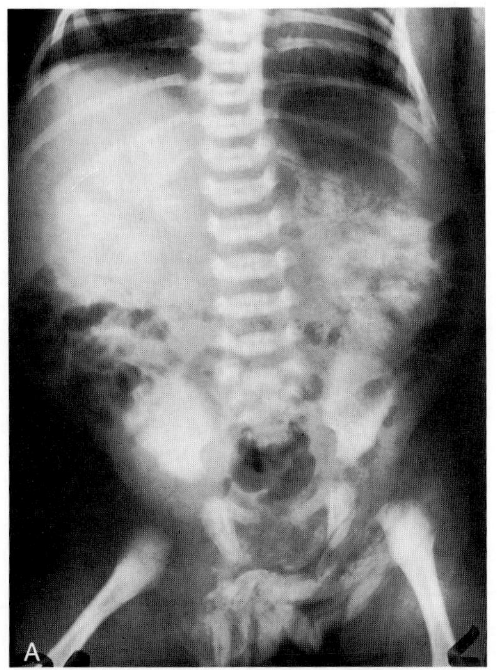

FIG. 2.9. Recessive polycystic disease. (A) Intravenous urogram on this 2-month-old performed for mildly enlarged kidneys reveals bilateral tubular ectasia as well as renal enlargement. The patient had minimal renal impairment. (B) High-resolution linear longitudinal scan reveals the kidneys to be echogenic and the small cysts throughout the cortices. The collecting system is well seen (Figure continues).

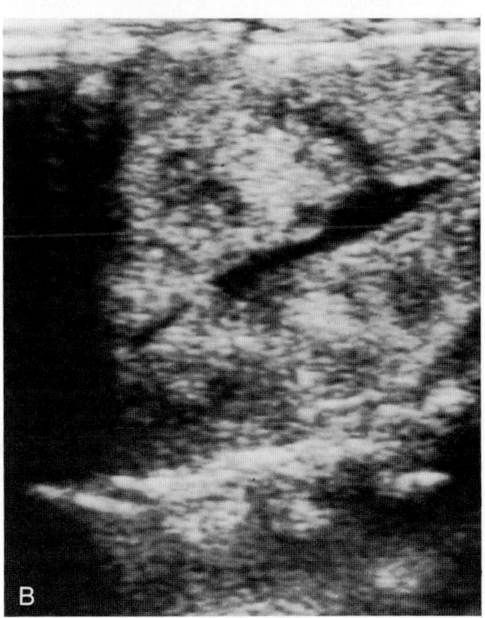

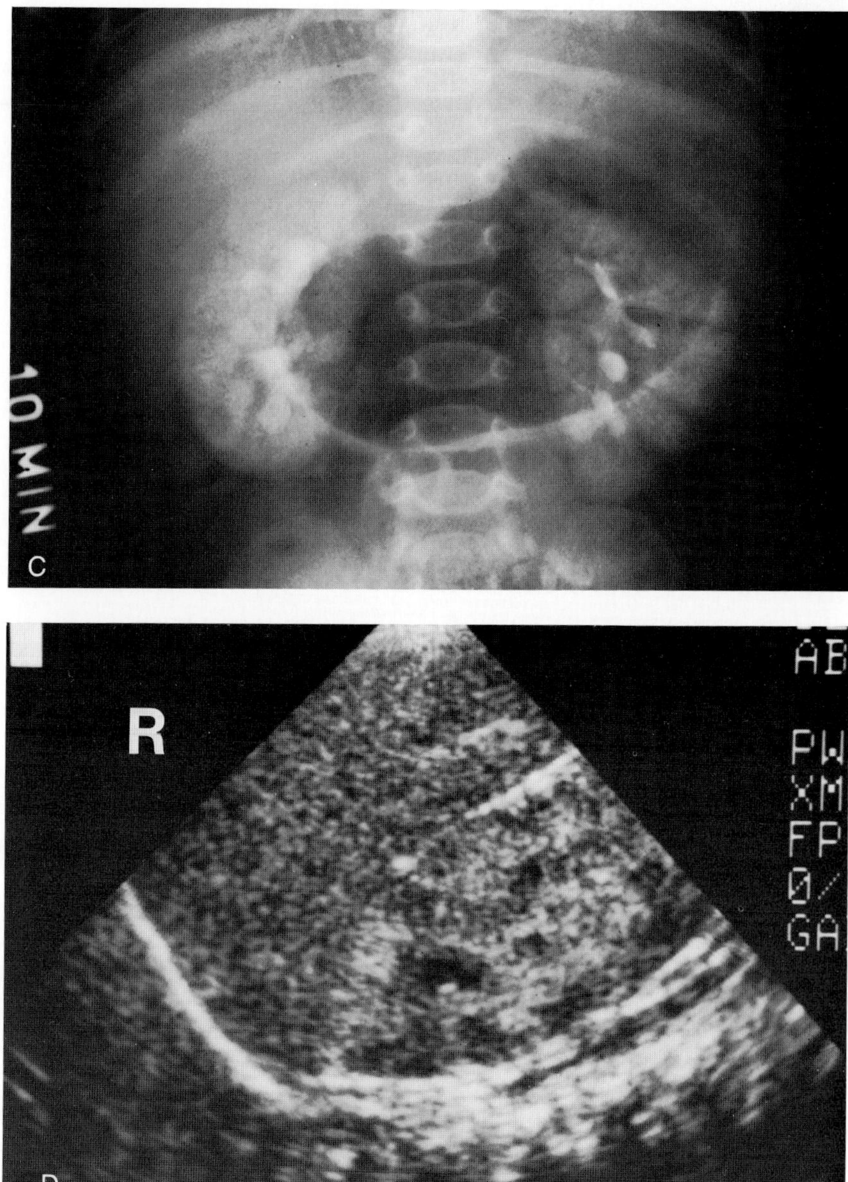

FIG. 2.9 (Continued). (C) This 2-month-old infant presented with failure to thrive and moderate renal impairment. The intravenous urogram shows the kidneys to be mild moderately enlarged with diffuse tubular ectasia and good visualization of the collecting system. (D) Longitudinal scan of the right kidney shows the echogenicity and abnormal architecture. There are small cysts scattered throughout the kidney. R = right (Figure continues).

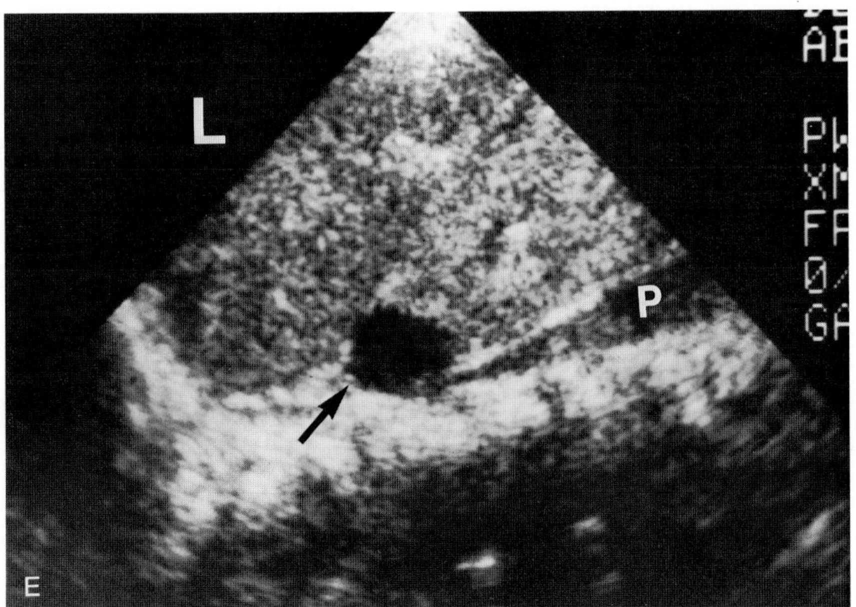

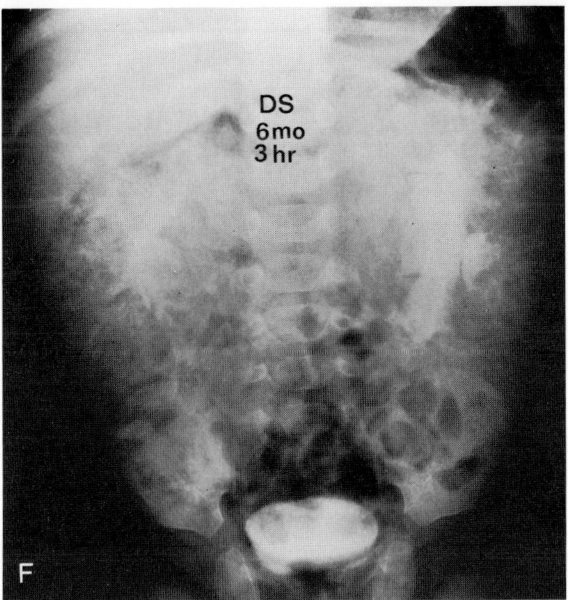

FIG. 2.9 (Continued). (E) Longitudinal scan of the left kidney reveals a large cyst (arrow) in the upper pole of the left kidney. The size of the cysts is not the determinate of the kind of cystic disease present or of the prognosis. P = psoas; L = left. (F) This intravenous urogram was done on a small for gestational age infant who at 6 months of age was found to have abdominal masses. The urogram shows a spoke-wheel appearance with the collecting ducts and tubules containing contrast. There is some dilatation of the renal pelvis, but the ureters and bladder are normal (Figure continues).

41

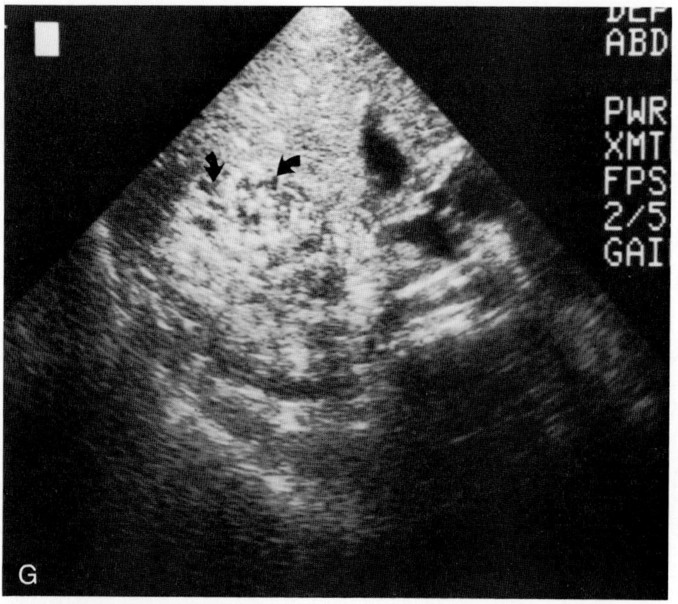

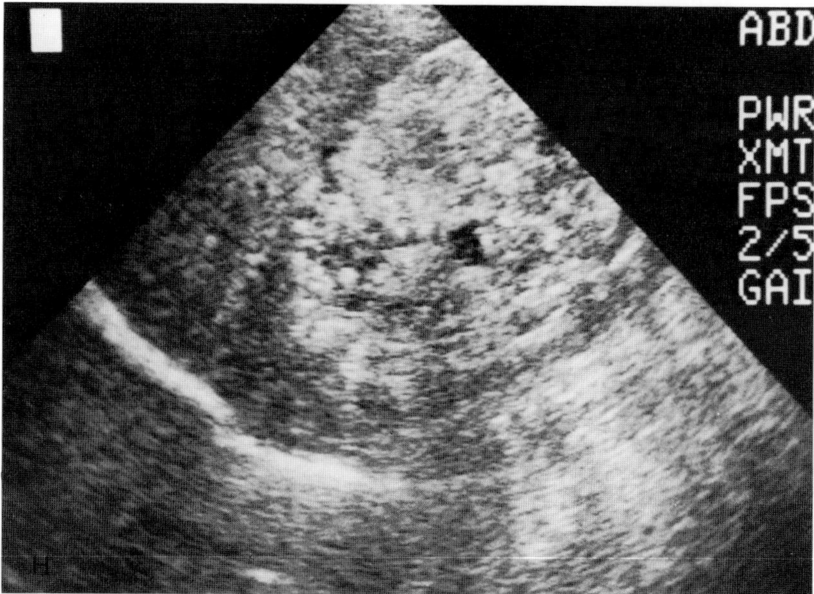

FIG. 2.9 (Continued). (G) Transverse ultrasound examination at 6 years of age reveals the enlarged echogenic right kidney with multiple cysts, most obvious in the anterior portion of the kidney (arrows). (H) Longitudinal scan of the right kidney shows the echogenicity and cystic structures.

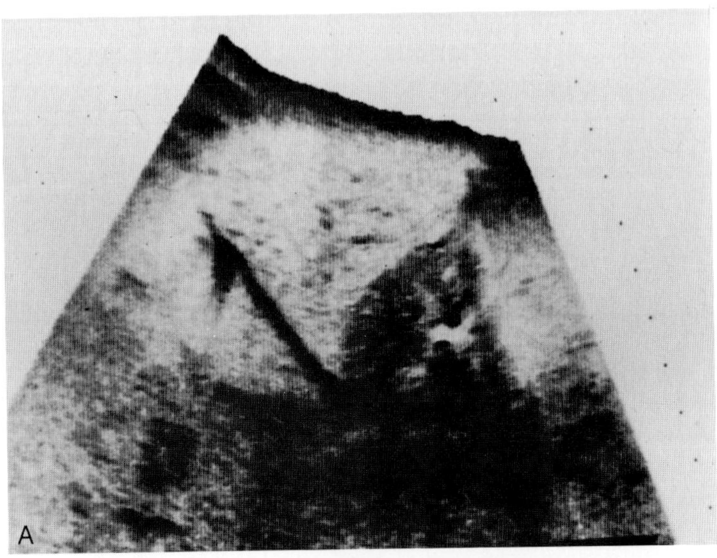

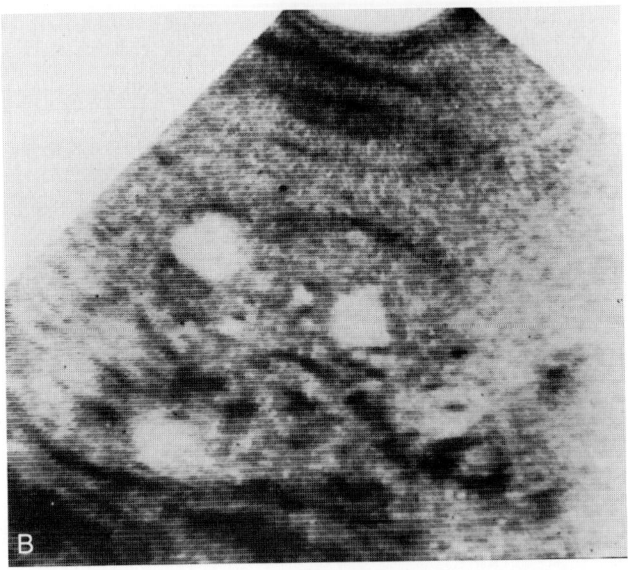

FIG. 2.10. Dominant polycystic disease. (A) Longitudinal scan of the newborn felt to have mildly enlarged kidneys. The kidney is quite echogenic without gross cysts. The collecting system is seen. (B) Evaluation of the patient's father reveals multiple cysts throughout the kidney (Figs. 2.10A and B are with permission of Dr. Beatrice Madrazo, Henry Ford Hospital, Detroit, Michigan.) (Figure continues).

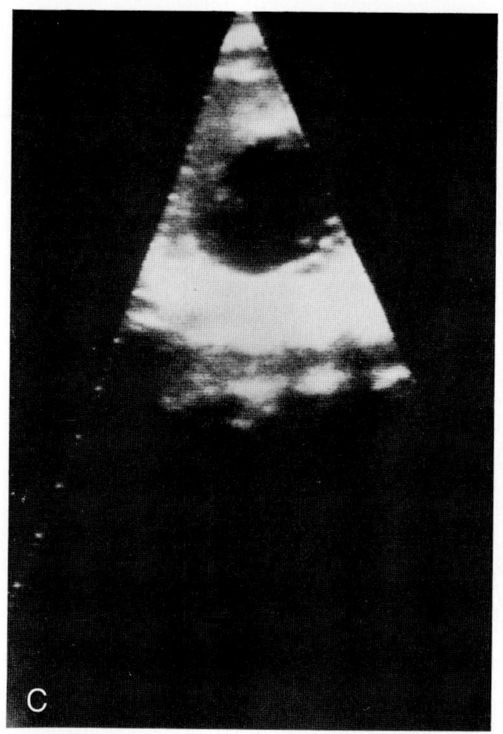

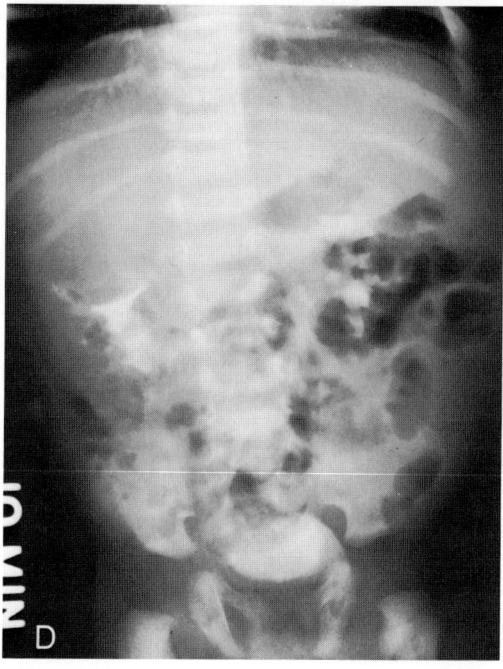

FIG. 2.10 (Continued).   (C) Longitudinal sonogram on a 14-day-old reveals a large upper pole cyst. There were cysts in both kidneys. (D) Intravenous pyelogram on the patient shows no evidence of tubular ectasia but rather mass effect of the cysts.

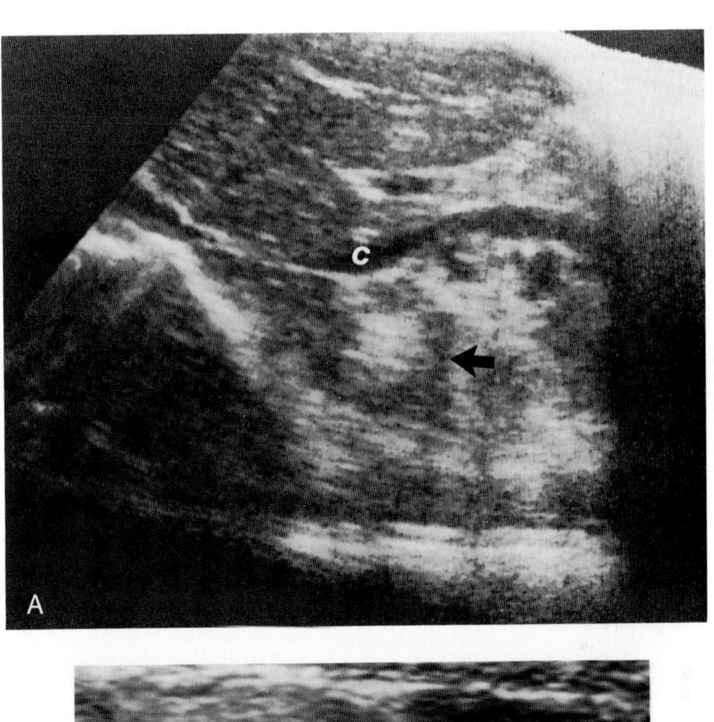

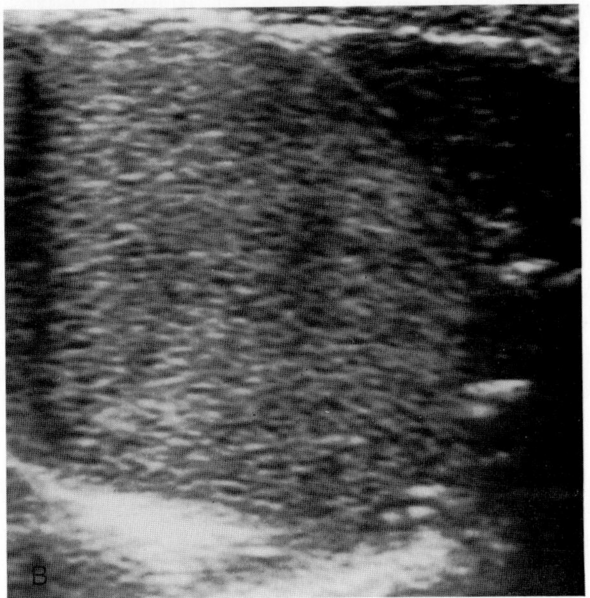

FIG. 2.11.   Neuroblastoma. (A) Longitudinal section of this child reveals the inferior vena cava (C) pushed superiorly by an inhomogeneous mass seen behind it. There was shadowing (arrow) indicating calcium. (B) A less typical picture of a neuroblastoma shows a homogeneous well-demarcated suprarenal mass. It was of even texture.

once beyond childhood, ultrasound is more diagnostic of dominant polycystic disease with large cysts present in any portion of the nephron. Sonographic familial renal screening has been performed in the older child.[34,35] Thus, in polycystic disease ultrasound alone is not diagnostic but it helps direct the workup (remember, we are starting with large renal masses) and is useful, although a histological diagnosis cannot be made by the sonographic architecture alone.

The histological diagnosis by sonography of renal and extrarenal masses has been debated.[36-39] Although in general the commonest extrarenal mass, a neuroblastoma, is more heterogenous than the commonest renal tumor, Wilms' tumor, there is a great deal of overlap. Wilms' tumor is more homogenous but may have necrosis and is most often clearly intrarenal; however, exophytic Wilms' tumor occurs, and conversely neuroblastomas can invade the kidney (Figs. 2.11 and 2.12).

Ultrasound does well when it identifies the viscera of origin (respiratory motion of the lesion with regard to the kidney is important on real-time scanning), directs the workup by examining the routes of spread of the most likely lesion, and leaves the histology to the pathologists.

In general, it is accepted that cystic lesions are more likely to be benign and solid ones malignant. A rare renal lesion contradicts this dictum.[40] The sonographic appearance of a multilocular renal cyst and "cystic" Wilms' tumor may be identical (Fig. 2.13). It is uncertain whether these cystic Wilms' tumor are areas of tumor necrosis or are malignant changes of a multilocular cyst (even the pathologists cannot always tell us). Once again, a histological diagnosis by sonography escapes us.

Two other cystic lesions can be quite indistinguishable on the sonogram alone—a simple renal cyst and an obstructed duplication.[41] Although the bilobed parenchymal outline and separation of the central sinus fat may suggest a duplication (both cyst and duplication have through transmission and posterior enhancement and are frequently found in the upper pole), the sine qua non is the identification of a dilated ureter. In fact, many small obstructed duplications have a small, not easily visualized, ureter, and a urogram is necessary to separate displaced calyces (duplication) from distorted ones (intrarenal mass, cystic or solid) (Fig. 2.1). Similarly, a giant hydrocalyx can present in the same manner. In these instances, both the urogram and sonogram are mandatory for the correct diagnosis.

Renal Trauma

Computed tomography (CT) has been shown to be the best single imaging modality for blunt abdominal trauma.[42-44] When CT is supplemented with contrast enhancement, it shows renal excretion, is equisitively sensitive to extravasation, and defines the full extent of the injury. Sonography fails to show function, and the retroperitoneal soft tissues are usually not well seen since gas (swallowed air, ileus, and so on) often obscures large areas of the retroperito-

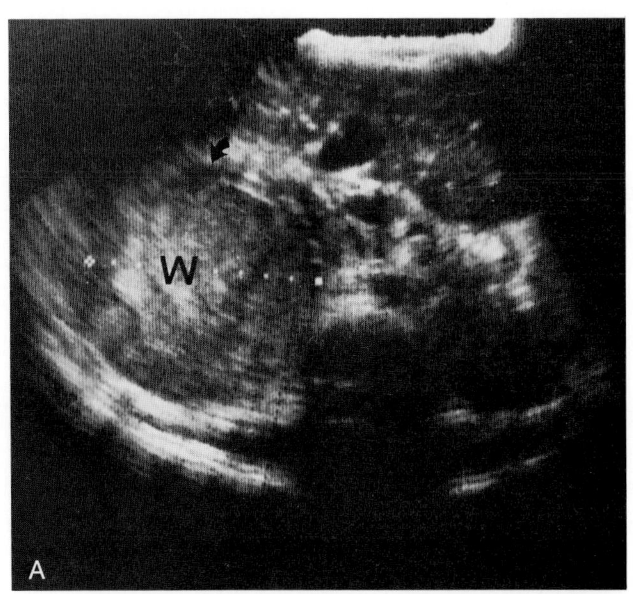

A

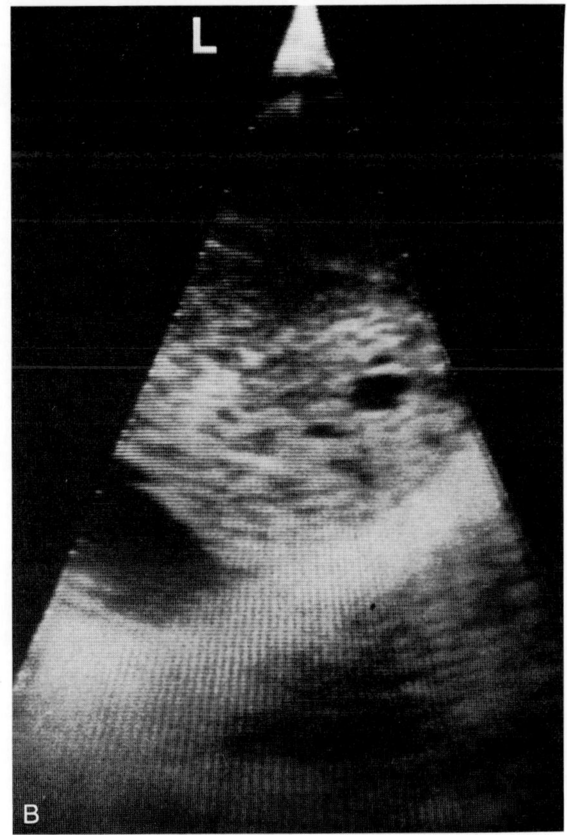

B

FIG. 2.12. Wilms' and other renal tumors. (A) Transverse scan in a typical Wilms' tumor (W). The tumor is homogeneous, and there is no through transmission. There is a pseudocapsule between the tumor and the liver (arrow). (B) It is not unusual to have multiple areas of necrosis within the tumor as seen in this left-sided Wilms' tumor. L = left (Figure continues).

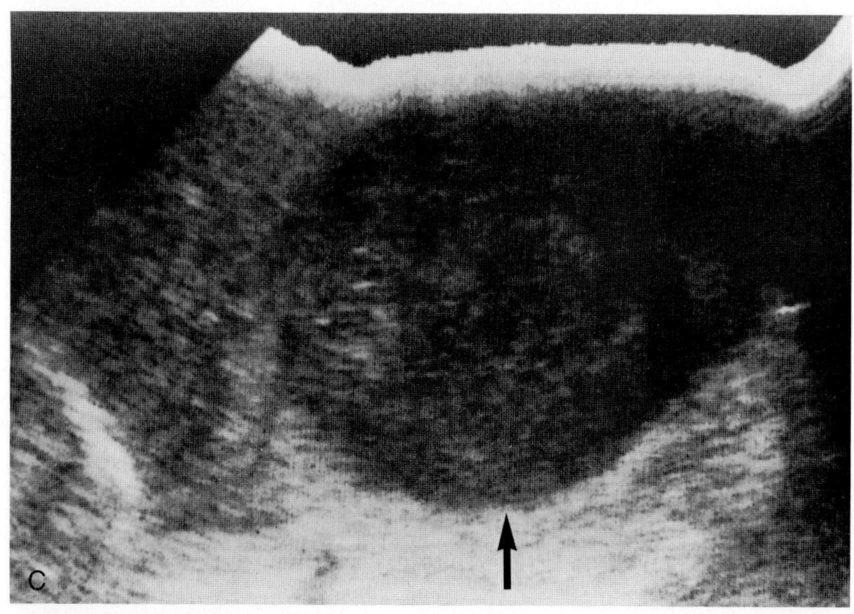

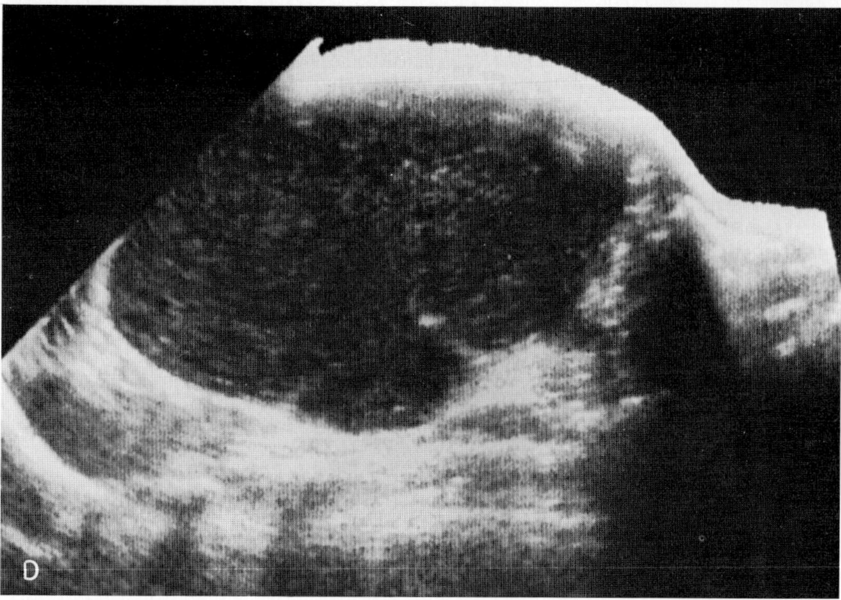

FIG. 2.12 (Continued). (C) Another Wilms' tumor, but this time with good transmission and good back wall (arrow). At surgery, this was a typical Wilms' tumor. (D) This renal tumor in a 13-year-old girl also had good through transmission and good posterior wall. It is much less echogenic than the typical case (A) and is similar to (C). This was proven to be a teratoma of the kidney (Figure continues).

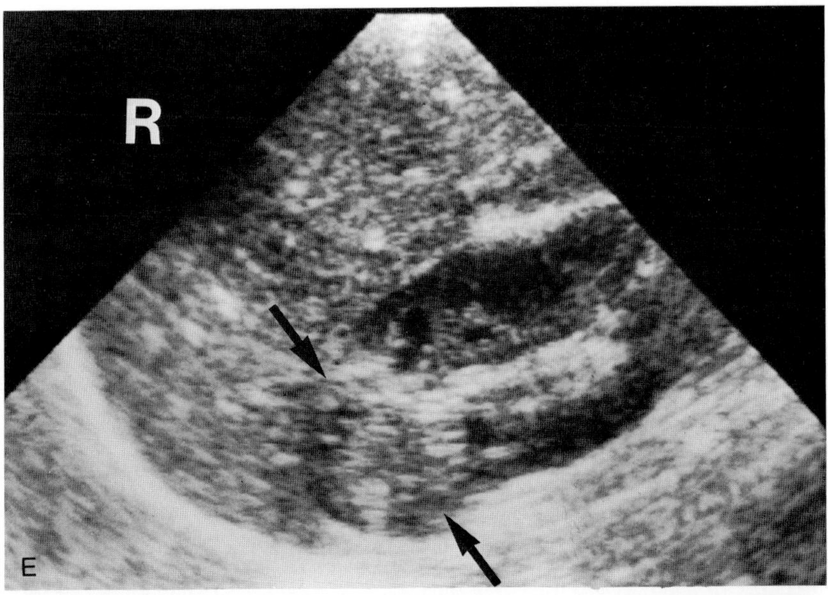
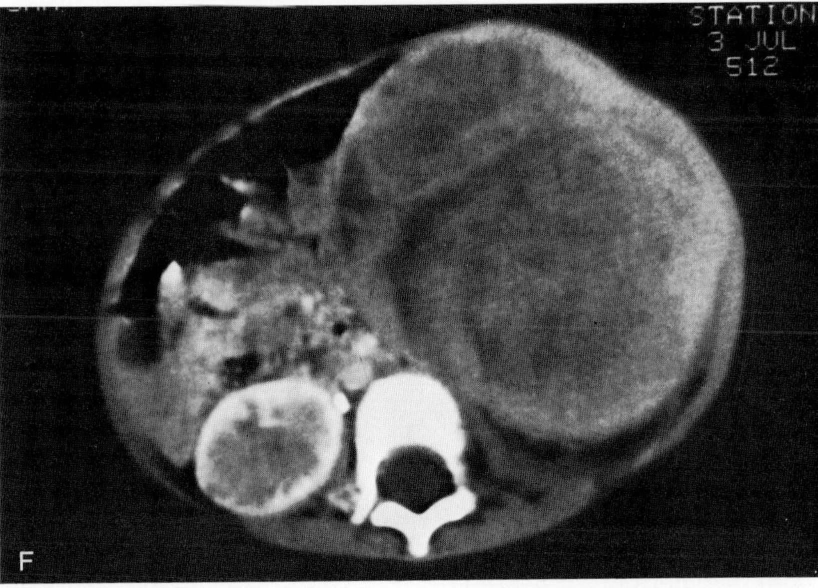

FIG. 2.12 (Continued). (E) This 18-month-old female presented with a huge left-sided mass. Ultrasound evaluation revealed a large echogenic mass with necrosis on the left, but this longitudinal scan of the right kidney was a surprise. There is a dense echogenic region in the upper pole (arrows) and similar lesions were found in the lower pole. (F) CT scan on the same patient reveals the large left tumor crossing the midline and a lesion in the right kidney. This child had bilateral Wilms' tumor.

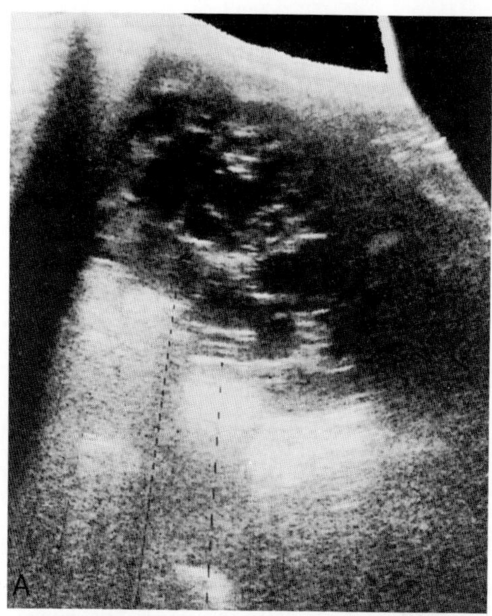

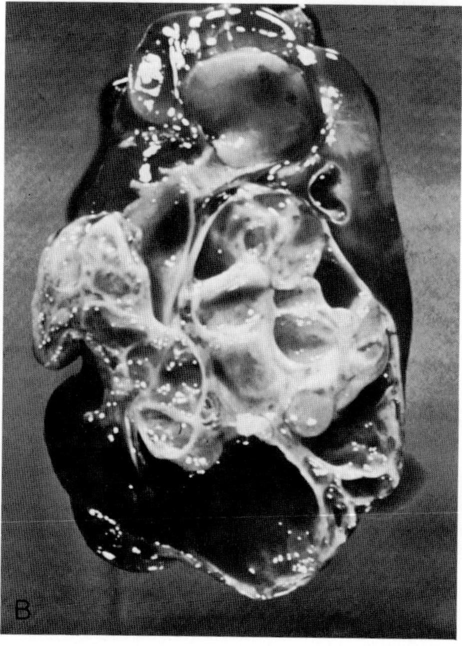

FIG. 2.13. Cystic masses of the kidney. (A) Female 18 months old presented with a large left flank mass. The longitudinal prone sonogram reveals multiple cystic structures with no solid component. The collecting system was distorted and not easily shown. (B) Gross specimen shows the multiloculated cyst in the center of the kidney distorting the normal collecting system and renal parenchyma (Figure continues).

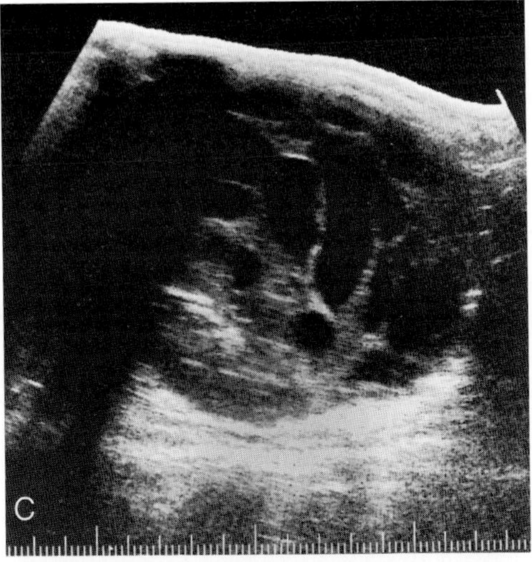

FIG. 2.13 (Continued). (C) A 5-year-old female presented with a large left flank mass. Ultrasound evaluation revealed multiple cystic areas distorting the entire kidney with no discernable collecting system visualized. (D) Gross specimen revealed a necrotic Wilms' tumor which is predominately cystic. Tumor was also found in the renal artery.

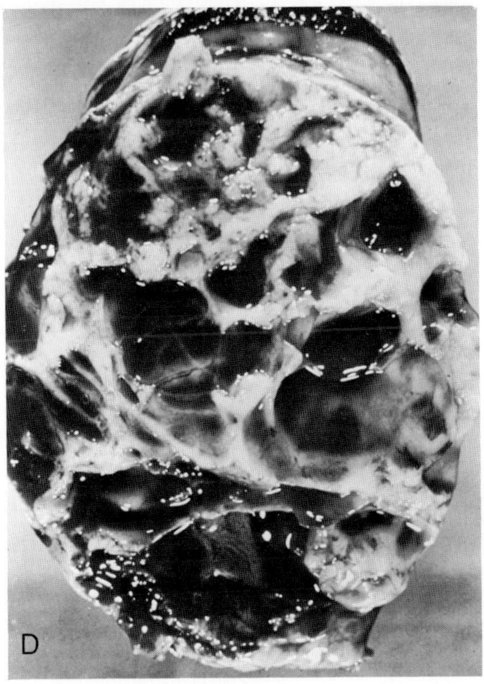

neum. Sonography, however, does have a role once the baseline injury is known.[42] Sonography directs the imaging follow-up by suggesting resolution or acute change that necessitates either a CT, nuclear study, or surgery.

Renal Calculi

The use of sonography as the *primary* imaging test to find renal calculi (not nephrocalcinosis) is fraught with dangers. The central sinus fat is quite echogenic, and this profusion of echoes may well mediate against detecting the stone. Whereas sonography is more sensitive for the detection of calcium, the plain film is more accurate in detecting renal pelvic and ureteral stones.[45] If the goal is detection of the etiology of flank pain, a plain film (to see the renal or ureteral stone) still seems most appropriate. Once a stone or questionable stone is identified on the plain film, the sonogram may confirm the presence of calculi and will accurately evaluate the degree of obstruction. If the patient is known to have calculi, the sonogram seems optimal for the detection of hydronephrosis and is less invasive than the urogram. However, if no calculi are detected and there is hydronephrosis, ultrasound should direct the workup to the cystogram and urogram to detect nonopaque calculi or refluxing system.

INTERVENTIONAL USES IN PEDIATRICS

At Children's Hospital of Michigan, ultrasound has been used for percutaneous guidance in 126 renal biopsies and 30 percutaneous drainage or aspiration procedures over the last 4 years. There have been no complications of these procedures, and in only 2 renal biopsies was there failure to obtain adequate tissue samples. Ultrasound prior to the biopsy has on occasion suggested potential dangers (calyces deep into the lower pole, gallbladder directly adjacent to the kidney, kidney high under the ribs, and so forth) which have necessitated an open biopsy.

After the initial ultrasound (frequently the day before the procedure), the patient is premedicated and brought to the ultrasound department with intravenous line in place. For renal biopsy, the patient is in the prone position and scanned with the static scanner *without* any angulation of the transducer. The skin surface is marked, and the depth to the center of the kidney determined. A True-cut biopsy needle (Travenol Laboratories) is used, and two biopsies are obtained.

For percutaneous drainage or biopsy of a lesion, a real-time examination is done, and the best access plane determined.[46–48] The procedure is monitored with real time, and for drainage procedures a 22-gauge spinal needle inserted. Once in the lesion, a guidewire is placed through the needle, the needle removed, and a catheter threaded over the guidewire. In most cases, contrast is placed in the lesion, and fluoroscopy is utilized to further define the lesion.

REFERENCES

1. Teele RL: Ultrasonography of the genitourinary tract in children. Rad Clin North Am 15:109, 1977

2. Slovis TL, Perlmutter AD: Recent advances in pediatric urological ultrasound. J Urol 123:613, 1980

3. Babcock DE: Medical diseases of the urinary tract and adrenal glands. p. 113. In Haller JO, Shkolnik A (eds.): Clinics in Diagnostic Ultrasound. Vol. 8. Churchill Livingstone, New York, 1981

4. Markle BM, Potter BM: Surgical diseases of the urinary tract. p. 135. In Haller JO, Shkolnik A (eds.). Clinics in Diagnostic Ultrasound. Vol. 8. Churchill Livingstone, New York, 1981

5. Cook JH, Rosenfield AT, Taylor KJ: Ultrasonic demonstration of intrarenal anatomy. Am J Roent 129:831, 1977

6. Haller JO, Berdon WE, Friedman AP: Increased renal cortical echogenicity: A normal finding in neonates and infants. Radiology 142, 1982

7. Hricak H, Slovis TL, Callen CW, Callen PW, Romanski RN: Neonatal kidneys: Sonographic anatomic correlation. Radiology 147:699, 1983

8. Bernstein J: Polycystic disease. p. 557. In Edelman CM Jr (ed.). Pediatric Kidney Disease. Vol. 40. 1978

9. Rosenfield AT, Taylor KJW, Crade M, DeGraaf CS: Anatomy and pathology of the kidney by gray scale ultrasound. Radiology 128:737, 1978

10. Wicks JD, Silver TM, Bree RL: Giant cystic abdominal masses in children and adolescents: Ultrasonic differential diagnosis. AJR 130:853, 1978

11. Sanders RC: The place of diagnostic ultrasound in the examination of kidneys not seen on excretory urography. J Urol 114:813, 1975

12. Shkolnick A:B-mode ultrasound and the nonvisualizing kidney in pediatrics. Am J Roent 128:121, 1977

13. Haller JO, Schneider M: Pediatric Ultrasound. Yearbook Medical Publishers, Chicago, 1980

14. Mitnick JS, Bosniak MA, Hilton S, Raghavendra BN, Subramanyam BR, Genieser NB: Cystic renal disease in tuberous sclerosis. Radiology 147:85, 1983

15. Foley LC, Atchawee L, Graviss ER, Campbell JB: Nephrocalcinosis: Sonographic detection in Cushing syndrome. AJR 139:610, 1982

16. Goh TS, LeQuesne QW, Wong KP: Severe Infiltration of the kidneys with ultrasonic abnormalities in acute lymphoblastic leukemia. AJDC 132:1204, 1978

17. Rosenfield AT, Glickman MG, Taylor KJW, Crade M, Hodson J: Acute focal bacterial nephritis (acute lobar nephronia). Radiology 132:553, 1979

18. Slovis TL, Babcock DS, Hricak H, Han BK, Rose G, McEnery P, Muz J, Chang C, Fleischmann LE, Corbett DP: Sonographic evaluation of children with renal transplants. Radiology, 153:659, 1984

19. Hricak H: Renal medical disorders: The role of sonography. p. 43. In Sanders RC, Hill MC (eds.). Ultrasound Annual. Raven Press, New York, 1982

20. Currarino G, Williams B, Dana K: Kidney length correlated with age: Normal values in children. Radiology 703, 1983

21. Haugstvedt S, Lundberg J: Kidney size in normal children measured by sonography. Scand J Urol Nephrol 14:251, 1980

22. Moskowitz PS, Carroll BA, McCoy JM: Ultrasonic renal volumetry in children. Pediatr Radiol 61, 1979

23. McCauley RGK, Leonides JC, Fretzayes AM, Klarber GC: To what extent can ultrasound replace excretory urography in children with UTI. Presented at The Society of Pediatric Radiology, Las Vegas, Nev., April 1984

24. Kangerloo H, Gold RH, Fine RN, Diament MJ, Boechat MI: Role of ultrasonography in evaluation of children with urinary tract infection. Radiology 154:367, 1984

25. Ben-Ami: The sonographic evaluation of urinary tract infections in children. Semin Ultrasound CT MR 5:19, March 1984

26. Mason WG Jr: Urinary tract infections in children: Renal ultrasound evaluation. Radiology 153:109, 1984

27. Radiation protection in pediatric radiology: NCRP Report No. 68. Washington, D.C., 1981

28. Kessler RM, Altman DH: Real time sonographic detection of vesicoureteral reflux in children. AJR 138:1033, 1983

29. Rosenfield AT, Siegel NJ: Renal parenchymal disease: Histopathologic-sonographic correlation. AJR 137:793, 1981

30. Hayden CK, Santa-Cruz FR, Ampro EG, Brouhard B, Swischuk LE, Ahrendt DK: Ultrasonographic evaluation of the renal parenchyma in infancy and childhood. Radiology 152:413, 1984

31. Mahony BS, Filly RA, Callen PW, Hricak H, Golbus MS, Harrison MR: Fetal renal dysplasia: Sonographic evaluation. Radiology 152:143, 1984

32. Bernstein J, Sedman A, Gabow P, Gardner KD, Drummond KN, Kissane JM: Non-neoplastic, genetic renal cystic disease, dialogues in pediatric urology. Glassberg KI (ed.). 1984

33. Hayden CK, Swischuk LE, Davis M, Brouhard BH: Puddling: A distinguishing feature of adult polycystic kidney disease in the neonate. AJR 142:811, 1984

34. Walker FC, Loney LC, Root ER, Meison GL, McAlister WH, Cole BR: Diagnostic evaluation of adult polycystic kidney disease in childhood. AJR 142:1273, 1984

35. Rosenfield A, Lipson MH, Wolf B, Taylor KJW, Rosenfield NS, Hendler E: Ultrasonography and nephrotomography in the presymptomatic diagnosis of dominantly inherited (adult-onset) polycystic kidney disease. Radiology 135:423, 1980

36. Jaffe MH, White SJ, Silver TM, Heidelberger KP: Wilms' tumor: Ultrasonic features, pathologic correlation, and diagnostic pitfalls. Radiology 140:147, 1981

37. White SJ, Stuck KJ, Blane CE, Silver TM: Sonography of neuroblastoma. AJR 141:465, 1983

38. Hartman DS, Sanders RC: Wilms' tumor vs. neuroblastoma: Usefulness of ultrasound in differentiation. J Ultrasound Med 1:117, 1982

39. Sanders RC, Hartman DS: The sonographic distinction between neonatal multicystic kidney and hydronephrosis. Radiology 151:621, 1984

40. Wood BP, Muurahainen N, Anderson VM, Ettinger LJ: Multicystic nephroblastoma: Ultrasound diagnosis (with a pathologic-anatomic commentary). Pediatr Radiol 12:43, 1982

41. Bartholomew TH, Slovis TL, Kroovand RL, Corbett DP: The sonographic evaluation and management of simple renal cysts in children. J Urol 123:732, 1980

42. Kaufman RA, Towbin R, Babcock DS, Gelfand MJ, Guice KS, Oldham KT, Noseworthy J: Upper abdominal trauma in children: Imaging evaluation. AJR 142:449, 1984

43. Berger PE, Munschauer RW, Kuhn JP: Computed tomography and ultrasound of renal and perirenal diseases in infants and children. Pediatr Radiol 9:91, 1980

44. Kay CJ, Rosenfield AT, Armm M: Gray-scale ultrasonography in the evaluation of renal trauma. Radiology 134:461, 1980

45. Erwin BC, Carroll BA, Sommer FG: Renal colic: The role of ultrasound in initial evaluation. Radiology 152:147, 1984

46. Pedersen JF, Cowan DF, Kristensen JK, Holm HH, Hancke S, Jensen F: Ultrasonically-guided percutaneous nephrostomy. Radiology 119:429, 1976

47. Winfield AC, Kirchner SG, Brun ME, Mazer MJ, Braren HV, Kirchner FK: Percutaneous nephrostomy in neonates, infants, and children. Radiology 151:617, 1984

48. Hruby W, Marberger M: Late sequelae of percutaneous nephrostomy. Radiology 152:383, 1984

3 Ultrasound of Renal Failure

DEBORA GREEN
BARBARA A. CARROLL

Sonography plays an important role in the clinical evaluation and management of patients with renal failure. Causes of renal failure can be categorized into prerenal (hypoperfusion due to shock, sepsis, or embolization or renal vein thrombosis), renal [parenchymal diseases including the glomerulonephritides, autoimmune diseases, acute tubular necrosis (ATN), and other diseases involving the interstitium], and postrenal (obstruction of the collection system).[1] Acute renal failure can occur promptly or develop over days to weeks. Chronic renal failure may ensue following prolonged renal involvement by most of the disease entities which produce acute renal failure. Chronic involvement frequently results in a small, echogenic kidney, "the end-stage kidney." Although this appearance is fairly characteristic of chronic nephropathy, the findings are nonspecific. The most important role of sonography in the evaluation of a patient with acute renal failure is accurate sonographic detection of hydronephrosis, distinguishing postrenal or obstructive causes of renal failure from other entities. In addition, this critical distinction can facilitate percutaneous nephrostomy tube placement or other interventional procedures to relieve the obstruction.

PRERENAL

Patients with prerenal-caused renal failure are normally recognized as such by clinical history and lab values. In two entities renal artery thrombosis and renal vein thrombotis sonographic findings have been described. Renal artery thrombosis is usually an acute process. The patient may present with acute flank pain and hematuria. Arterial thrombosis may be diagnosed sonographically when echogenic material is present within the renal arterial lumen.[2] Doppler analysis may show absent renal arterial flow. Areas of prior infarction may appear as wedge-shaped atrophic scars or echogenic foci within the renal cortex due to fibrosis and/or fatty infiltration.[3]

Renal vein thrombosis may present as an acute or chronic process. Acute

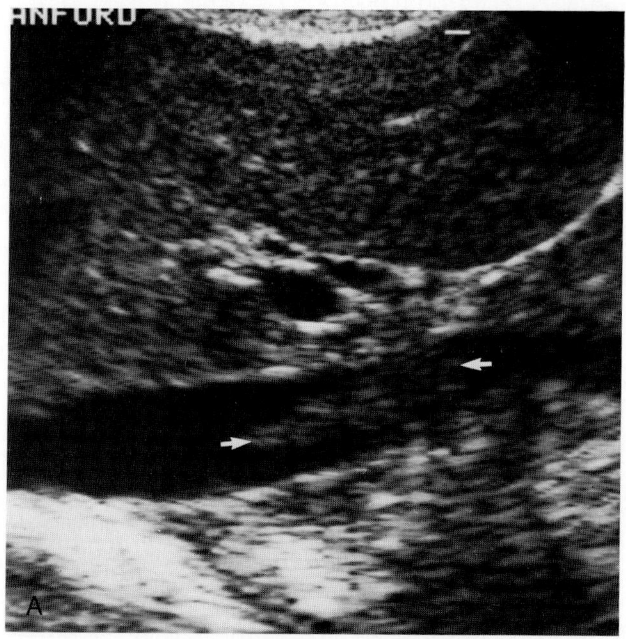

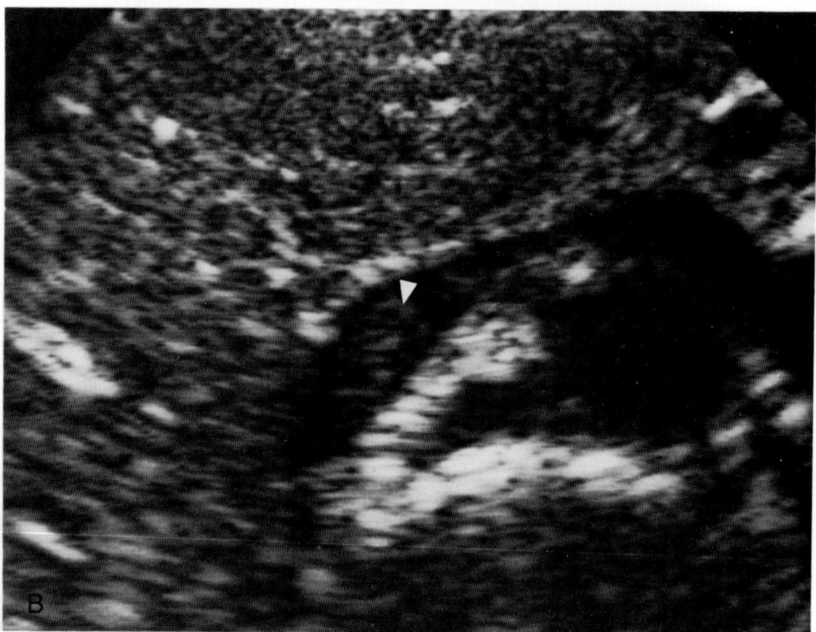

FIG. 3.1. (A) A right sagittal scan demonstrates thrombus in the inferior vena cava (arrows) in a case of renal vein thrombosis. (B) The transverse scan of the same patient shows extension of clot into the left renal vein (arrowhead) (Figure continues).

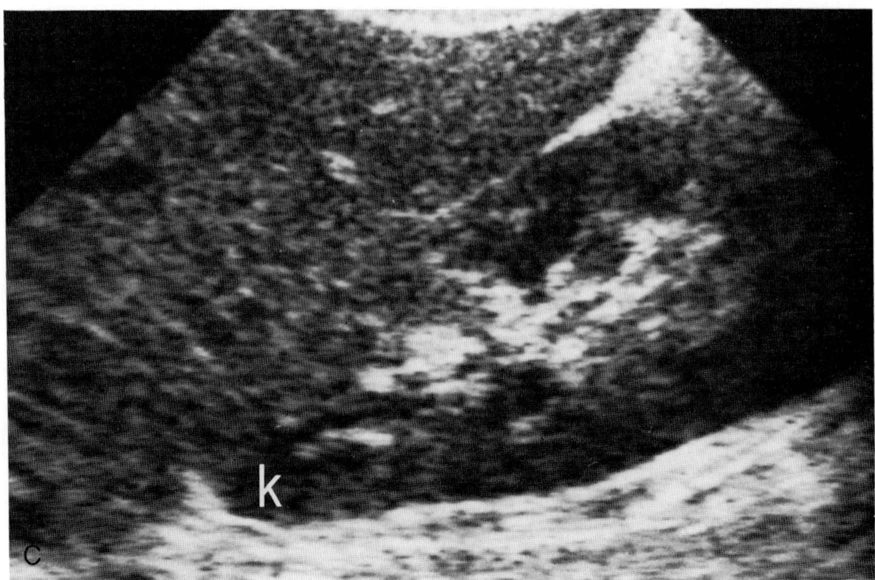

FIG. 3.1 (Continued).   (C) A mildly echogenic right kidney (K) is seen in this case of acute renal vein thrombosis.

symptoms include pain or hematuria; however, such findings are nonspecific.[4] Patients with renal cell carcinoma, retroperitoneal tumors, trauma, dehydration, amyloidosis, inferior vena cava thrombosis, and membranous glomerulonephritis have increased risk for the development of renal vein thrombosis. A similar predisposition is found in patients with nephrotic syndrome, renal transplants, and infants of diabetic mothers.[4,5] Early stages of acute renal vein thrombosis show histopathological changes of hemorrhagic infarction or edema. These changes progress to cellular infiltration and subsequent fibrosis. Similar findings have been noted in dogs following surgical ligation of the renal vein.[5]

Early sonographic changes of acute renal vein thrombosis include increased renal size and decreased echogenicity due to renal edema.[1,4,5] Echogenic material can be identified in the renal vein and/or inferior vena cava (Fig. 3.1A,B). Such echogenic foci are indistinguishable sonographically from tumor or infected thrombus. Real-time ultrasound readily distinguishes these intravascular masses from extravascular tumors which indent the vena cava. In addition, transmitted venous pulsations from the inferior vena cava may be absent on real-time examination. As renal vein thrombosis progresses (10 days to 3 weeks following the initial insult), renal cortical echogenicity increases (due to cellular infiltration) (Fig. 3.1C). Corticomedullary definition is preserved in most cases, and the kidney shows progressive decrease in size. In late stages (more than 3 weeks after renal vein thrombosis), the kidney undergoes further shrinkage with continued increase in echogenicity and loss of corticomedullary definition due to parenchymal fibrosis.[1,4,5] The differential diagnosis of an enlarged hypoechoic kidney in a patient with acute symptoms which might suggest renal vein thrombosis should include acute pyelonephritis and possibly acute renal arterial thrombosis. Chronic processes such as xanthogranulomatous pyelonephritis and malacoplakia may have a similar appearance.[4]

RENAL

Acute renal parenchymal (medical) disease may show no sonographic abnormalities and usually requires clinical correlation and biopsy for definitive diagnosis. However, cases of primary renal disease may demonstrate increased cortical echogenicity and accentuated corticomedullary definition, similar to the appearance of the normal neonatal kidney. Normal adult renal parenchyma should be less echogenic than normal liver or spleen, and medullary pyramids can be identified in more than half of normal patients as wedge-shaped structures, which are less echogenic than the renal cortex.[1,6] In the normal newborn, however, the kidneys are often isoechogenic with the liver and spleen, and in normal premature babies renal echogenicity may exceed that of these adjacent organs (Fig. 3.2).[7]

Acute Tubular Necrosis

Acute tubular necrosis (ATN), the most common cause of acute renal failure, describes many forms of renal failure which result from a variety of toxic and ischemic insults leading to widespread tubular epithelial cell destruction.[1] Toxins responsible for such changes include heavy metals and drugs (including antibiotics, anesthetics, and solvents). The renal insufficiency which develops in such cases is abrupt; however, the process may be reversible. Histologically, there is necrosis of tubular cells, and cellular casts are present in the collecting tubules. The kidneys are often swollen and edematous. Most patients with ATN have sonographically normal kidneys; no changes in renal architecture, cortical echogenicity, cortical thickness, or the appearance of medullary pyramids will be identified.[1,8-10] Occasionally, increased cortical echogenicity and accentuated corticomedullary definition will be observed, as well as a slight increase in renal size.

Acute Cortical Necrosis

Acute cortical necrosis is a rare form of acute renal failure which occurs most commonly in patients with shock, sepsis, hemorrhage, burns, renal vein thrombosis, hemolytic uremic syndrome, toxemia of pregnancy with abruptio placenta, and cases of severe dehydration.[11,12] The actual mechanism responsible for acute cortical necrosis (ACN) is uncertain, but it may be due to capillary damage and vasospasm secondary to intravascular thrombus or toxin production, resulting in ischemic necrosis.[12] Histological findings are those of acute

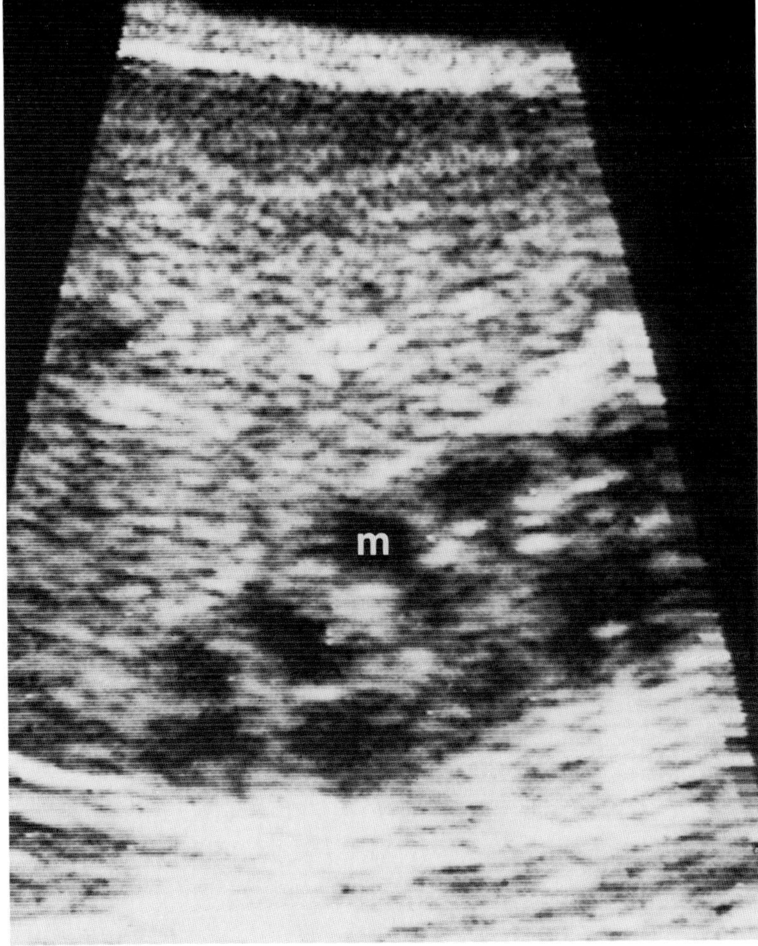

FIG. 3.2. A right sagittal scan through the kidney of a premature neonate shows increased cortical echogenicity and prominent medullary pyramids (m).

ischemic infarction limited to the cortex, with necrosis of tubular cells and cellular infiltration into the interstitium. The medulla and a thin rim of subcapsular tissue, which derives its blood supply from capsular vessels, remain intact. Punctate or linear calcifications may be seen as early as 24 hours after infarction at the junction of necrotic and viable tissue or diffusely throughout the renal cortex.[11]

Initially, the renal cortex may be hypoechoic on ultrasound. Subsequently, there is often increased renal cortical echogenicity due to calcific depositions (such changes are more commonly seen in the chronic stages of this disease process) (Fig. 3.3). Increased echogenicity is directly related to the degree of calcification and collagen deposition in the renal cortex. Follow-up studies have shown progressive decreases in renal size and increased echogenicity.

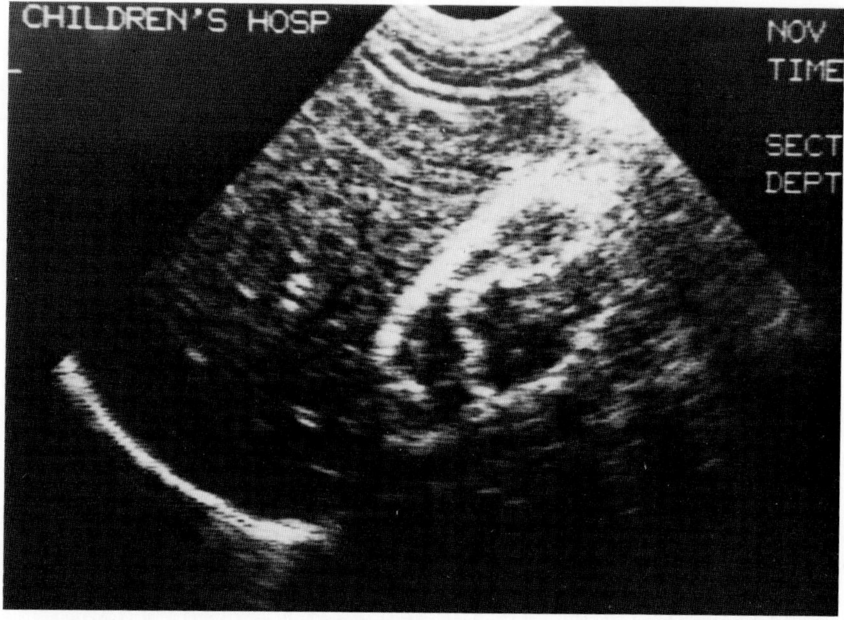

FIG. 3.3. Longitudinal sonogram of the right kidney shows the renal cortex is intensely echogenic compared with the liver parenchyma in a case of renal cortical necrosis in hemolytic uremic syndrome. (Sty JR, Starshak R, Hubbard A: Acute renal cortical necrosis in hemolytic uremic syndrome. J Clin Ultrasound 11:175, 1983.)

Myoglobinuria

Myoglobinuria is the cause of acute renal failure in 5 to 7 percent of patients; conversely, as many as 33 percent of patients with myoglobinemia develop acute renal failure.[13] Other patients with lower levels of myoglobinemia and myoglobinuria may develop chronic renal failure. Myoglobinemia results from myoglobin release into the tissues and blood stream following rhabdomyolysis due to a number of causes including alcohol and drug addiction, crush injuries, strokes, toxins, fever, or myositis. Myoglobin is normally cleared in the liver by metabolism to bilirubin.[13] Myoglobinuria occurs when the blood levels exceed the renal threshhold of 1.5 mg/dl. The cause of renal failure is uncertain but is thought to be secondary to nephrotoxicity with tubular obstruction.[13] Histological findings include acute tubular necrosis, brown casts, interstitial edema, and cellular infiltration. There may be engorgement of medullary and glomerular vessels. Chronic changes include atrophy and fibrosis.

The sonographic appearance of kidneys affected by this entity is variable as the histological changes would indicate. The kidneys may appear completely normal in cases where the histological changes are those characteristic of ATN, or be enlarged and echogenic in cases where the histological changes reflect cellular interstitial infiltration. On some occasions, the medullary pyramids may be prominent and hypoechoic due to enlarged, distended medullary vessels. The kidneys may also be shrunken and echogenic in end-stage fibrosis.[13]

Acute Glomerulonephritis

Acute renal inflammation may be categorized into two basic areas: (1) the glomerulonephritides which represent a renal inflammatory response caused by an autoimmune reaction resulting in glomerular damage in such diseases as lupus, and (2) interstitial nephritis which is an entity caused by infectious organisms, exposure to toxins and drugs, or infiltration of inflammatory cells into the renal interstitium.[14]

Patients with acute glomerulonephritis (AGN) typically present with hematuria, hypertension, azotemia, and red cell casts in the urine. The disease may reverse or progress to end-stage renal disease. Streptococcal glomerulonephritis is caused by immune complexes interacting with glomerular basement membranes. Histologically, there is proliferation of endothelial and mesangial cells in glomeruli and exudate of white blood cells.[15] Other forms of AGN include Goodpasture's syndrome, which appears similar histologically, rapidly progressive glomerulonephritis, and collagen vascular disease.

Sonographically, the kidneys appear enlarged, although they may be normal in size early in the disease process. Marked increased echogenicity similar to that of the renal sinus is frequent, and the medullary pyramids, which remain sonolucent, may appear quite prominent (Fig. 3.4).[16,17] Follow-up examinations show progressive decrease in renal size. Echogenicity may return to a more normal appearance with reversal of azotemia. No definite histological entity responsible for the increased echogenicity has been identified.[17]

Bacterial Interstitial Nephritis (Pyelonephritis)

Interstitial nephritis caused by infectious organisms is termed "pyelonephritis." This is usually a unilateral process and therefore rarely a cause of renal failure. Such renal infections usually result from urinary or hematogenous spread, with an increased incidence seen in renal obstruction due to urinary stasis. These kidneys are usually normal on ultrasound, although local or diffuse renal enlargement and decreased echogenicity may be seen. Complications including lobar nephronia and abscess formation may be identified; lobar nephronia usually appears as a focal hypoechoic mass, whereas abscesses present as irregular cystic collections within the kidney.

Other Interstitial Nephritides

Acute bacterial nephritis is a more severe acute infectious interstitial process occurring most often in diabetics. Histologically, there is marked infiltration of parenchyma by inflammatory cells and edema. Sonographically, there is

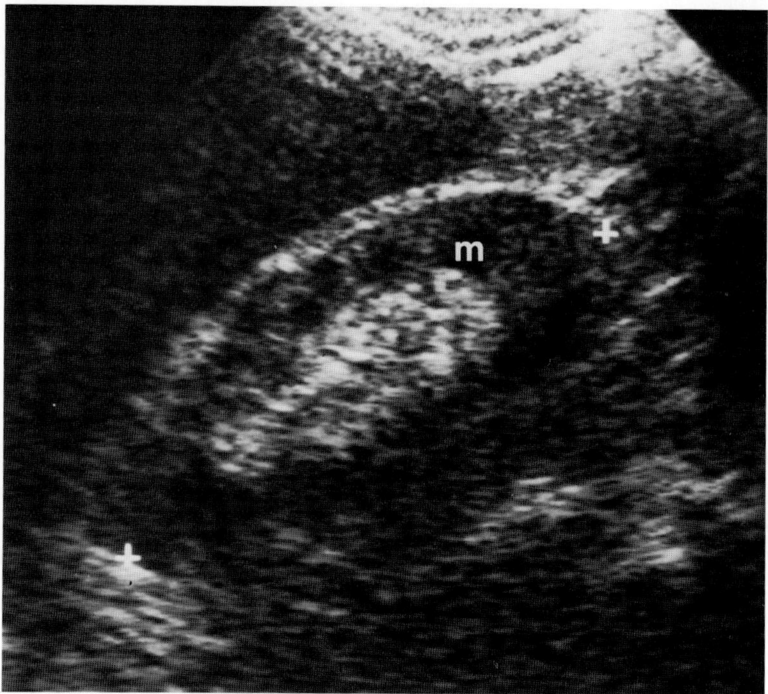

FIG. 3.4. A patient with renal failure and systemic lupus erythematosis demonstrates an enlarged kidney (+) with prominent medullary pyramids (m).

enlargement and increased renal echogenicity.[14] Interstitial nephritis secondary to systemic infections, drug hypersensitivity, and analgesic abuse also demonstrate interstitial white cell infiltration.[15] Although the sonographic appearance of such kidneys has not been reported, presumably they would appear echogenic.

Xanthogranulomatous Pyelonephritis

Xanthogranulomatous pyelonephritis is usually associated with chronic infections, struvite stone formation, and obstruction secondary to staghorn calculi. *Proteus* is the most common inciting organism, and there is an increased incidence in middle-aged females and diabetics. Pathologically, the kidney is enlarged with yellowish nodules containing lipid-filled macrophages and granulomata, calculi, and pyelonephrosis. Twenty-seven to eighty percent of these kidneys have diffuse involvement and are nonfunctioning. A renal mass may be evident in cases of focal disease involvement in as many as 62 percent of cases, and calculi are present in the majority of these kidneys. Sonographically, the kidneys are enlarged with uniform or heterogeneous hypo or anechoic masses and echogenic foci.[18,19] Echogenic central staghorn calculi with posterior acoustic shadowing are usually demonstrated. The differential diagnosis includes renal cell carcinoma, particularly in cases of more focal xanthogranulomatous pyelonephritis, lymphoma, and tuberculosis, although this is less likely to produce a renal mass.

Renal Tuberculosis

Renal tuberculosis occurs following hematogenous dissemination of the pulmonary tubercle bacillus.[20] Screening studies reveal that 2.3 to 5 percent of patients with pulmonary tuberculosis (TB) have concurrent renal TB, although renal TB may occur in the absence of active pulmonary foci. The peak age of presentation is the third decade, but patients may present at any age.[21] The patients may be asymptomatic or relate frequency, dysuria, and hematuria; in addition, chronic renal failure, uremia, and pyuria may be noted on initial presentation.

Bacilli seed the cortex via a hematogenous route inducing abscesses and granuloma formation, caseation necrosis, fibrosis, and cortical destruction. Such fibrosis may progress even while on chemotherapy.[20] Cortical lesions may extend to involve the medullary pyramids, ulcerate and discharge bacilli into collecting structures, seeding the renal pelvis, ureters, and bladder. This results in granuloma formation, edema, and fibrosis, and ultimately stricture formation.[20,21] On IV urogram, the most common abnormalities are calyceal distortion and dilatation due to stricture formation; these changes are present in 68 percent of cases.

In diffuse renal tuberculosis, renal echogenicity may be entirely normal. Areas of caseous necrosis adjacent to collecting structures may be difficult to differentiate from clubbed calyces filled with echogenic debris. Focal echogenic areas with shadowing may be seen in diffuse or focal involvement secondary to calcification. Renal tuberculosis may also present with tumefactive masses similar in appearance to those seen in xanthogranulomatous pyelonephritis (Fig. 3.5).[20] Sonography could be expected to detect focal irregularities and thickening of the bladder, as well as bladder calcifications associated with tuberculosis. The differential diagnosis of this process includes xanthogranulomatous pyelonephritis and renal cell carcinoma. Clubbed calyces and scarring due to tuberculosis may result in changes indistinguishable from those seen in chronic pyelonephritis secondary to bacterial infection, papillary necrosis, or occasionally calyceal diverticula.

Amyloidosis

Amyloidosis is one cause of nephrotic syndrome that often progresses to renal failure. Histological changes include extensive amyloid deposits in glomeruli, arterioles, and the interstitium. It is commonly associated with abnormal serum proteins including Bence Jones proteins, and occurs in such disease processes

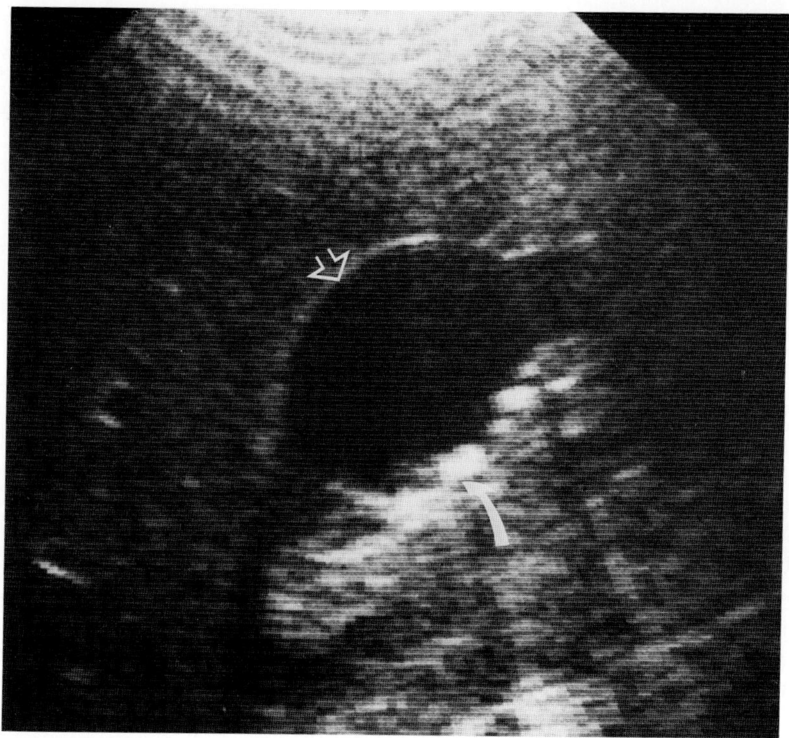

FIG. 3.5. A right sagittal scan shows a dilated hydronephrotic scarred calyx (open arrow) associated with renal calcification (curved arrow) in a case of renal tuberculosis.

as multiple myeloma, or Waldenström's macroglobulinemia. It may also occur in response to chronic infections or inflammation; in such cases, the disease entity is referred to as reactive systemic amyloidosis.[22] Rheumatoid arthritis is the most common cause of reactive systemic amyloidosis; at postmortem, 14 to 26 percent of patients have pathological evidence of amyloidosis. This usually occurs several years after the clinical onset of symptoms of rheumatoid arthritis and is manifested by proteinuria, renal insufficiency, and hepatosplenomegaly.[22] Amyloidosis is also a common complication of juvenile rheumatoid arthritis. It occurs in 4 percent of these patients, and accounts for 44 percent of deaths when the disease is over 10 years in duration.[22,23]

Other immunological diseases, including ankylosing spondylitis, Reiter's syndrome, rheumatic heart disease, scleroderma, dermatomyositis, and systemic lupus erythematosis (SLE), may be complicated by amyloidosis. Tuberculosis is the most common cause of systemic amyloidosis due to chronic infectious processes; however, a longstanding chronic disease such as syphilis, colitis, or osteomyelitis may be associated with the development of reactive amyloido-

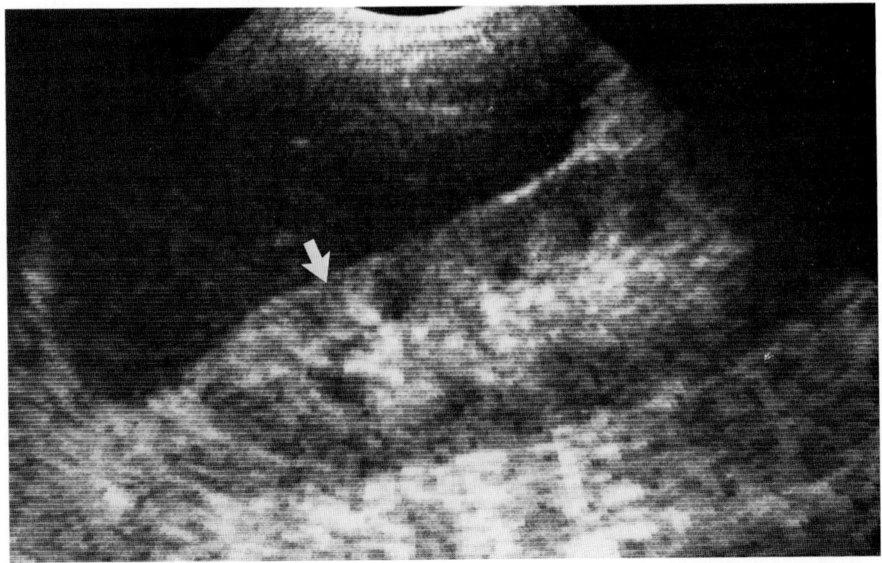

FIG. 3.6.   An enlarged, echogenic right kidney (arrow) with prominent pyramids is seen in this case of acute renal failure secondary to amyloidosis.

sis. Some tumors, particularly renal cell carcinoma and Hodgkin's disease, have a high incidence of associated amyloidosis.

Primary amyloidosis is a disease of uncertain etiology and is unrelated to other underlying disease processes.[24] Primary amyloidosis is present in 0.2 to 0.5 percent of routine autopsies. Secondary amyloidosis is found in 10 to 15 percent of patients with multiple myeloma, 20 to 25 percent of patients with rheumatoid arthritis, and 26 to 40 percent of patients with familial Mediterranean fever. Over half of patients with chronic tuberculosis will demonstrate histopathological evidence of amyloid deposits. In addition, histological evidence of amyloid increases with age.

Although sonographic abnormalities associated with amyloidosis have been described as mainly those of increased echogenicity and diffuse renal enlargement, recent observations have shown that renal enlargement occurs predominantly in acute stages of amyloidosis, with progressive decrease in renal size as the disease advances (Fig. 3.6). Eventually an "end-stage" shrunken kidney results.[23,24] Thus, the kidneys may appear large, normal, or small in size, depending upon the disease stage. Increased cortical echogenicity and accentuated corticomedullary definition are more pronounced in chronic stages of the disease. Although such findings are nonspecific and may result from any number of diffuse medical renal processes, such findings in a patient with abnormal renal function and a history of collagen vascular disease or chronic illness should raise the possibility of amyloidosis.

Diffuse Infiltrative Disease

Renal involvement by leukemia is a frequent finding in leukemic patients at autopsy. One study reports 60 percent of patients in remission at the time of autopsy had microscopic evidence of renal leukemic infiltration.[25] Renal involvement is seen in 3 to 5 percent of pediatric patients with acute lymphatic leukemia; however, such leukemic infiltration rarely causes renal failure, even when disease is extensive. Renal infiltration resulting in uremia occurs in only 1 percent of patients with leukemia and renal involvement.[25] Such renal failure due to leukemia must be differentiated from azotemia due to other causes related to the disease or therapy, including urate nephropathy and drug toxicity; metabolic abnormalities, including hypercalcemia or hypokalemia; obstruction due to adenopathy or stones; side effects of x-ray therapy; or disseminated intravascular coagulopathy.[25-27]

Leukemic cortical infiltration produces nephromegaly. Such infiltration is usually diffuse and bilateral, but may affect the kidneys in an asymmetric fashion with resultant discrepancies in renal size. Less commonly, infiltration is focal and nodular. The degree of infiltration correlates well with the degree of increase in renal size in the majority of patients.[28] However, 15 to 30 percent of patients with leukemia will have mild renal enlargement without histological evidence of leukemic involvement. The etiology of this organomegaly is uncertain, and the extent of renal enlargement seen in this entity is usually not as great as that seen with leukemic infiltration. The degree of renal infiltration does not correlate well with renal function.

Sonographic findings include renal enlargement with normal or increased parenchymal echogenicity.[29] The nodular form of leukemic involvement may show multiple hypo- or anechoic masses, often associated with an irregular outline. Sonography is a useful method to follow reduction of renal size and return to normal echogenicity following radiation and chemotherapy. Similarly, it may be the first means of detection of changes indicative of recurrent disease. Complications of leukemia including unilateral or bilateral hydronephrosis secondary to calculi or tumor masses can also be identified.

Renal lymphoma is usually secondary to hematogenous dissemination or direct extension from local pathological nodes.[30,31] With the exception of the hematopoietic system, the urinary tract is the most common site of metastatic lymphomatous involvement.[32] Primary renal lymphoma is exceedingly rare, possibly because the kidneys do not normally contain lymphoid tissue. In Burkitt's lymphoma in children and occasional non-Hodgkin's lymphomas, renal involvement may be present at the time of initial diagnosis. However, renal lymphoma occurs more commonly in non-Hodgkin's lymphomas at the later stages of disease. Although 33 to 65 percent of patients with lymphoma have renal involvement at autopsy (bilateral involvement in 74 percent of cases), only 7.5 to 14 percent of patients with non-Hodgkin's lymphoma and renal involvement have clinical evidence of disease, because lymphomatous involvement rarely causes renal insufficiency or other symptoms.

The sonographic appearance varies with the form of parenchymal involve-

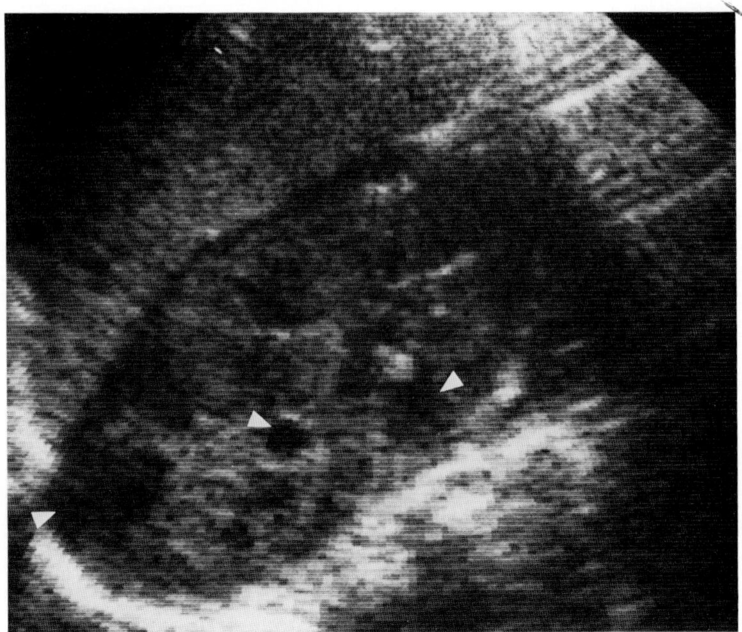

FIG. 3.7. Diffusely enlarged kidneys were seen bilaterally in this patient with lymphoma and renal failure. Focal anechoic masses coexist (arrowheads) with diffuse renal infiltration.

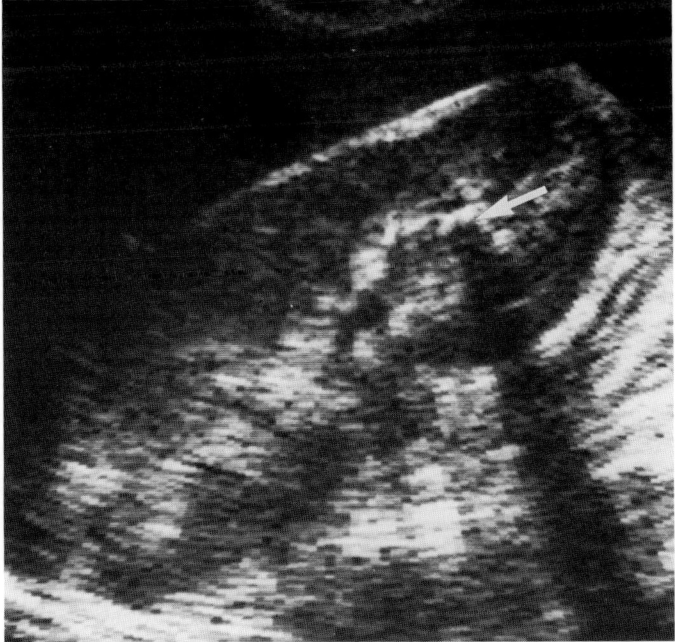

FIG. 3.8. Diffuse lymphomatous infiltrates produced renal enlargement without focal masses in this patient. Renal stone formation (arrow) secondary to hypercalcemia was also noted.

ment. Most commonly, renal lymphoma presents with focal solitary or multiple anechoic or hypoechoic lesions, although echogenic lymphoma masses have been reported. Enhanced posterior sound transmission behind these renal masses may suggest a cyst. However, the margins of these lesions are usually not as discretely defined as those seen in a renal cyst, and they more closely resemble renal abscesses.[33] Diffuse renal infiltration by lymphomatous cells results in renal enlargement, obliteration of corticomedullary definition, and increased echogenicity (Figs. 3.7, 3.8).[27,31-33] Direct renal extension from contiguous abnormal retroperitoneal nodes, ureteral or renal pelvic obstruction by adenopathy, or encasement of the renal collecting system may be identified. It is of interest that the degree of hydronephrosis secondary to lymphomatous adenopathy is often less than anticipated due to adenopathy secondary to other forms of neoplasms.

Sonographic evaluation of changes in renal size and echogenicity or the size of renal masses can be used to monitor response to therapy. Changes in mass echogenicity are less reliable indicators of response to treatment than decrease in mass size. The differential diagnosis of focal lymphomatous involvement includes renal cysts (although this is usually not a difficult distinction to make), necrotic tumors, abscesses, polycystic kidney disease, or xanthogranulomatous pyelonephritis.

Adult Polycystic Disease

Adult polycystic disease (APKD) is a form of primary renal disease transmitted as an autosomal dominant trait with 100 percent penetrance. APKD is a common disease of unknown etiology and occurs in 1 out of every 1,000 births.[17] Although adult polycystic disease can present in infancy and childhood, typically the disease becomes clinically evident in middle age (30 to 40 years), often after the patient has had children.[17,34,35]

Typically, patients present with bilateral renal enlargement, deteriorating renal function, and hypertension. The rate of progression of renal failure is variable, and in some instances the level of renal function may permit a normal life span. Differential diagnosis of bilateral enlarged kidneys with renal failure includes polycystic disease, infiltrative processes, and bilateral renal vein thrombosis. Urographic or sonographic findings of cysts which distort the pelvocalyceal system confirm the diagnosis of polycystic disease. Associated hepatic cysts occur in 25 to 33 percent of patients and pancreatic cysts in 15 percent.[17] Berry aneurysms of the circle of Willis are seen in 11 to 20 percent of patients.

Ultrasound demonstrates large kidneys replaced by multiple bilateral renal cysts of varying sizes. There is often increased echogenicity of the underlying renal parenchyma (Fig. 3.9). Renal cysts are not confluent and therefore can be distinguished from renal hydronephrosis. Kidneys in APKD usually maintain reniform configuration in contradistinction to multicystic dysplastic kidneys which do not. Ultrasound also readily identifies hepatic or pancreatic abnormalities when present. Sonography has been advocated as a means of screening

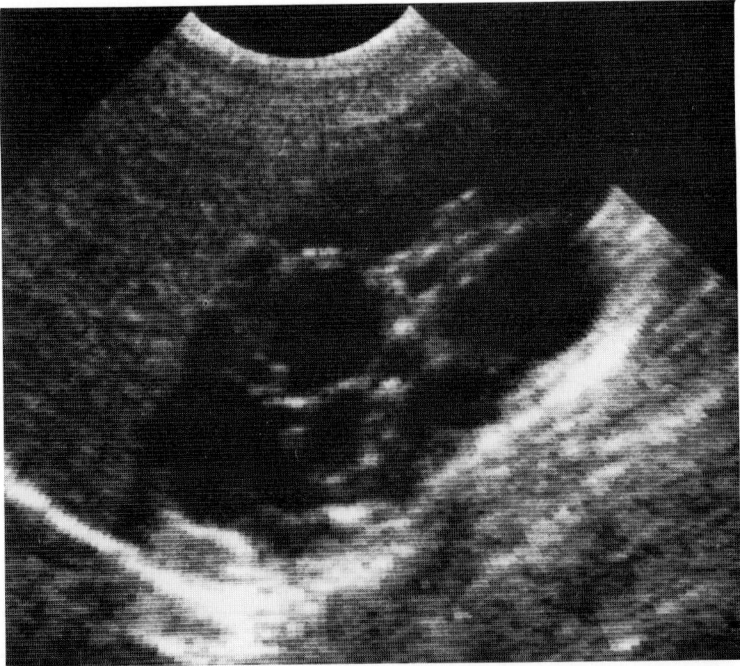

FIG. 3.9. Multiple renal cysts replace most of the normal renal parenchyma in this case of adult polycystic renal disease and uremia. The enlarged right kidney retains its reniform shape on this longitudinal scan.

asymptomatic progeny of patients with a family history of polycystic disease. A recently reported study of such patients ranging in age from 14 months to 32 years revealed renal cysts and some hepatic cysts on the initial exam in 37 percent of asymptomatic patients screened. Such information can be useful in genetic counseling in such patients.[34] This is particularly true as sequential ultrasound examinations can be repeated without risk of ionizing radiation or contrast exposure.

Infantile Polycystic Disease

Infantile polycystic disease is an autosomal recessive trait which occurs with varying degrees of severity. The most severe form of disease causes death early in infancy due to pulmonary insufficiency. Histologically, this disease consists of a proliferation of dilated renal tubules, leading to small cyst formation and renal enlargement. Sonographically, the kidneys are enlarged bilaterally and echogenic, often with enhanced posterior sound transmission.[36-38] The increased echogenicity is thought to arise from the multiple specular echoes which occur at the interfaces of the ectatic tubules. There is loss of normal cortico-

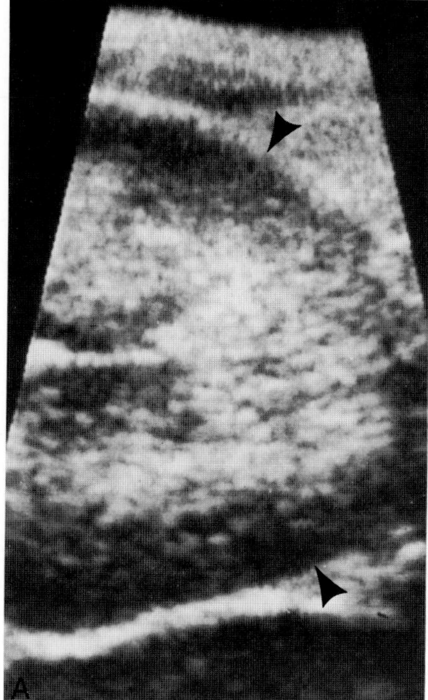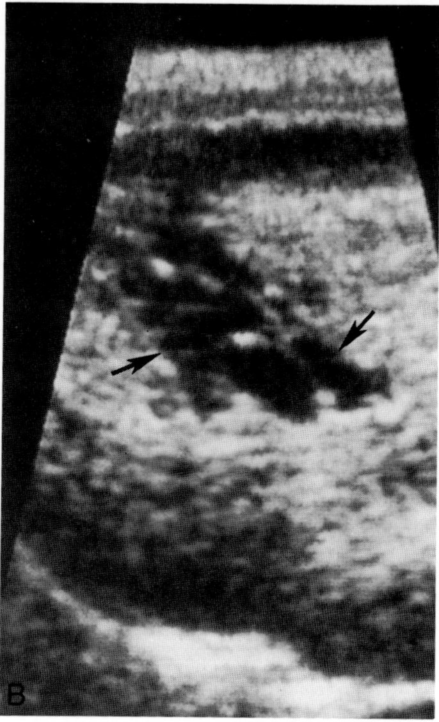

FIG. 3.10.   (A) Longitudinal scans through the lower pole of the left kidney in a neonate with infantile polycystic kidney disease show a markedly enlarged echogenic kidney (lower pole) (arrowheads) with loss of the normal hypoechoic medullary pyramids. (B) A transverse scan through the right kidney of the same infant shows an echogenic, enlarged kidney with scattered macrocysts (arrows).

medullary definition, although the kidneys are reniform in shape. Macrocysts can occur in kidneys involved by infantile polycystic disease, although these are less common than in adult polycystic disease (Fig. 3.10A,B).[17] Similarly, associated hepatic cysts may be seen in patients with infantile polycystic disease. More commonly, however, hepatic fibrosis leading to liver failure occurs in those patients with infantile polycystic disease who survive beyond early childhood.[17] Such abnormalities of the liver are manifested sonographically by increased echogenicity in the hepatic parenchyma. Occasionally, APKD may manifest in infancy, and its appearance may be similar to that of either infantile polycystic disease or adult polycystic disease. A positive family history will usually help distinguish between these two types of polycystic renal disease. Also helpful is the fact that adult polycystic disease results in minimal renal dysfunction in the infant. Infantile polycystic disease can be detected in utero and is often associated with oligohydramnios.

Medullary Cystic Disease and Nephronophthisis

Medullary cystic disease is an autosomal dominant entity which typically affects children and young adults. It occurs rarely in middle age and in older patients.[17] Patients present with a classic triad of symptoms including azotemia, anemia, and salt-losing nephropathy.[39] There is a high incidence of associated renal osteodystrophy. Sonographic findings include small shrunken kidneys with anechoic cysts located at the corticomedullary junction. If these cysts are tiny, the medullary pyramids may appear echogenic, as in infantile polycystic disease resulting in "fluffy" medullary echoes.[17,39] Clinically, the differential diagnosis of azotemia and salt-losing nephropathy includes chronic interstitial nephritis secondary to analgesic abuse, bilateral renal hypoplasia or dysplasia, postobstructive atrophy or chronic obstruction. The sonographic features of medullary cystic disease should be distinctly different from those in these other entities. The fact that the kidneys are small and the cysts are medullary in location is useful in differentiating this entity from polycystic disease.

Nephronophthisis is similar to medullary cystic disease except that it is autosomal recessive in inheritance and effects a younger age group. Occasionally, these patients may benefit from salt replacement. Thus, differentiation of this process from chronic renal failure of other causes may be useful for purposes of genetic counseling and therapy. Although nephronophthisis effects a younger age group, it may represent a variant of medullary cystic disease, as the pathological changes are similar to those seen in this entity. Sonography usually shows decreased renal size, loss of corticomedullary definition, and increased echogenicity; medullary cysts may also be identified. Demonstration of medullary cysts in a child with renal failure is virtually pathognomonic of nephronophthisis or medullary cystic disease, as such medullary cysts are rare in other forms of childhood renal failure.[40] Cystic changes associated with chronic renal failure can also occur in a rare syndrome called the Laurence-Moon Biedl syndrome; however, the symptoms in this disease entity are significantly different from those in nephronophthisis.

Nephrocalcinosis

Renal parenchymal calculi can be a cause of renal failure when they are diffuse, result in bilateral renal obstruction, or obstruction of a solitary functioning kidney. The most common cause of acute bilateral obstruction due to calculi is urate stones. Such stones are often not radiopaque, but can be readily identified by ultrasound. Causes of nephrocalcinosis include hypercalcuria and hypercalcemia due to any pathological process. Malignancy is the most common cause of hypercalcemia due to bone metastases or ectopic hormone production. When hypercalcemia exceeds the renal tubular threshold for calcium resorption, there is deposition of calcium in renal tissues. Classically, this calcification occurs at the corticomedullary junction, but such deposits may occur anywhere

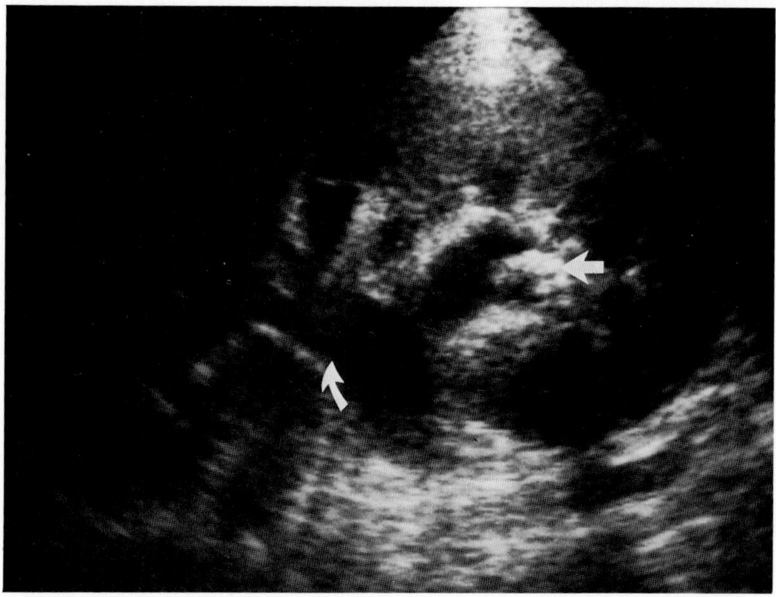

FIG. 3.11.   A patient with a lower pole renal calculus (arrow) also demonstrates mild hydronephrosis (curved arrow).

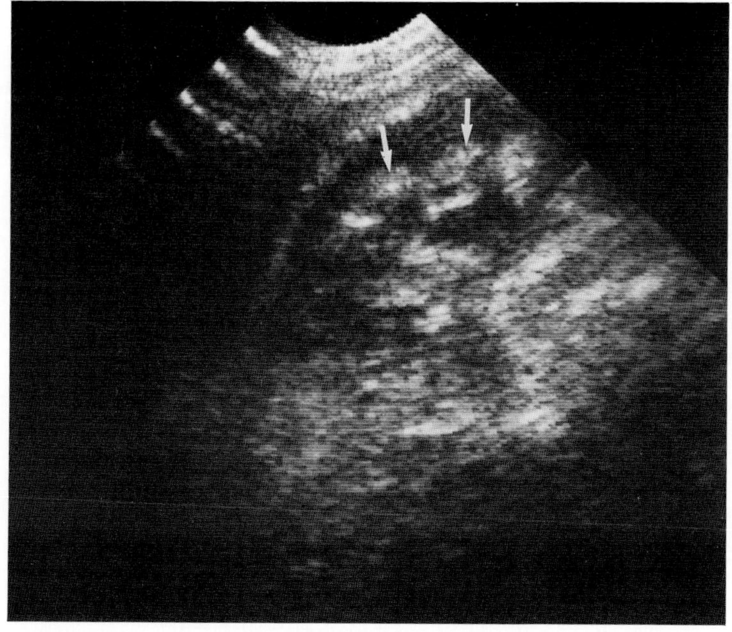

FIG. 3.12.   A right coronal scan in a patient with medullary sponge kidney and renal failure shows echogenic medullary pyramids (arrows) secondary to medullary calcification.

in the renal parenchyma.[41] Other causes of nephrocalcinosis include dehydration, excessive excretion of calcium, abnormalities of urine PH, and endocrine abnormalities including gout, excess urate excretion, and hyperoxaluria.

Solitary renal calculi are identified sonographically as focal echogenic structures with posterior acoustic shadowing. The appearance is similar regardless of stone composition.[42,43] Stones as small as 1 1/2 × 1 1/2 mm are readily visualized providing that the proper transducer frequencies, focal zones, and gain settings are utilized (Fig. 3.11).

Diffuse nephrocalcinosis appears markedly different from focal renal calculi in most instances.[44,45] In the normal kidney, the medullary pyramids are decreased in echogenicity relative to the cortex or can be difficult to differentiate from normal cortical echoes. Conversely, in cases of medullary nephrocalcinosis, medullary pyramids become highly echogenic relative to the adjacent renal cortex, and there may be posterior acoustic shadowing emanating behind the pyramids. Visualization of arcuate arteries at the base of the renal pyramids confirms the localization of echogenicity to the medulla. Such medullary calcifications are also readily identified by their triangular shape and their position relative to the renal sinus and columns of Bertin. Echogenic medullary pyramids are virtually pathognomonic for medullary nephrocalcinosis and may be seen even when there is no evidence of calcification on a radiographic plain film or tomogram (Fig. 3.12).

Other etiologies of echogenic renal pyramids have been cited; however, most of these occur in the neonate and are relatively uncommon. These include polycystic kidney disease of the infantile form and transient anuria of the newborn due to tubular precipitation of TAM-Horsfall proteins.[46]

Primary hyperoxaluria, a rare metabolic hereditary disorder, results in calcium oxalate nephrocalcinosis and nephrolithiasis.[47-49] Extrarenal oxalate depositions, oxalate calculi, and progressive renal failure occur in this entity. This disorder results in cortical rather than medullary calcifications. Sonographically, these kidneys are of normal size, but have a highly echogenic cortex with obliteration of the corticomedullary junction. Although some authors report that this entity has a highly specific ultrasound appearance, increased cortical echogenicity in normal-size kidneys has also been described in the absence of hyperoxaluria and may occur in the absence of any renal dysfunction. Cortical nephrocalcinosis may also be seen after acute renal cortical necrosis. In such instances, the kidneys may remain normal in size. Hypercalcemia secondary to carcinoma may also produce diffuse cortical nephrocalcinosis. Occasionally, the increased cortical echogenicity seen in end-stage kidney disease may be marked and difficult to distinguish from nephrocalcinosis on the basis of the sonographic findings alone.

POSTRENAL RENAL FAILURE (OBSTRUCTION)

Bilateral renal obstruction accounts for only 5 percent of cases of acute renal failure; however, it is one of the major correctable causes of renal failure.[1] Bilateral obstruction can be encountered in patients with chronic renal failure

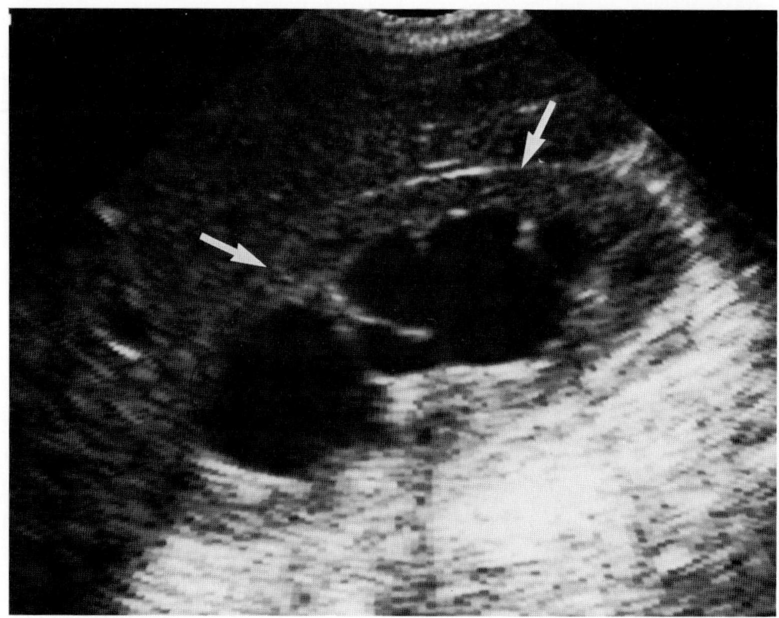

FIG. 3.13.   A right coronal scan in a patient with renal failure and bilateral hydronephrosis secondary to a pelvic mass shows moderate hydronephrosis and slightly increased cortical echogenicity (arrows).

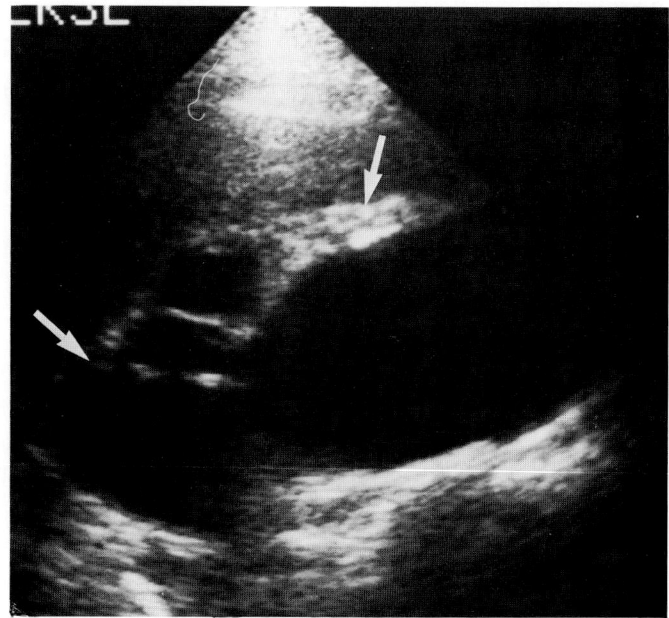

FIG. 3.14.   A patient with longstanding, intermittent obstruction demonstrates marked hydronephrosis with atrophic, echogenic renal cortex (arrows).

as well. The most common cause of bilateral obstruction in adults is a pelvic tumor.[50,51] Bilateral ureteral calculi are uncommon (should this occur, the most common type of stone is a uric acid stone). Since renal obstruction can be relieved by a variety of methods of drainage, including ultrasound-guided percutaneous nephrostomy, it is important to exclude hydronephrosis as a cause of acute or chronic renal failure in any patient.

The normal renal sinus is an echogenic area composed of peripelvic fat and many interfaces including vascular and collecting structures.[6] Hydronephrosis produces separation of the normal renal sinus echoes by an anechoic fluid collection with posterior acoustic enhancement. Hydronephrosis can be graded as mild (slight separation of central sinus echoes by an anechoic fluid collection within the dilated renal pelvis), moderate (further separation of central echoes), and marked (evidence of thinning of the renal parenchyma associated with the central fluid collection) (Figs. 3.11, 3.13, 3.14).[51-53] Severe hydronephrosis may be difficult to differentiate from a large cystic mass; however, real-time sonography should demonstrate continuity of multiple cystic structures with a dilated central renal pelvis.[54] Visualization of a dilated renal pelvis and calyces as well as ureter provides the most reliable indicator of renal obstruction. Although the thickness of overlying renal cortex may be useful in determining the chronicity of obstruction and as a prognostic indicator of future renal function following relief of obstruction,[17] renal cortical thickness is not always a reliable indicator of renal function, and radionuclide studies provide more accurate information in such situations.

Real-time ultrasonography demonstrates urographically confirmed obstruction in 97 to 100 percent of cases.[1] Static scanning is slightly less accurate. False-positive diagnoses may occur in up to 10 to 26 percent of cases. Most commonly, this is due to interpreter variability in diagnosing mild hydronephrosis in cases of minimal separation of central renal sinus echoes.[52,55] Additionally, anatomical and physiological causes of dilatation such as congenitally large collecting systems, prominent extrarenal pelves (Fig. 3.15),[7] marked bladder filling with delayed calyceal emptying, congenital megacalyces and calyceal diverticuli may be misinterpreted as hydronephrosis.[1,52,53] In patients who are well hydrated and actively diuresing, real-time ultrasound will demonstrate a dynamic filling of the collecting system which may be quite prominent followed by rhythmic contractions and emptying of the renal pelvis at anywhere from two to six contractions per minute (Fig. 3.16A,B). Jets of urine extending from the region of the ureteral orifice to the center of the bladder lasting for a few seconds can be visualized and may be useful in excluding obstruction in questionable cases.[56,57] The intravesicle echoes which arise from the ureteral orifices may be due to turbulent flow, differences in specific gravity, or other factors. The presence of these jets can be useful in determining whether there is an excreting kidney as well as ruling out potential reflux. Physiological states where there is increased urine output causing distension of the collecting system without obstruction include diabetes insipidus, overhydration, or diuresis due to drugs or following an IV urogram and postobstructive diuresis in cases of renal failure in the nonoliguric phase.

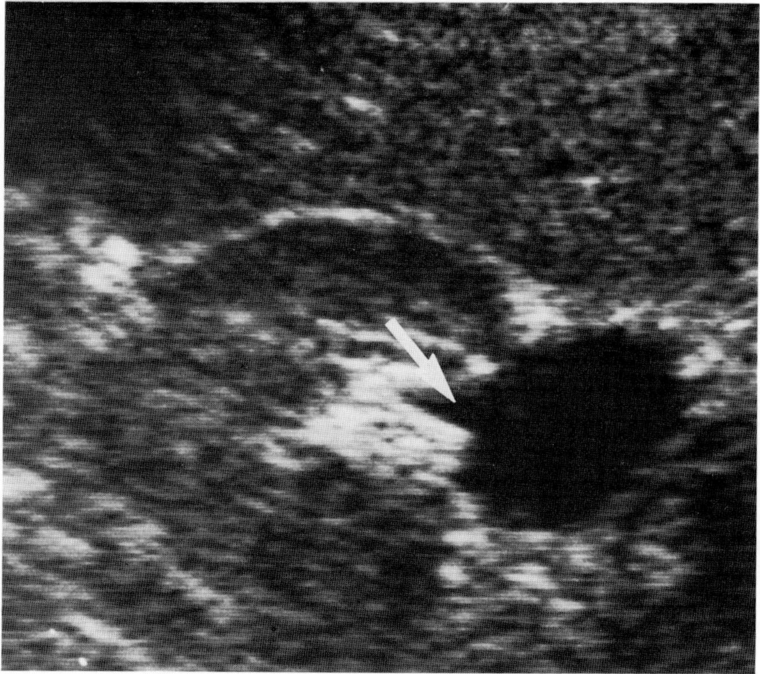

FIG. 3.15. A transverse scan demonstrates a prominent, distended extrarenal pelvis (arrow) but no evidence of calyceal dilatation. Transverse scans help distinguish such an anatomical variant from pathological obstruction.

Pathological entities which mimic diffuse hydronephrosis include chronic pyelonephritis with blunted scarred calyces, tuberculosis with focal areas of stricture and calyceal dilatation, papillary necrosis, and ureterocalyceal dilatation in cases of acute pyelonephritis. Residual calyceal dilatation may also be seen in the postobstructive phase following relief of hydronephrosis and may persist for some months to years. In addition, pelvocalyceal dilatation may be seen in cases of severe reflux without obstruction.[17] Multiple confluent renal cysts, peripelvic cysts, and arteriovenous malformation may be mistaken for hydronephrosis.[58,59] However, careful real-time examination will show that these cysts have neither intercommunication nor branching patterns to suggest a dilated collecting structure.[1,58]

False-negative diagnoses are infrequent, occurring less than 1 percent of the time.[52] This misdiagnosis occurs most frequently in the setting of minimal dilatation and interpreter variability. Dilated calyces are misinterpreted rarely as medullary pyramids. Other causes of false-negative diagnoses include staghorn calculi with posterior acoustic shadowing which obscures dilated collecting structures, acute obstruction which has not yet resulted in dilatation, decompression of the system by tubular backflow or calyceal rupture (Fig. 3.17), and renal obstruction associated with longstanding renal failure. One may also

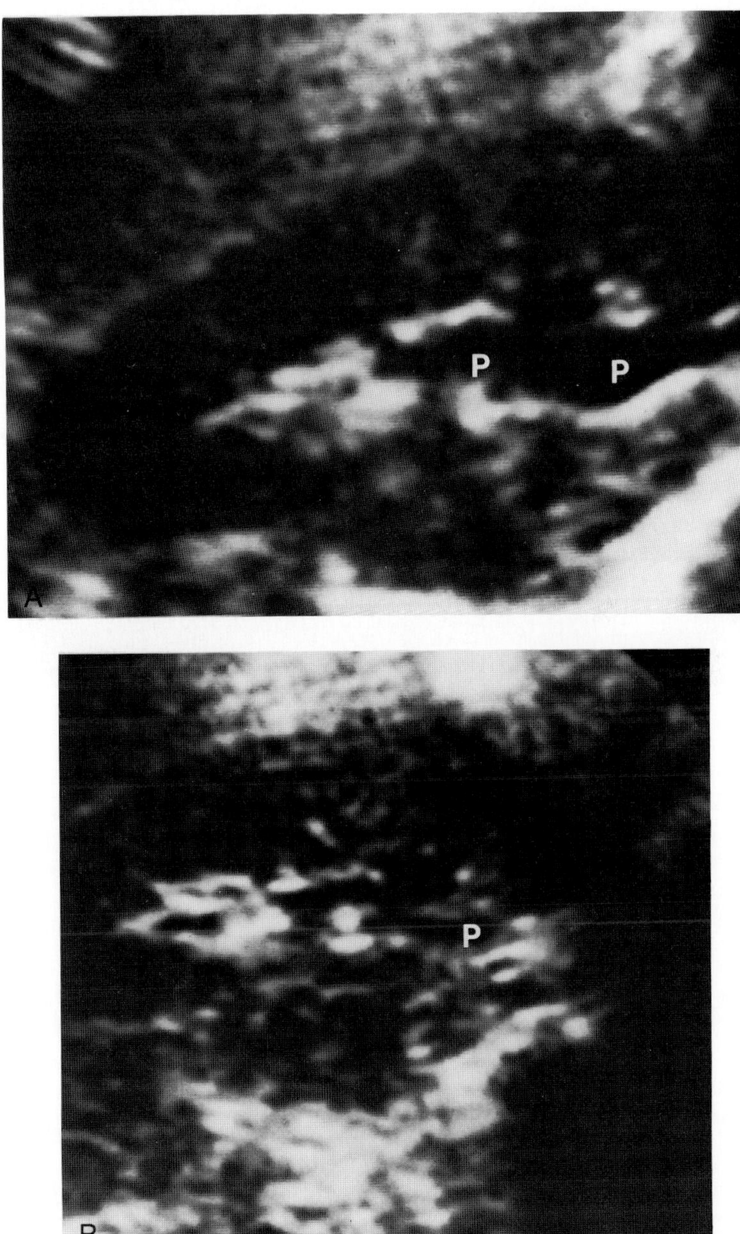

FIG. 3.16. (A) A transverse scan through the renal pelvis in a well-hydrated patient shows a prominent renal pelvis (p). (B) Immediately following a normal peristaltic contraction, the renal pelvis is significantly smaller (p).

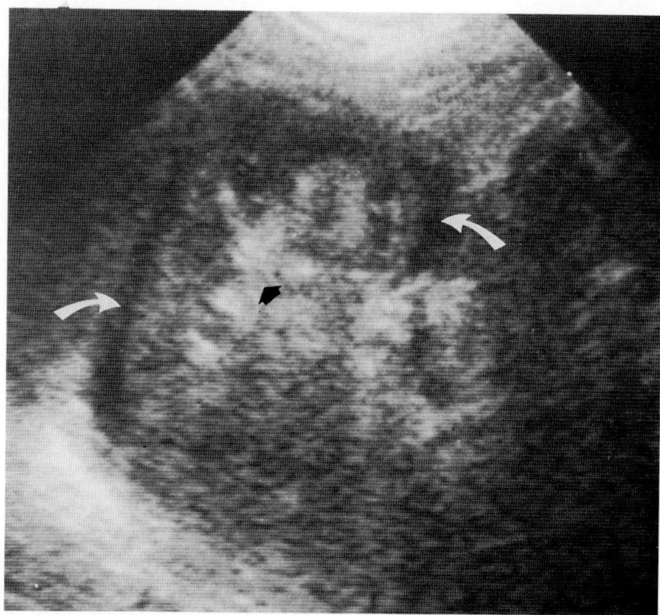

FIG. 3.17.   A patient without evidence of left hydronephrosis on a coronal scan (arrow) has renal obstruction which has been decompressed through a ruptured fornix with resultant perinephric urinoma (curved arrows).

fail to see hydronephrosis in patients that are severely dehydrated or who have only partial intermittent obstruction. In minimal dilatation nephropathy, secondary to longstanding retroperitoneal fibrosis, impaired renal function associated with decreased urine output may result in mild-to-absent hydronephrosis in the presence of significant renal obstruction.[50] All routine radiographic techniques used to rule out obstruction will have similar difficulties diagnosing this entity. Causes of minimal dilatation nephropathy include an anatomical variant of intrarenal collecting system, retroperitoneal fibrosis, periureteral or perirenal tumor, or encasement of the ureters.[50,60] Superimposed infection and ureteric edema may cause complete obstruction in the setting of underlying chronic partial obstruction. The inability to detect hydronephrosis or hydro-ureter is probably the result of periureteric fibrosis or compression of a long-standing nature, resulting not only in decreased renal function but in the inability of the ureter to be distended. In patients with signs and symptoms of longstanding obstructive nephropathy, a kidney which is of normal size and echogenicity with a normal-appearing collecting system or demonstrating only mild dilatation, the possibility exists that there is significant obstruction due to one of the previously mentioned causes. An IV urogram and/or retrograde or antegrade ureterogram with subsequent drainage may prove that obstruction is really present. On rare occasions, obstruction in end-stage kidneys may be difficult to detect due to a difficulty visualizing the distorted collecting system, decreased urine output, or inability to visualize the kidney due to patient obesity and bowel gas.

Hydronephrosis Due to Renal Calculi

Ultrasound offers a viable alternative to the intravenous urogram in the initial evaluation of patients with renal colic.[61] Using the ultrasound criteria for a positive examination of either a visualized calculus within the ureter or unilateral hydronephrosis or hydroureter on the side of symptoms, one can correctly identify patients in whom renal colic secondary to stone exists. Although obstruction secondary to calculi is rarely a cause of renal failure, this can occur in cases of a solitary functioning kidney or rarely in cases of bilateral obstruction. Adequate patient hydration results not only in a full bladder through which the distal ureters and ureterovesicle junction can be observed (the most common site for a stone to be lodged is the ureterovesicle junction), but also accentuates renal obstruction and hydronephrosis. In cases of renal obstruction, the normal rhythmic ureteral activity may be disrupted for long periods, and this aperistalsis can be demonstrated on ultrasound. In addition, mounds of periureteric edema surrounding the obstructing renal calculus are frequently present. The detection of ureteric jets into the bladder can be used to infer the presence of a nonobstructive renal calculus.

Pregnancy

One common physiological state which results in dilatation of the collecting structures is pregnancy. The incidence of ureteral dilatation in pregnancy is at least 65 to 80 percent and is more marked on the right side. In this condition, ureters are of normal caliber below the pelvic inlet. Dilatation of the renal system should return to normal within several weeks post partum.[62,63] The etiology of this hydronephrosis is probably due to mechanical pressure on the ureters by the enlarged uterus as the degree of hydronephrosis and the right-sided predominence of ureteral dilatation is similar to that seen in pelvic masses. Other etiologies may include relaxation of the ureters due to hormonal factors. Ureteropelvicalyceal dilatation described as mild to moderate is seen by 10 to 20 weeks' gestation in more than 60 percent of women and often increases in severity as the pregnancy progresses, peaking at 24 to 28 weeks.[62] It is important to be aware of the range of normal dilatation in pregnancy in order to be able to evaluate the pregnant woman with symptoms suggestive of acute obstruction. Measurements of the renal pelvis in the anterior-posterior diameter in pregnant women in both the prone and prone oblique position have been recorded in a study of several hundred pregnant women compared with controls. Maximum measurements were 1.1 cm on the right and 0.9 cm on the left in nonpregnant controls; 1.8 cm on the right and 1.5 cm on the left in the first trimester and 2.7 cm on the right and 1.8 cm on the left in the last two trimesters. These statistics may provide useful guidelines in evaluating the pregnant patient with symptoms of acute urinary obstruction. There may be variability among patients and, when necessary, sequential ultrasound examinations can be done to exclude rapidly increasing dilatation.[62]

Pyonephrosis

The fluid in the hydronephrotic collecting system is usually anechoic. However, in patients in whom there is pyonephrosis, a common complication of renal obstruction and stasis, internal echoes within the fluid, many of which are dependent and mobile, can be identified. These echoes may be due to tissue and cellular debris or hemorrhage and may be diffusely dispersed or layer dependently in the collecting system (Fig. 3.18).[14,64-66] The echogenicity of such debris is variable. In some instances infected urine may be extremely echogenic; however, increased posterior sound transmission and an absence of posterior acoustic shadowing should readily distinguish such debris from renal calculi. Hemorrhage, and fungus balls may appear similar to pyonephrosis.[5] Increased echogenicity in the renal pelvis associated with posterior acoustic shadowing is usually due to stones. Occasionally, however, this may be due to air within the collecting system secondary to infection by gas-

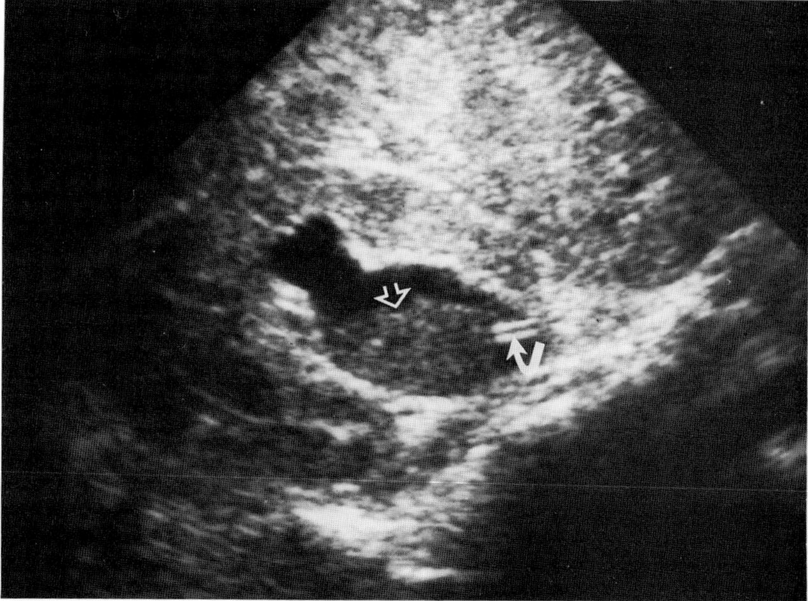

FIG. 3.18.   A patient with pyonephrosis secondary to obstruction demonstrates dependent, echogenic debris (open arrow) following retrograde ureteral stint placement (curved arrow).

forming organisms or recent instrumentation. In cases of large gas collections, multiple reverberations behind the echogenic collection may be useful in distinguishing gas from calcification. Tumors in the renal sinus may also appear as masses of low-level echogenicity within the collecting system. They should not demonstrate posterior enhancement, nor should they change in position. Sonography is particularly valuable in the study of the pyonephrotic kidney because these kidneys are rarely visualized at urography. In patients with symptoms of infection, absence of internal echogenicity in the hydronephrotic fluid is virtually exclusive of infection, whereas discovery of internal echoes within the obstructed kidney (provided the gain settings are properly set) is more than 90 percent accurate for the detection of pyonephrosis.[65] Occasionally false positives may be seen due to debris secondary to hemorrhage. Ultrasound can direct aspiration of these dilated renal pelves, and examination of the fluid should reveal the presence of infection, thus facilitating subsequent percutaneous drainage and antibiotic therapy. (See Chapter 6.)

Ultrasound is a useful screening procedure to exclude obstruction. It provides rapid, accurate evaluation of the collecting system and can be done in the face of elevated creatinine and decreased renal function without the use of contrast or ionizing radiation. It can also provide a useful means of directing subsequent drainage procedures.[51,55,67]

END-STAGE RENAL DISEASE

End-stage renal disease can result from a variety of entities including nephrotic syndrome, glomerulonephritis, collagen vascular disease, diabetes, hypertension, nephrosclerosis, analgesic nephropathy, and chronic pyelonephritis. Because the kidney has only a limited number of ways to respond to various insults, the end-stage kidney usually has a similar appearance pathologically and sonographically regardless of the etiology of renal failure.[37,68,69] Researchers have attempted to predict the underlying disease process and severity of disease on the basis of ultrasound characteristics. This has proven unrewarding except for a few differentiating findings. There is no definite correlation that has been found between the type and severity of glomerular disease and the renal echogenicity on ultrasound.[68,70] Possibly this is due to the minimal space occupied by glomeruli in the renal cortex relative to tubules and interstitium. There is, however, a definite correlation between cortical echogenicity on ultrasound and severity and distribution of interstitial disease histologically.[68-70] Cortical echogenicity has been positively correlated with disease entities leading to global sclerosis, focal tubular atrophy, hyalin casts, and interstitial and cellular infiltration.[68] Again, this is nonspecific, as causes of increased cortical echogenicity are numerous, including glomerulonephritis, amyloidosis, hypertensive nephrosclerosis, leukemic infiltration and atherosclerotic diseases, renal vein thrombosis, and chronic obstructions. The degree of blood urea nitrogen (BUN) and creatinine elevation often correlates with the degree of increased echogenicity; however, a wide range of variability has been found, and patients with high BUN and creatinines may have kidneys with fairly normal echogenicity.[68-70]

Focal disease processes responsible for chronic renal failure include pyelonephritis, tuberculosis, papillary necrosis, and obstructive atrophy.[68,70-72] These diseases usually produce less uniform increased echogenicity than diffuse renal diseases. Renal cortical thickness and renal length can be rough indicators of residual renal function; however, since ultrasound is an anatomical rather than a physiological imaging tool, a more accurate assessment of renal function is usually obtained by a radionuclide study or a radiographic contrast study. Renal lengths less than 10 cm are considered abnormal in the adult. Such decrease in renal size can be positively correlated with longstanding diffuse renal processes; however, there is no significant correlation between the type of disease and the degree of decrease in renal length.[68] No well-defined correlation can be detected between the appearance of the renal sinus and the type or severity of renal disease. Detectability of medullary pyramids or distinctiveness of the corticomedullary junction is also an unreliable way of defining the type or severity of disease in cases of chronic renal failure. Of note is the fact that the normal pediatric kidney may have increased cortical echogenicity equal to that of the liver or spleen up to 6 months of age. This has been attributed to nephron heterogeneity and hypotonicity of medullary fluid.[70] Premature infants may routinely have kidneys which are more echogenic than the adjacent liver or spleen associated with well-preserved corticomedullary definition and normal renal size. Such changes are not indicative of primary renal pathology.[7]

Chronic pyelonephritis is usually a more focal pathological process than other forms of chronic renal failure and involves the full cortical thickness overlying a calyx leading to focal areas of increased echogenicity and cortical thinning.[59,71] The involved calyx is retracted and distorted, resulting in extension of the echogenic collecting structures into the parenchyma and/or focal areas of sonolucency associated with areas of calyceal dilatation and scarring. In addition to detecting echogenic scars within the parenchyma and/or focal dilatation of clubbed calyces, sonography may also detect irregularities of the renal cortex associated with scar formation.

Renal papillary necrosis may be focal or diffuse. It has a variety of causes including diabetes, renal obstruction, sickle cell disease, alcoholism, pyelonephritis, analgesic abuse, ATN, and renal vein thrombosis. Necrosed papillae may detach and remain in situ, or they may be sloughed. When papillae are sloughed, sonography reveals an anechoic space peripheral to the renal sinus representing the deformed calyx similar to that described in chronic pyelonephritis.[71] If multiple, these abnormal papillae will appear as multiple round or triangular hypoechoic or cystic spaces in the region of the medullary pyramids.[72] Occasionally, the arcuate arteries can be identified as echogenic foci peripheral to these anechoic fluid collections, confirming the absence of the papilla. In diffuse papillary necrosis, these cystic spaces may completely ring the renal sinus (Fig. 3.19). The overlying renal cortex will demonstrate abnormalities compatible with the underlying renal pathology. Entities with a sonographic appearance similar to diffuse papillary necrosis include postob-

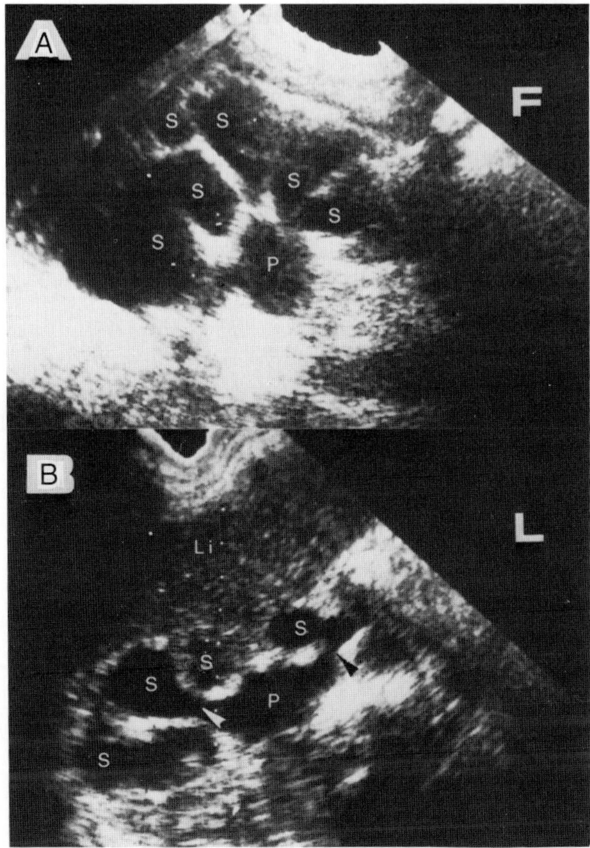

FIG. 3.19. Papillary necrosis in an analgesic abuser. (A) Longitudinal sonogram in the right side up position shows multiple large fluid-filled spaces (S) within the kidney arranged in a spoke-wheel distribution about the renal pelvis (P) which is also mildly distended. (F = toward the patient's feet.) (B) Transverse sonogram in the same position demonstrates the narrow infundibuli (arrows) between the fluid-filled clubbed calyces (S) and the renal pelvis (P). (Li = liver, L = toward the patient's left.) (Hoffman J, Schmur M, Koenigsberg M: Demonstration of renal papillary necrosis by sonography. Radiology 145:785, 1982.)

structive atrophy and congenital megacalyces. The medullary areas are thinned in both abnormalities, and peripheral fluid collections are present. Differentiating factors, however, include normal renal function in congenital megacalyces and a dilated renal pelvis in postobstructive changes.

In summary, except for those few entities described above, the ultrasound findings in chronic renal failure are not disease specific. While the findings of a small shrunken echogenic kidney are quite definitive for end-stage renal disease, this end point may be caused by a variety of pathological processes.

RENAL TRANSPLANTATION

Ultrasound has become a primary method of evaluating the transplanted kidney in order to evaluate potential changes of early transplant rejection. Other causes of transplant kidney failure can also be distinguished on ultrasound including renal obstruction and perinephric fluid collections potentially representing infections. This topic will receive attention in a separate chapter in this volume.

NATIVE KIDNEYS IN PATIENTS WITH RENAL FAILURE

Sonography is not only a useful method of evaluating kidneys in patients with renal failure, but it can also be used in the continued assessment of those kidneys when the patient is placed on chronic hemodialysis or has a renal transplant. The development of bilateral renal cysts, adenomas, and adenocarcinomas in the native kidneys of patients with chronic renal failure who undergo hemodialysis or transplantation is common.[73-75] It is not clear whether these cysts result from an underlying renal pathological process or from the chemical effects of hemodialysis. These cysts reported in more than 43 percent of patients on dialysis for 3 years and more than 79 percent of patients on dialysis for more than 5 years are thought to form by dilatation of tubules and collecting ducts due to obstruction by oxalate crystals and fibrosis.[73,75] Cystic changes have been detected in 30 to 50 percent of patients with uremia and no family history of APKD. They have been subsequently shown to increase in size while the patient is on dialysis and persist in patients who have a viable renal transplant. It is thought that hemodialysis and renal transplantation promote the cyst formation by allowing such patients longer survival.[74] Cysts are located throughout the kidney involving cortex, corticomedullary junction, and medulla.[73-75] Histological changes in the kidneys also include atypical hyperplasia of tubular epithelium and neoplasia. Neoplasms arise in close association with or within the cysts and occur in 10 to 40 percent of patients with cystic changes.[73-75]

Sonographically, the kidneys are small and echogenic with cysts seen throughout the parenchyma (Fig. 3.20). Cysts may range in size from 0.5 to 3 cm, and progressive growth may result in increase in renal size. Many parenchymal cysts may be too small to be visualized discretely, and the overall distortion of these shrunken kidneys may make it difficult to visualize small tumors. Hemorrhage into cysts causing pain and hematuria results in echogenic collections within the cysts on sonography. Such hemorrhagic cysts may be indistinguishable in appearance from neoplasms. In addition, neoplasms may actually arise adjacent to or within cysts; such tumors may also be anechoic but usually do not demonstrate posterior acoustic enhancement. Matrix stones similar in appearance to other renal calculi may also form within these cysts. The differential diagnosis of such cystic changes within the kidneys of patients on dialysis should include polycystic disease (however, such kidneys usually are large) and hydronephrosis, which usually can be readily differentiated from cystic changes with real-time ultrasound.

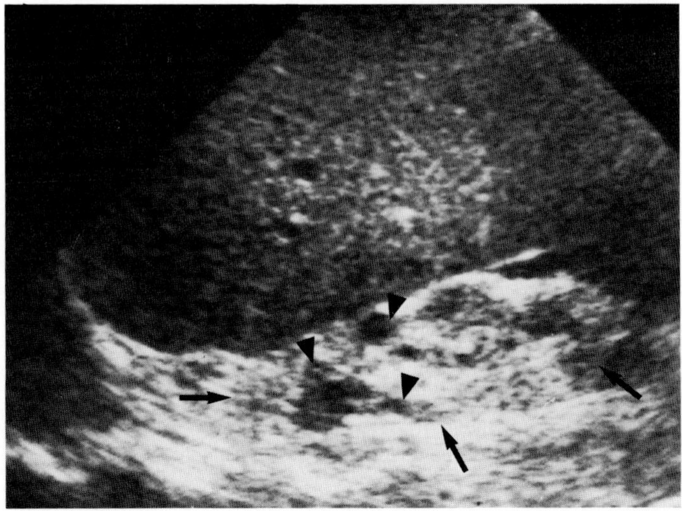

FIG. 3.20.   A patient with chronic renal failure on dialysis shows a small, echogenic end-stage kidney (arrows) with small cysts and solid tumors (arrowheads).

REFERENCES

1. Jeffrey R, Federle M: CT and ultrasonography of acute renal abnormalities. Radiol Clin North Am 21:515, 1983

2. Barber-Riley P, Patel A: Ultrasonic demonstration of renal artery thrombosis. Br J Radiol 54:351, 1981

3. Erwin B, Carroll B, Walter J et al.: Renal infarction appearing as an echogenic mass. AJR 138:759, 1982

4. Rosenfield A, Zeman R, Cronan J et al.: Ultrasound in experimental and clinical renal vein thrombosis. Radiology 137:735, 1980

5. Braun B, Weilemann L, Weigand W: Ultrasonographic demonstration of renal vein thrombosis. Radiology 138:157, 1981

6. Rosenfield A, Taylor K, Crade M et al.: Anatomy and pathology of the kidney by gray scale ultrasound. Radiology 128:737, 1978

7. Erwin B, Carroll B: Renal cortical echogenicity in the newborn. J Ultrasound Med 4:217, 1985

8. Hricak H, Toledo-Pereyra L, Eyler W et al.: Evaluation of acute post-transplant renal failure by ultrasound. Radiology 133:443, 1979

9. Makland N, Wright C, Rosenthal S: Gray scale ultrasonic appearances of renal transplant rejection. Radiology 131:711, 1979

10. Fried A, Woodring J, Lon F et al.: The medullary pyramid index: An objective assessment of prominence in renal transplant rejection. Radiology 149:787, 1983

11. Sefczek R, Beckman I, Lupetin A et al.: Sonography of acute renal cortical necrosis. AJR 142:553, 1984

12. Sty J, Starshak R, Hubbard A: Acute renal cortical necrosis in hemolytic uremic syndrome. J Clin Ultrasound 11:175, 1983

13. Pardes J, Auh Y, Kazam E: Sonographic findings in myoglobinuric renal failure and their clinical implications. J Ultrasound Med 2:391, 1983

14. Wicks J, Thornbury J: Acute renal infections in adults. Radiol Clin North Am 17:245, 1979

15. Robbins S: Pathologic Basis of Disease. W.B. Saunders, Philadelphia, 1974

16. Behan M, Wexson D, Kazam E: Sonographic evaluation of the nonfunctioning kidney. J Clin Ultrasound 7:449, 1979

17. Ralls P, Halls J: Hydronephrosis, renal cystic disease and renal parenchymal disease. Semin Ultrasound:49, 1981

18. Van Kirk O, Go R, Wedel V: Sonographic features of xanthogranulomatous pyelonephritis. AJR 134:1035, 1980

19. Malek R, Elder J: Xanthogranulomatous pyelonephritis: A critical analysis of 26 cases and of the literature: J Urol 119:589, 1978

20. Schaffer R, Becker J, Goodman J: Sonography of the tuberculous kidney. Urology 22:209, 1983

21. Naranya A: Overview of renal tuberculosis. Urology 19:231, 1982

22. Glenner G: Amyloid deposits and amyloidosis the B-fibrilloses (part 2). N Engl J Med 302:13, 1980

23. Subramanyam B: Renal amyloidosis in juvenile rheumatoid arthritis: sonographic features. AJR 136:411, 1981

24. Ekelund L: Radiologic findings in renal amyloidosis. AJR 129:851, 1977

25. Lundberg W, Cadman E, Finch S et al.: Renal failure secondary to leukemic infiltration of the kidneys. Am J Med 62:636, 1977

26. Gore R, Shkolnik A: Abdominal manifestations of pediatric leukemias:sonographic assessment. Radiology 143:207, 1982

27. Kaude J, Lacy G: Ultrasonography in renal lymphoma. J Clin Ultrasound 6:295, 1978

28. Goh T, LeQuesne G, Wong K: Severe infiltration of the kidneys with ultrasonic abnormalities in acute lymphoblastic leukemia. Am J Dis Child 132:1204, 1978

29. Krensky A, Keddish J, Teele R: Causes of increased renal echogenicity in pediatric patients. Pediatrics 72:840, 1983

30. Heiken J, Gold R, Schnur M et al.: Computed tomography of renal lymphoma with ultrasound correlation. J Comput Assist Tomogr 7:245, 1983

31. Hartman D, Davis C, Goldman S et al.: Renal lymphoma: Radiologic-pathologic correlation of 21 cases. Radiology 144:759, 1982

32. Shirkoda A, Staab E, Mittelstaedtl C: Renal lymphoma imaged by ultrasound and gallium-67. Radiology 137:175, 1980

33. Carroll B, Ta H: Ultrasonic appearance of extranodal abdominal lymphoma. Radiology 136:419, 1980

34. Rosenfield A, Lipson M, Wolfe B et al.: Ultrasonography and nephrotomography in the presymptomatic diagnosis of dominantly inherited (adult-onset) polycystic kidney disease. Radiology 135:423, 1980

35. Rosenfield A, Curtis A, Putman C et al.: Gray scale ultrasonography, computerized tomography and nephrotomography in evaluation of polycystic kidney and liver disease. Urology 9:436, 1977

36. Habif D, Berdon W, Yeh M: Infantile polycystic kidney disease: in utero sonographic diagnosis. Radiology 142:475, 1982

37. Krensky A, Reddish J, Teele R: Causes of increased renal echogenicity in pediatric patients. Pediatrics 72:840, 1983

38. Grossman H, Rosenberg E, Bowie J et al.: Sonographic diagnosis of renal cystic diseases. AJR 140:81, 1983

39. Rego J, Laing F, Jeffrey F: Ultrasonographic diagnosis of medullary cystic disease. J Ultrasound Med 2:433, 1983

40. Garel L, Habib R, Pariense D et al.: Juvenile nephronophthisis: sonographic appearance in children with severe uremia. Radiology 151:93, 1984

41. Shuman W, Mack L, Rogers J: Diffuse nephrocalcinosis: hyperechoic sonographic appearance. AJR 136:830, 1981

42. Brennan R, Curtis J, Kurtz A et al.: Use of tomography and ultrasound in the diagnosis of nonopaque renal calculi. JAMA 244(6):594, 1980

43. Wolfman MG, Thornbury JR, Braunstein EM: Nonobstructing radiopaque ureteral calculi. Urol Radiol 1:97, 1979

44. Cacciarelli A, Young N, Levine A: Gray-scale ultrasonic demonstration of nephrocalcinosis. Radiology 128:459, 1978

45. Glazer G, Callen P, Filly R: Medullary nephrocalcinosis: sonographic evaluation. AJR 138:55, 1982

46. Sty J, Starshak R, Hubbard A: Medullary nephrocalcinosis in a newborn: real-time, ultrasound evaluation. J Clin Ultrasound 11:326, 1983

47. Sauvegrain J, Garel L, Pariente D: Sonography of nephrocalcinosis in Cushing syndrome. AJR 140:833, 1983

48. Brennan J, Diwan R, Makker S et al.: Ultrasonic diagnosis of primary hyperoxaluria in infancy. Radiology 145:147, 1982

49. Wilson D, Wenzl J, Altshuler G: Ultrasound demonstration of diffuse cortical nephrocalcinosis in a case of primary hyperoxaluria. AJR 132:659, 1979

50. Curry N, Gobien R, Schabel S: Minimal-dilation obstructive nephropathy. Radiology 143:531, 1982

51. Malave S, Neiman H, Spies S et al.: Diagnosis of hydronephrosis: comparison of radionuclide scanning and sonography. AJR 135:1179, 1980

52. Amis E, Cronan J, Pfister R et al.: Ultrasonic inaccuracies in diagnosing renal obstruction. Urology 19:101, 1982

53. Lee J, Baron R, Melson L et al.: Can real-time ultrasonography replace static B-scanning in the diagnosis of renal obstruction? Radiology 139:161, 1981

54. Ralls P, Esensten M, Boger D et al.: Severe hydronephrosis and severe renal cystic disease: ultrasonic differentiation. AJR 134:473, 1980

55. Ellenbogen P, Scheible F, Talner L et al.: Sensitivity of gray scale ultrasound in detecting urinary tract obstruction. AJR 130:731, 1978

56. Kremer H, Dobrinski W, Mikyska M et al.: Ultrasonic in vivo and in vitro studies on the nature of the ureteral jet phenomenon. Radiology 142:175, 1982

57. Dubbins PA, Kurtz AB, Darby J et al.: Ureteric jet effect: The echographic appearance of urine entering the bladder. Radiology 140:513, 1981

58. Hidalgo H, Dunnick N, Rosenberg E et al.: Parapelvic cysts: appearance on CT and sonography. AJR 138:667, 1982

59. Rosenfield A, Taylor K, Dembner A et al.: Ultrasound of renal sinus: New observations. AJR 133:441, 1979

60. Rascoff J, Golden R, Spinowitz B et al.: Nondilated obstructive nephropathy. Arch Intern Med 143:696, 1983

61. Erwin B, Carroll B, Sommer F: Renal colic: The role of ultrasound in initial evaluation. Radiology 152:147, 1984

62. Fred A, Woodring J, Thompson D: Hydronephrosis of pregnancy: A prospective sequential study of the course of dilatation. J Ultrasound Med 2:255, 1983

63. Fried A: Hydronephrosis of pregnancy: Ultrasonographic study and classification of asymptomatic women. Am J Obstet Gynecol 135:1066, 1979

64. Subramanyam B, Raghavendra B, Bosniak M et al.: Sonography of pyonephrosis: A prospective study. AJR 140:991, 1983

65. Coleman B, Arger P, Mulhern C et al.: Pyonephrosis:Sonography in the diagnosis and management. AJR 137:939, 1981

66. Stuck K, Silver T, Jaffe M et al.: Sonographic demonstration of renal fungus balls. Radiology 142:473, 1981

67. Curatola G, Mazzitelli G, Monzani P: The value of ultrasound as a screening procedure for urological disorders in renal failure. J Urol 130:8, 1983

68. Hricak H, Cruz C, Romanski R et al.: Renal parenchymal disease: Sonographic-histologic correlation. Radiology 144:141, 1982

69. Hricak H, Slovis T, Callen P et al.: Neonatal kidneys: Sonographic anatomic correlation. Radiology 147:699, 1983

70. Rosenfield A, Siegel N: Renal parenchymal disease: Histopathologic-sonographic correlation. AJR 137:793, 1981

71. Kay C, Rosenfield A, Taylor K et al.: Ultrasonic characteristics of chronic atrophic pyelonephritis. AJR 132:47, 1979

72. Hoffman J, Schnur M, Koenigsberg M: Demonstration of renal papillary necrosis of sonography. Radiology 145:785, 1982

73. Kutcher R, Amodio J, Rosenblatt R: Uremic renal cystic disease: Value of sonographic screening. Radiology 147:833, 1983

74. Scanlon M, Karasick S: Acquired renal cystic disease and neoplasia: Complications of chronic hemodialysis. Radiology 147:837, 1983

75. Anderson B, Curry N, Gobien R: Sonography of evolving renal cystic transformation associated with hemodialysis. AJR 141:1003, 1983

4 Renal Infections

EWA KULIGOWSKA

INTRODUCTION

The evaluation and management of patients with renal infection continues to be a serious clinical problem for clinicians and radiologists. Renal inflammatory disease covers a wide spectrum of pathological conditions. The process may be acute, subacute, or chronic. It may be localized, or it may involve the kidney diffusely. The disease may also extend into the perirenal space, or it may be confined to the collecting system, producing pyohydronephrosis.

Since the advent of the cross-sectional imaging methods, gray scale ultrasound[1-3] and computed tomography,[4] there have been changes in the approach to the radiological diagnosis of acute renal infection. Until recently, excretory urography (EU) was preferred as the initial radiographical examination. It gave disappointing results. Excretory urography studies were completely normal in 75 percent of patients with documented acute renal infection.[5,6]

Ultrasonography provides an excellent modality for assessing the internal renal architecture.[7] Abnormalities can be recognized early in the course of disease. Ultrasound can differentiate between focal and diffuse renal inflammatory disease, and it can clearly demonstrate extension of the infection to the adjacent retroperitonal space. Furthermore, ultrasound imaging is not affected by renal function or allergy to contrast material. Serial examinations are easily performed and allow the clinician to monitor the resolution of disease without exposing the patient to ionizing radiation or intravenous contrast agents. This is particularly important in the evaluation of women in childbearing age who are the patients most affected by persistent urinary tract infection.

This chapter summerizes the pathological, clinical, and ultrasonographic features of inflammatory renal disease, gives analysis of the diagnostic imaging techniques, the role of needle aspiration in making an early diagnosis, and the subsequent use of percutaneous catheter drainage for treatment (see Chapter 7). Prompt diagnosis and early therapeutic intervention result in cure for many patients and avoid the need for general anesthesia and surgery.

THE PATHOPHYSIOLOGY OF RENAL INFECTION

Bacterial infections of the kidney proceed through a series of pathological stages affecting primarily the interstitium (Table 4.1). They can be viewed as pathological continuum. A spectrum of changes from edema to extensive necrosis can be traced with ultrasound.

Acute bacterial renal infection is a combination of parenchymal, calyceal, and pelvic inflammation resulting from the spread of pathogenic organisms to the kidney. The three pathways by which bacteria can gain access to the urinary tract and cause infection[8] are listed next.

Infection by the Ascending Route

Most clinical and experimental evidence clearly supports the ascending pathway in the vast majority of kidney infections. These infections are commonly caused by normal intestinal flora, which include coliform and other enteric bacteria. Any interference with normal voiding, incompletely emptying, stasis, or instrumentation will produce residual urine in the bladder and enhance bacterial multiplication.[9] Bacteria must then ascend to the kidney against the ureteral flow of urine.[10]

In children, vesicoureteric reflux is commonly present and carries bacteria into the upper urinary tract.[11-13] In adults, ascending infections also occur, although reflux is rarely demonstrated. It is postulated that organisms may be able to ascend the ureter when ureteric peristalsis is disordered or ureteric tone is diminished as occurs in pregnancy and in patients with neurogenic bladder.[10,12,14]

TABLE 4.1 Spectrum of bacterial renal infections

Acute renal inflammation	Acute pyelonephritis
	Focal bacterial nephritis (lobar nephronia)
	Diffuse bacterial nephritis
Acute renal abscess	Confined to the kidney
	Spread to perirenal or pararenal tissue
	Superimposed infection in preexisting renal lesions (cysts and tumor)
Pyohydronephrosis	
Subacute chronic renal abscess	
Chronic renal infection	Chronic atrophic pyelonephritis
	Xanthogranulomatous pyelonephritis

Hematogenous Infection

The kidney may also become infected when bacteremia produces a hematogenous dissemination of bacteria from remote primary sites such as the skin infections, osteomyelitis, or endocarditis. *Staphylococcus aureus* is frequently the causative organism.

Infection by Lymphatic Spread

Another mechanism of infection which has been postulated, but not proven, is the spread of bacteria to the kidneys by the lymphatic system. This cause of pyelonephritis is based on indirect evidence derived from animal studies which demonstrate lymphatic connections between the upper and lower urinary tracts and the possible existence of lymphatic channels between the colon and the right kidney.[8]

The patient's immune response and ability to eliminate bacterial infection determine whether a focus of infection will become established or not once bacteria have gained access to the kidney. Diabetics and other immunocompromised patients have a greater tendency to develop renal infection than patients with normal immune defenses. The virulence of the invading organisms is another factor which contributes to the development of urinary tract infection.

SPECTRUM OF BACTERIAL RENAL INFECTIONS

Acute Renal Inflammation

Acute inflammation may involve the kidney either diffusely or focally (see Table 4.1). The extent of the involvement of the kidney is determined by the virulence of the infecting organism, host immunity, and other local factors. The histopathological appearance of *acute pyelonephritis* is diffuse edema that produces renal enlargement (Fig. 4.1) with foci of intense inflammation which may lead to microabscess formation throughout the involved interstitial tissue.[8]

This process may be localized and form a wedge-shaped phlegmonous lesion called "acute focal bacterial nephritis or lobar nephronia" (Fig. 4.2). In this entity, one specific segment or lobe of the kidney is infected, generally by *Escherichia coli.*[8,14] No true abscess exists since there is no liquefaction or necrosis. These lesions may be single or multiple, unilateral or bilateral (Fig. 4.3, 4.14). As the process becomes more extensive, inflammatory changes and tissue necrosis may spread to involve the entire kidney to produce *acute diffuse bacterial nephritis,* also called "acute suppurative pyelonephritis"[8,16] (Figs. 4.4, 4.5). Acute diffuse bacterial nephritis is a more virulent form of pyelonephritis caused by gram-negative organisms including *Klebsiella, Proteus,* and fungi (Fig. 3.5). This severe

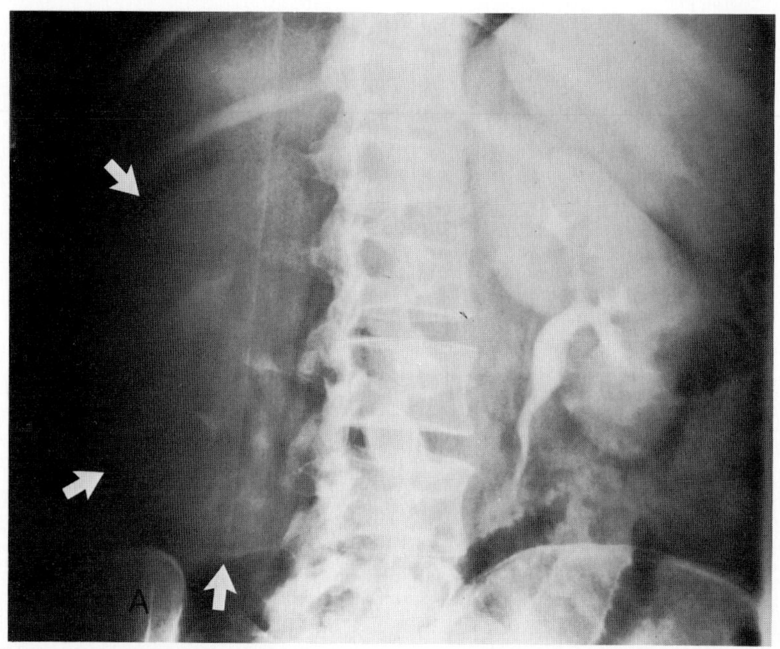

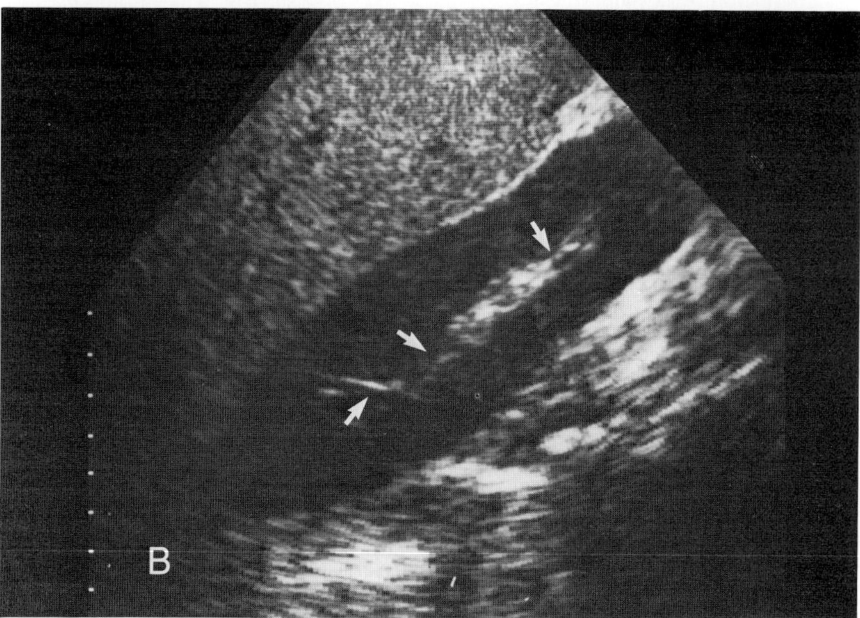

FIG. 4.1.   Acute pyelonephritis in a 17-year-old paraplegic girl with fever and leukocytosis. (A) Excretory urography shows right renal enlargement (arrows). (B) Longitudinal sonogram revealed diffusely enlarged swollen right kidney. The echogencity of the renal parenchyma is homogeneous and decreased. Echogenic sinus is still present but compressed (arrows).

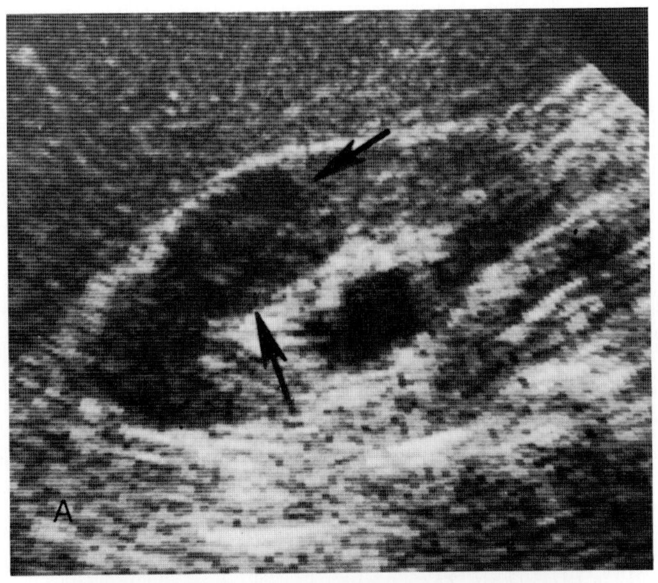

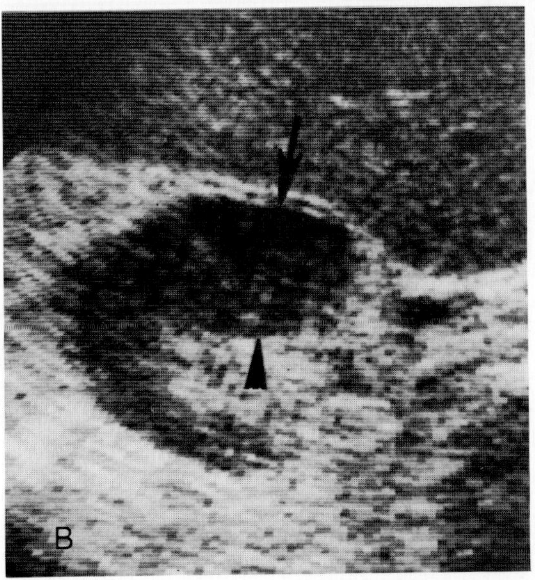

FIG. 4.2. A 82-year-old man with *Klebsiella* urosepsis. (A) Longitudinal coronal sonogram of the right kidney shows hypoechoic mass (arrows) disrupting the corticomedullary junction. (B) Transverse scan of the right kidney demonstrates the characteristic lesion of lobar nephronia (arrow). Note mass impression on the collecting system (arrowhead).

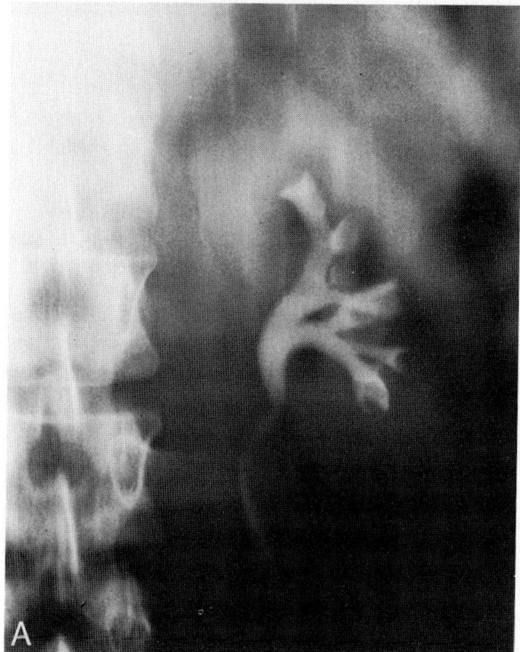

FIG. 4.3. A 70-year-old man with clinical diagnosis of renal infection. Lack of response to antibiotics led to further investigations. (A) Excretory urography; left kidney entirely normal. (B) Prone longitudinal scan of left kidney shows hypoechoic mass corresponding to focal bacterial nephritis (asterisk). Subsequently the mass resolved completely on antibiotic therapy.

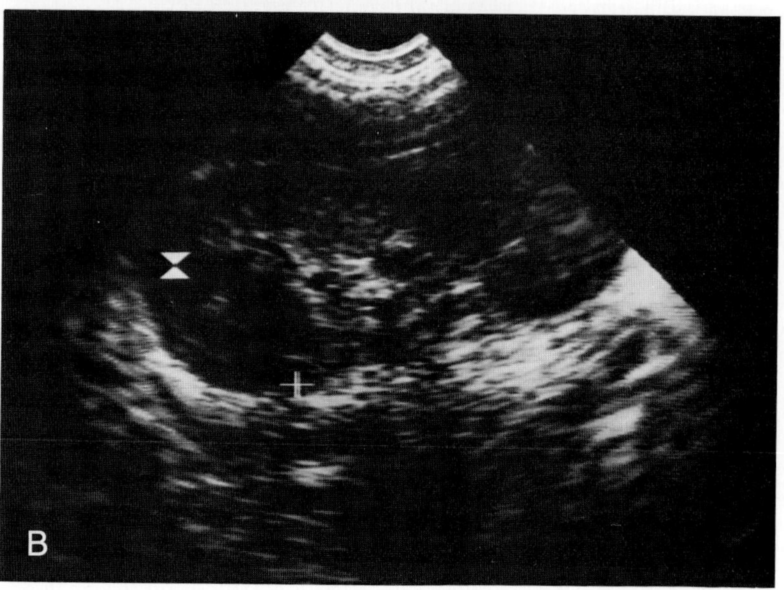

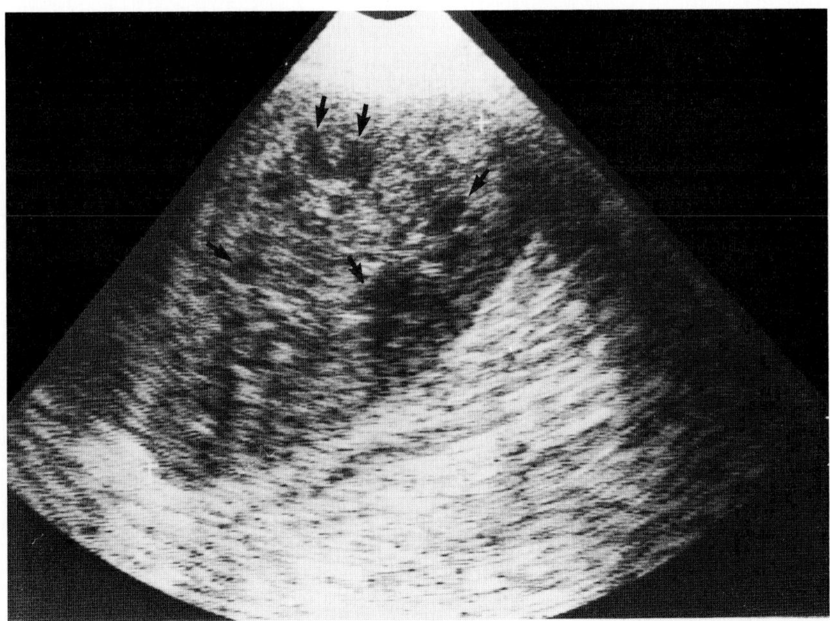

FIG. 4.4.   Acute diffuse bacterial nephritis in 20-year-old diabetic man with septicemia and acute renal failure. Blood culture was positive for *Klebsiella* and *Proteus*. Coronal sonogram of the right kidney shows extensive inflammatory changes and tissue necrosis involving the entire kidney. Note the disorganized parenchymal pattern in the enlarged, bulky kidney. Multiple hypoechoic fosi represent macroabscesses (arrows). The center renal sinus echo blends with the abnormal parenchyma.

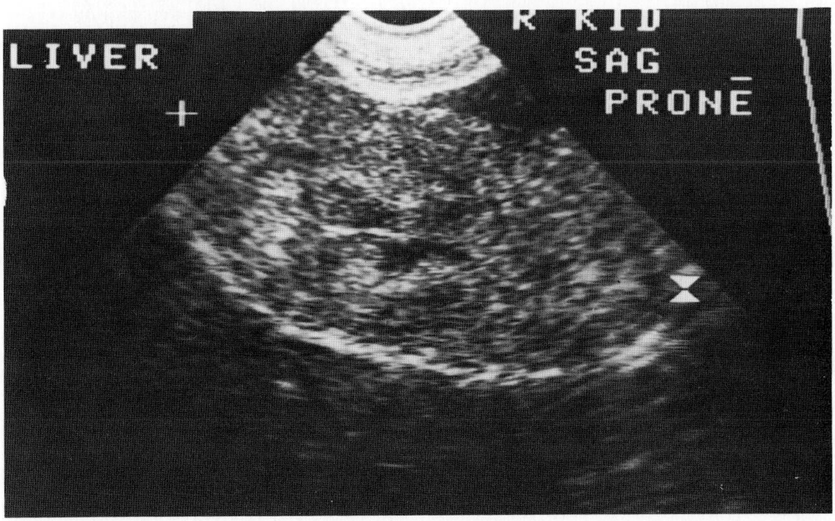

FIG. 4.5.   A 30-year-old diabetic paraplegic man with acute diffuse bacterial nephritis due to *Candida* infection. Prone longitudinal sonogram shows nonhomogeneous, enlarged kidney. A normal echogenic renal sinus is not seen.

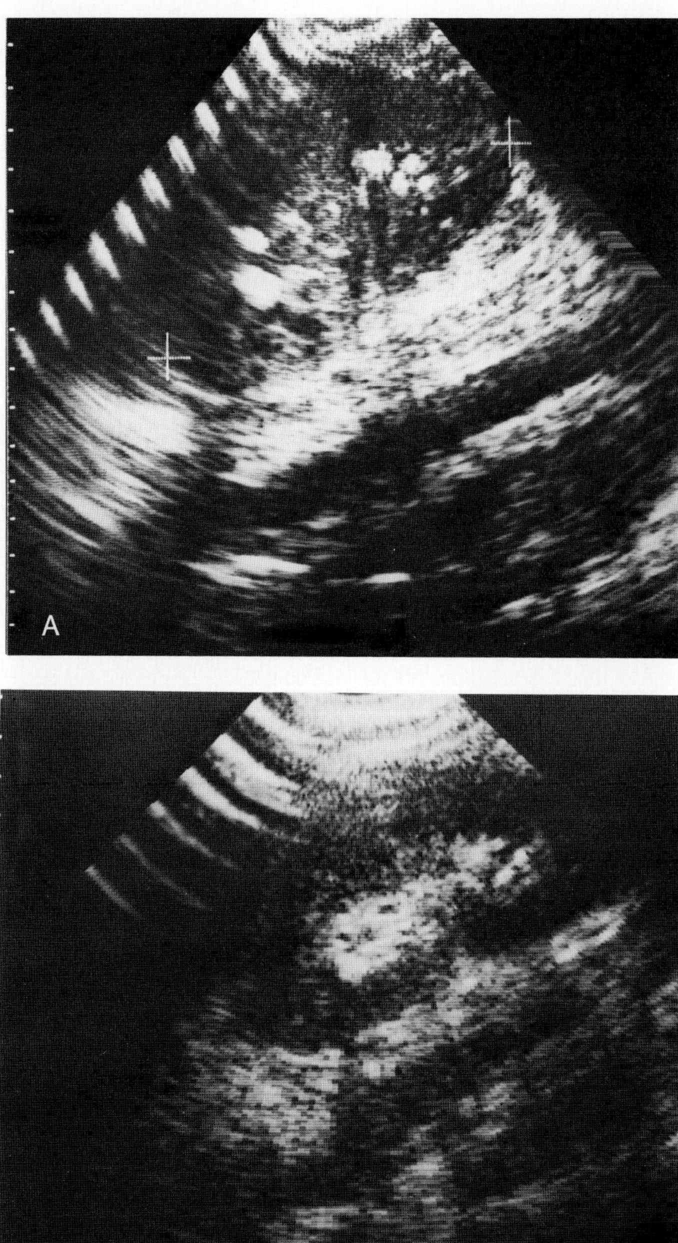

FIG. 4.6.   A 55-year-old man with diabetes and *Candida* septicemia developed acute diffuse bacterial nephritis. (A) Enlarged left kidney with multiple hypoechoic fosi (macroabscesses). Several stones are present in collecting system. These stones were obscured on previous examination 3 months before, (B) by a normal echogenic renal sinus, which is now no longer visible.

form of renal infection is almost exclusively seen in immunocompromised patients.[4,17]

Acute Renal Abscess

Untreated acute focal bacterial nephritis can progress to abscess formation. When this occurs, the early stage of infection with edema and multiple microabscesses may subsequently coalesce to form a large suppurative intrarenal abscess with frank liquefaction or necrosis. This suppuration may remain within the kidney (Fig. 4.7), or it may break through the renal capsule to involve the perirenal space, where it tends to localize in fat tissue which is posterolateral to the kidney. The thick layer of Gerota's fascia usually presents a barrier to the further spread of infection, except in fulminant cases. Acute progression to an abscess or extension beyond the renal capsule occurs in patients with predisposing risk factors, such as urinary tract obstruction, immunosuppression, trauma, or intravenous drug abuse.[8,16] The commonest organism found in renal abscesses in the past was *S. aureus* spread by the hematogenous route. Today, gram-negative bacteria, especially *E. coli, Pseudomonas,* and *Proteus,* are with increasing frequency found to be the cause of renal abscesses spread to the kidney either hematogenously or by the ascending route.[8,16,17] If renal infection develops in a kidney containing a preexisting abnormality (Fig. 4.8), such as a cyst or renal tumor, the wall and lumen may become infected, producing an abscess (Fig. 4.9).

Pyonephrosis

Obstruction of the renal collecting system predisposes to infection. The obstruction may be the result of a congenital anomoly, calculus disease, or a stricture. Pyonephrosis is a serious complication of hydronephrosis that may develop as a consequence of urinary stasis and secondary infection. Pyohydronephrosis may result from ascent and trapping of infected urine in a hydronephrotic kidney or by extension of an infection from an intrarenal focus to an obstructed collecting system. Purulent exudate collects in the dilated pelvocalyceal system. Pathologically the purulent exudate is composed of sloughed urothelium and a variety of inflammatory cells[18] (Fig. 4.10).

Subacute Chronic Renal Abscess

The eventual outcome of acute renal infection depends on the virulence of the organism, the host response, and sensitivity to antibiotic therapy. Complete resolution may occur, or the lesion may progress. Untreated or partially treated intrarenal abscesses become progressively more localized by the formation of a thick wall of granulation tissue. The chronic renal abscess is a necrotic mass

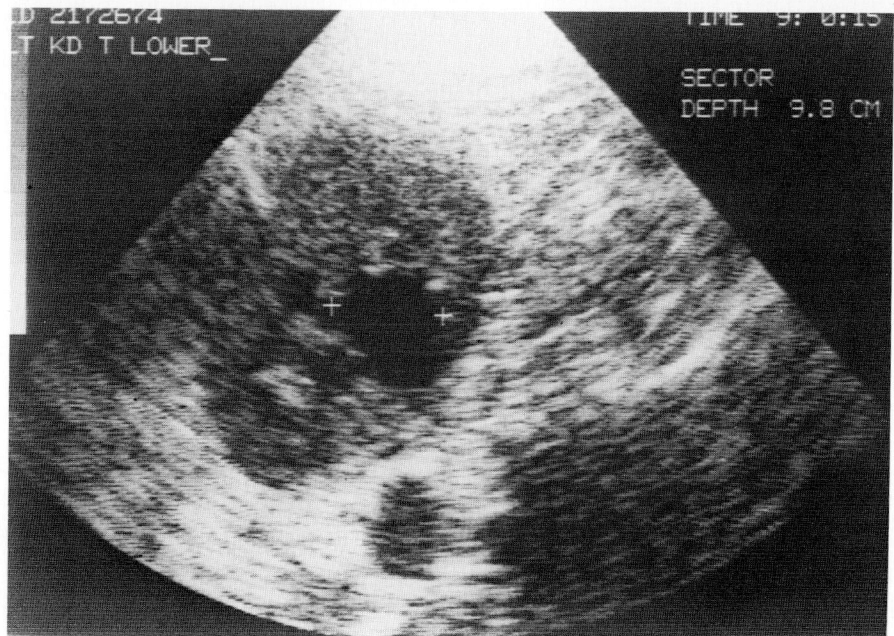

FIG. 4.7.   A 55-year-old man with positive urine culture for *Staphylococcus aureus.* Excretory urography was reported as normal. Transverse ultrasound shows an anechoic solid mass with an irregular margin, located in the renal parenchyma compatible with renal abscess.

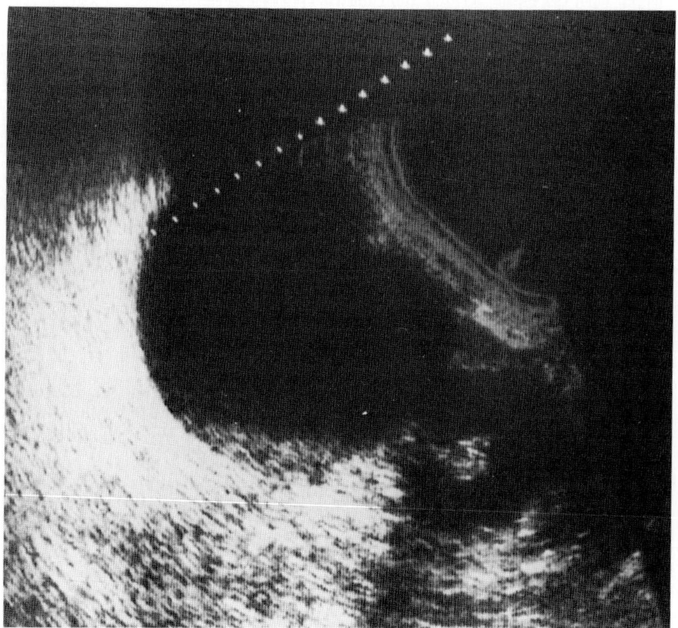

FIG. 4.8.   A 30-year-old woman with *Staphylococcus aureus* septicemia was found to have infected cyst in the left kidney. Coronal section of the left kidney shows large cystic mass with fluid debris level in the dependent portion. Drainage was performed by percutaneous placement of a 12 French trocar catheter; 450 cc of purulent material was drained.

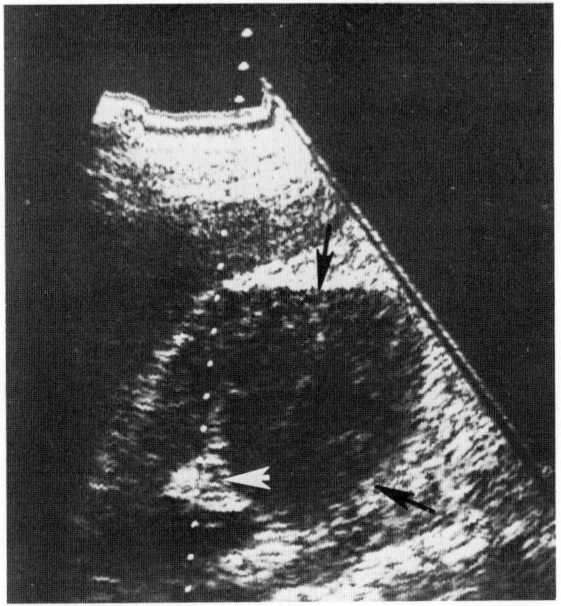

FIG. 4.9.   A 65-year-old diabetic man with flank pain, hematuria, and fever. Coronal sonogram of the left kidney shows a 10 × 8 cm hypoechoic mass (arrows) producing effacement of the collecting system (arrowheads). Diagnostic needle puncture revealed purulent specimen. Cystology discovered abnormal cells suggesting tumor, which was subsequently confirmed by surgery.

surrounded by a broad zone of granulation tissue and may persist for many months.[8]

Chronic Renal Infection

Chronic Atrophic Pyelonephritis

During the resolution of acute pyelonephritis, neutrophils are replaced by a chronic inflammatory infiltrate consisting of macrophages and lymphocytes. Granulation tissue forms slowly and causes retraction and subsegmental scarring. Childhood infections frequently cause gross renal scarring. Most of the severe damage leading to the changes associated with chronic pyelonephritis occur in the preschool age.[11-14] Adult infections result in visible scarring much less frequently.

Xanthogranulomatous Pyelonephritis

Xanthogranulomatous pyelonephritis is a rare form of infection that is usually seen in patients with obstruction secondary to longstanding calculi as well as a sequela to multiple renal infections.[8,20] Xanthogranulomatous pyelonephritis may involve the kidney in two ways: (1) focal (Fig. 4.11A) and (2) diffusely (Fig. 4.11B). The pathological process of focal or diffuse involvement is the same. The renal parenchyma is replaced by xanthogranulomatous masses.[16,20] They have the gross appearance of yellow nodules scattered throughout the

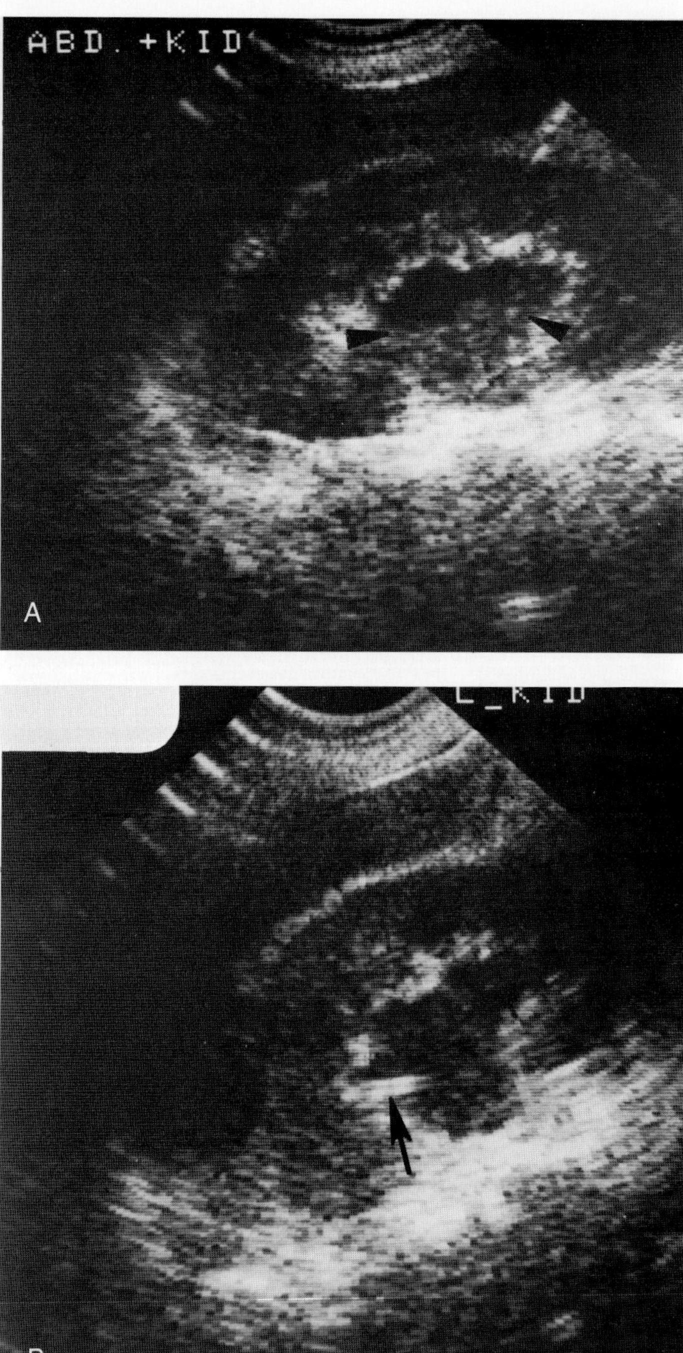

FIG. 4.10. A 65-year-old woman with carcinoma of the bladder presented with fever and bilateral hydronephrosis. (A) Coronal sonogram of left kidney shows moderate dilatation of collecting system with urine debris level (arrowheads). (B) Percutaneous catheter (arrow) is seen within collecting system after ultrasonically guided placement.

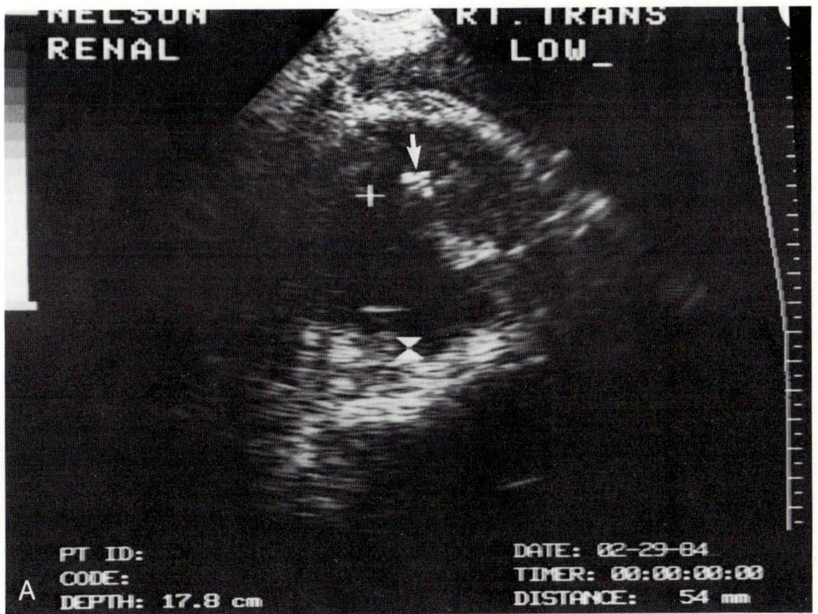

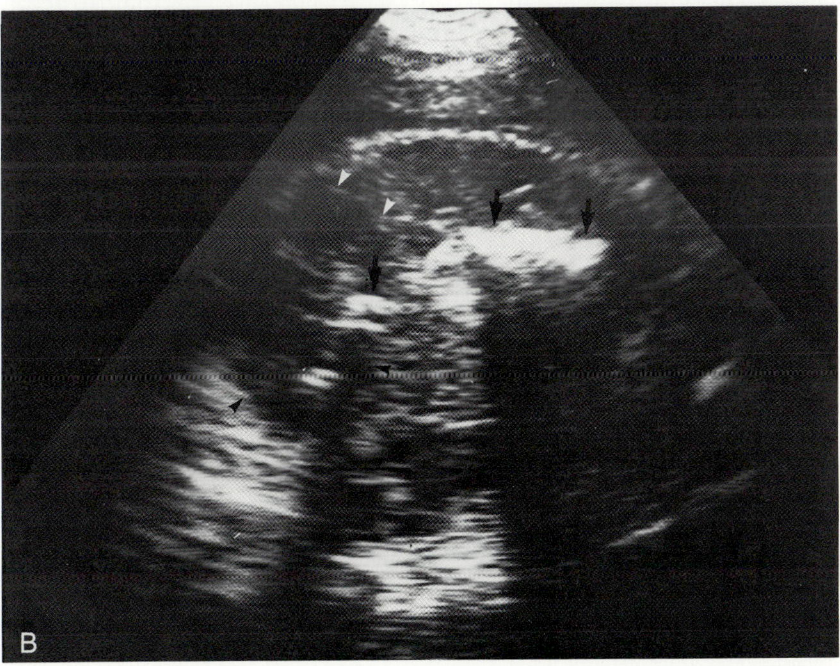

FIG. 4.11. Two diabetic patients with xanthogranulomatous pyelonephritis. (A) Focal renal involvement; hypoechoic mass with irregular border, good through transmission representing an abscess (asterisk). Staghorn calculi seen in collecting system (arrow). (B) Diffuse form of xanthogranulomatous pyelonephritis. Staghorn calculi in collecting system with posterior accoustic shadows (arrows). Small macroabscesses in renal parenchyma (arrowheads).

involved portion of the kidney. Female and diabetic patients seem to be more susceptible. *Proteus mirabilis* is the organism most often implicated.

CLINICAL MANIFESTATIONS OF INFLAMMATORY RENAL DISEASE

The classic clinical manifestations of upper tract involvement include fever, sometimes accompanied by chills, flank pain, flank tenderness, and often by lower tract symptoms of frequency, urgency, and dysuria. Most patients with symptomatic urinary tract infection are women of childbearing age. Almost all patients have positive urine cultures, and many have bacteremia as well. *E. coli* is the predominant causative organism.[8]

Patients with renal abscess, unlike patients with acute bacterial pyelonephritis, often present with a nonspecific clinical syndrome. In acute abscess, signs and symptoms of septicemia may be present without specific symptoms referrable to the urinary tract. The more chronic the infection the more nonspecific the clinical and laboratory findings tend to be. Flank pain, low-grade fever, leukocytosis, and occasional weight loss may be found in these patients. It is not unusual in our experience for patients with renal abscesses to have negative urinalysis and cultures (up to 25 percent of cases). This is most likely due to the effectiveness of the abscess wall in localizing the renal infection.

ANALYSIS OF IMAGING TECHNIQUE

We believe that ultrasonography is the imaging modality of choice for evaluating the acute renal infection. Diagnostic accuracy is dependent on skillful and thorough ultrasound examination of the entire renal parenchyma, in two projections at right angles to each other.

In the past, intravenous urography and renal angiography were used to study patients in whom renal inflammation was suspected. Angiography is no longer performed in our institution for that purpose. Sonography and computed tomography are important diagnostic methods in the diagnosis and management of these patients. Gallium isotope imaging can be used as an adjunct to these diagnostic studies. In our experience, as well as that of other authors, ultrasound alone is sufficient in most cases for establishing the diagnosis and for following the response to appropriate therapy.

Excretory Urography

The excretory urogram is still preferred as the initial examination in many centers. Positive findings on excretory urography are seen in about 25 percent of patients with acute pyelonephritis.[5,6] A positive excretory urogram is usually nonspecific for renal inflammatory disease. Depending of the stage and extent of the renal inflammatory process, the following radiographical findings can be observed:[21] (1) renal enlargement, (2) abnormal nephrogram density (mottled or striate), (3) decreased opacification of collecting system, (4) pelvocalyceal displacement or dilatation, (5) obliteration of renal outline, (6) extrarenal mass effect, (7) loss of ipsilateral psoas margin, and (8) immobility of kidney during respiration. The most common radiographical appearance of acute renal infection is that of a normal kidney (75 percent) (Fig. 4.3). The most common abnormal appearance is delayed excretion and dilatation of collecting system. A nonexcreting kidney is very rarely found in acute pyelonephritis. Small inflammatory renal masses often cannot be demonstrated on excretory urography. The number of positive urograms increases as the abnormal masses become larger and more defined.

In the diffuse form of xanthogranulomatous pyelonephritis, plain films will show an enlarged kidney with a staghorn calculus. Excretory urography may demonstrate a nonexcreting kidney. In focal xanthogranulomatous pyelonephritis, the kidney shows normal excretion on excretory urography and a mass effect is seen.[22] The mass may distort the collecting system or renal outline and usually is indistinguishable radiologically from a renal neoplasm or chronic renal abscess.

In pyohydronephrosis the affected kidney frequently demonstrates decreased or absent excretion due to marked parenchymal atrophy resulting from long-standing hydronephrosis.

Radionuclide Studies

Radionuclide cortical imaging used in the evaluation of renal inflammatory lesions is a complementary technique.[1-3] In order to increase specificity, many radiologists now obtain a technetium renogram followed by a gallium citrate scan. The gallium citrate scan is not always specific because other diseases such as lymphoma and primary or metastatic tumor can give positive results.[23]

Positive findings on gallium scan are characterized by focal areas of increased uptake which must correlate with "cold" areas on the static technetium scan.[24] Diffuse increased gallium uptake by renal parenchyma is compatible with diffuse pyelonephritis.[25] Although the gallium scan increases the specificity, there is a delay of 72 hours in imaging and in confirmation of the diagnosis. In several instances, small lesions less than 2 cm which are detectable by ultrasound may not be imaged on radionuclide studies because of the limited resolution of this modality. Gallium scanning as recommended in the past is now only used in confusing cases.

Computed Tomography

Computed tomography (CT) has proven to be an accurate and valuable modality for evaluating acute inflammatory renal abnormalities. The CT findings in acute infection depend on the severity, stage, and extension of the inflammatory process.[2-4,26,27]

Precontrast scans are normal in most cases of renal infection; however, they may occasionally reveal areas of slightly lower density surrounded by normal renal parenchyma.

Homogenious enlargement of an affected edematous kidney can often be demonstrated as the only abnormality.

Postcontrast scans are more informative. They demonstrate segmental, wedge-shaped, low-density areas with internal striation. These focal striations, similar to those which are occasionally noted on excretory urography, may be identified as a zone situated in the parenchyma extending from the collecting system toward the periphery of the cortex. This zone of abnormal enhancement most likely represents nonfunctioning nephrons which have become obstructed or ischemic from the infection.[2-4,26]

Intrarenal abscesses have a lower attenuation value than normal renal parenchyma on noncontrast study. They either do not enhance after administration of the intravenous contrast material or may rarely enhance in a patchy nonhomogenous pattern. The wall of an abscess usually enhances on a contrast scan.

Perirenal extension of infection causes increased density in the perirenal fat, thickening of Gerota's fascia, and displacement of the affected kidney. The renal fascia can also be thickened by focal bacterial nephritis or more commonly by renal abscess.[28]

Gas-forming renal infection can be readily identified by the presence of gas in the abnormal renal parenchyma (Fig. 4.12B) subcapsular region, or may even extend through the renal capsule into the perirenal or pararenal spaces.

Advantages

Computerized tomography may be the only imaging modality capable of diagnosing acute renal infection in patients' who have massive obesity, a large amount of gas in the upper abdomen, or surgical wounds with multiple catheters.

Disadvantages

Exposure of patients to ionizing radiation is a disadvantage of computerized tomography which may be especially important for children and individuals in childbearing ages.

Distinguishing focal inflammation from abscess and abscess from benign or malignant tumor may be difficult with computerized tomography. Microbiological cultures and cytological study of a specimen obtained by needle aspiration may be required to clarify the diagnosis in these situations.

CT with intravenous contrast injection is essential for establishing a diagnosis of inflammatory renal disease. Whenever an element of renal failure is present, especially in diabetic patients, the use of contrast material may be contraindicated and, therefore, the use of CT scan as a diagnostic modality may be limited.

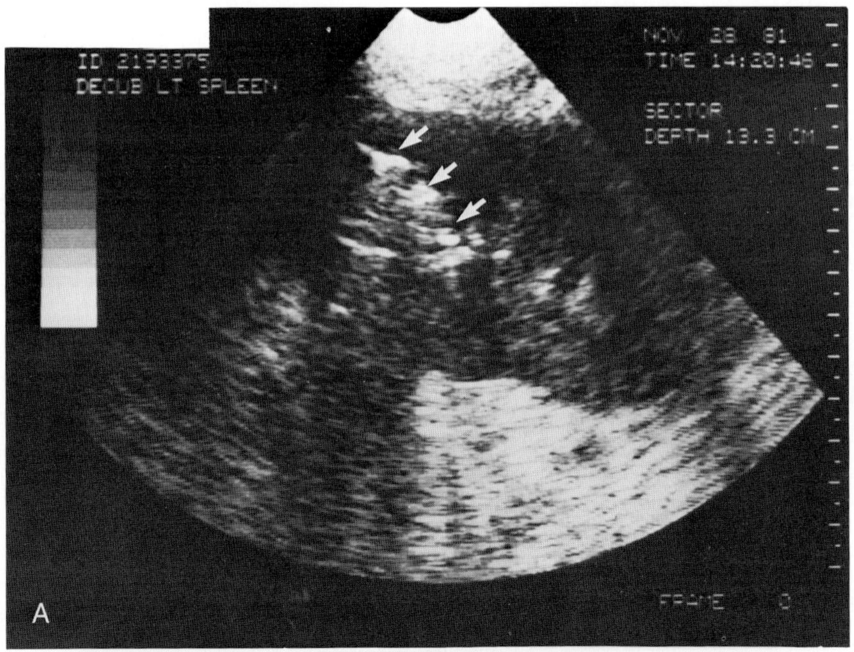

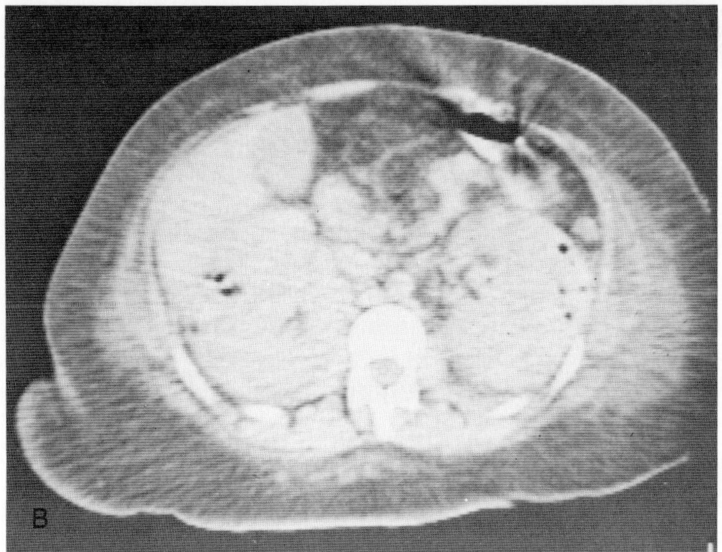

FIG. 4.12. A 20-year-old woman with 2-year history of insulin-dependent diabetes mellitus and a long history of alcohol abuse, developed enphysematous pyelonephritis bilaterally. (A) Coronal scan of left kidney demonstrates diffuse renal enlargement. The multiple punctuate highly echogenic fosi represent small collections of gas in parenchyma (arrows). (B) Precontrast CT scan confirms the ultrasound findings.

Renal Ultrasonography

State of the art ultrasound evaluation of renal architecture requires meticulous examination using high-resolution real-time instruments. The primary goal of renal ultrasonography is the imaging of all renal and perirenal tissue with maximum possible resolution. The standard examination of the kidney includes multiple coronal, longitudinal, and transverse sections. When necessary, scanning in the prone position can be added to adequately visualize the renal parenchyma and psoas muscle. The resolution obtained with current gray scale ultrasonography exquisitely defines renal parenchymal structures.[29] The cortex is usually composed of uniform, closely spaced, relatively low-level echoes of an intensity less than either normal liver or spleen parenchyma. The medullary pyramids are displayed as rounded triangular zones between the cortex and renal sinus. These are separated from each other by bands of cortical tissue called columns of Bertin, which also extend inward to the renal sinus. Intense punctate echoes may be seen at the boundary between cortex and medulla. These echoes represent the arcuate arteries and veins. The renal capsule is seen by ultrasound as a strong continuous echogenic reflection surrounding the cortex. The dense central pelvocalyceal echo complex (the renal sinus) is produced by numerous interfaces of vessels, ureteral lining, and renal pelvic fat.

ECHOGRAPHIC SPECTRUM OF RENAL INFLAMMATION

Indications

Ultrasound is usually performed when there is inadequate clinical response to antibiotic therapy or suspicion of an underlying lesion predisposing to infection such as obstruction by a urinary tract anomoly. The presence or absence of these entities is effectively established by ultrasound examination.

Ultrasound is an imaging modality which can be used to identify the different phases of renal infection as described below (see Table 4.1).

Acute Renal Inflammation

Acute Bacterial Nephritis (Pyelonephritis)

Acute pyelonephritis produces a diffusely enlarged swollen kidney.[30] The echogenicity is homogenious and decreased overall compared with normal renal parenchyma (Fig. 4.1B). We have observed alterations in appearance of the renal sinus structure. Changes in the central echo pattern of the renal sinus are a sensitive indicator of the severity of the inflammatory process. In the early stage of infection, the echogenic sinus is present but compressed and less intense than normal (Fig. 3.1B). As the infection progresses, the central echo complex blends into the homogenous edematous parenchyma and disappears completely (Figs. 4.4–4.6).

Acute Focal Bacterial Nephritis

Acute focal bacterial nephritis or lobar nephronia appears as an indistinct hypoechoic solid mass without definable walls (Figs. 4.2A, B, 4.3B). This focal mass disrupts normal corticomedullary differentiation and contains scattered low-level echoes.[31,32] No through transmission can be demonstrated.

Acute Diffuse Bacterial Nephritis

Acute diffuse bacterial nephritis (also called "acute suppurative nephritis") involves the entire kidney and produces a patchy disorganized parenchymal pattern in an enlarged bulky kidney.[1,4,8] The central renal sinus echo blends with abnormal parenchyma and later may completely disappear in a manner similar to pyelonephritis (Figs. 4.4–4.6).

Acute Renal Abscess

Intrarenal Abscess

Renal abscess appears as a nearly anechoic mass with an irregular margin which is better defined than focal bacterial nephritis (Fig. 4.7). Some degree of through transmission is noted. Occasionally it may be highly echogenic (Fig. 4.13). Increased echogenicity in the renal parenchyma implies early inflammation by gas-producing organisms.[33]

The Perirenal or Pararenal Tissue

Perinephric extension of the disease is shown by a hypoechoic zone around the kidney confined by Gerota's fascia or with extension to the psoas muscle. When an abscess is confined to the psoas muscle, it often produces elevation of the affected kidney.

Superimposed Infection in Preexisting Renal Lesion

An infected cyst may be recognized by the presence of fine, low-amplitude echoes within a well-defined simple cystic structure. Fluid levels or debris in the dependent portion of the cyst can also be identified (Fig. 4.8).

Infected tumor can be a diagnostic problem because the ultrasound appearance is usually identical to renal abscess. A hypoechoic mass with good through transmission and an irregular wall or capsule is seen in both entities (Fig. 4.9).

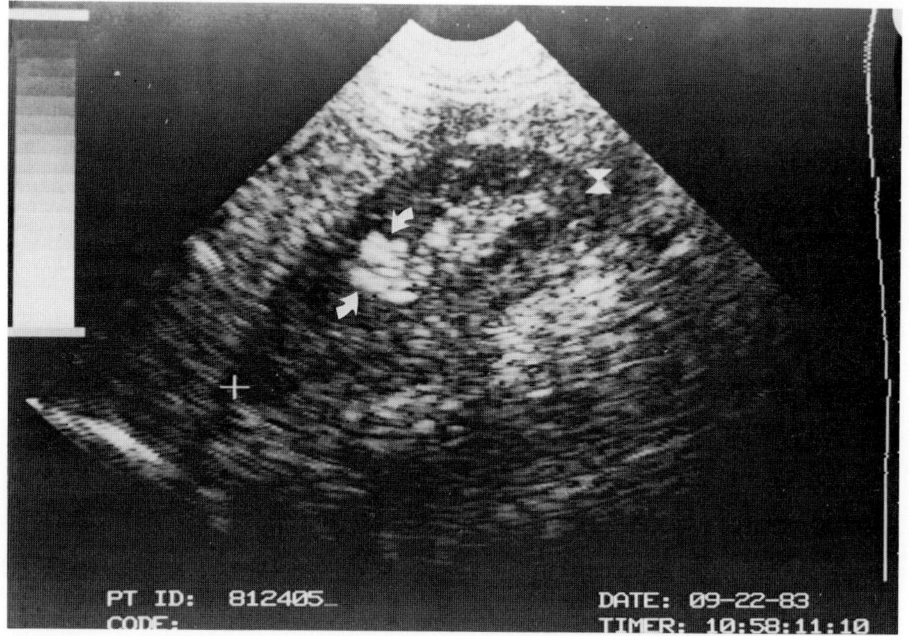

FIG. 4.13.   A 9-year-old girl with *E. coli* septicemia. Echogenic focus in the midportion of the right kidney represents early abscess formation with gas-producing organism. A 22-gauge needle aspiration revealed a few drops of purulent specimen. Patient was successfully treated with antibiotic therapy alone.

Pyohydronephrosis

Pyonephrosis and pyohydronephrosis are often used synonymously to refer to an obstructive uropathy with superimposed infection. A sonographic diagnosis of pyonephrosis depends on the presence of tissue and cellular debris which produce low-level echoes within the dilated collecting system.[34,35] The internal echoes may be dependent and seen as a fluid debris level (Fig. 4.10A). The variable nature of the purulent exudate in pyonephrosis depends on the stage and duration of inflammation and the extent of proteolysis of the purulent exudate.[18] These factors explain why pyonephrosis may occasionally be totally anechoic on ultrasound and simulate hydronephrosis (see Chapter 4). Ultrasound-guided needle aspiration may be used in selected cases of abnormal fluid collections for establishing the diagnosis (see Chapter 6).

Subacute Chronic Renal Abscess

Untreated or partially treated intrarenal abscesses become progressively more localized as a thick wall is formed by granulation tissue. Chronic abscesses tend to resemble acute renal abscesses; however, they often have more pronounced irregular thick walls or capsules.

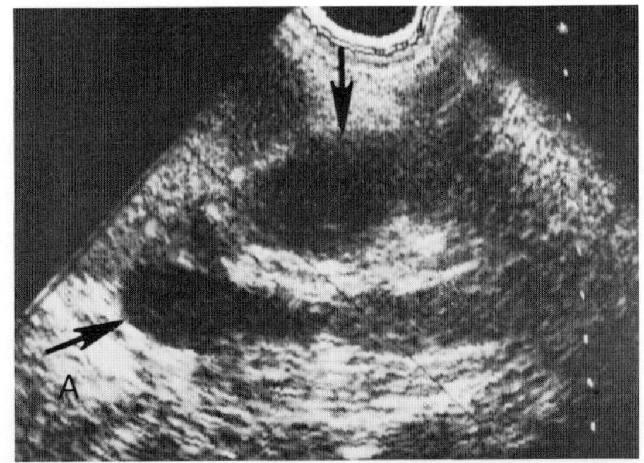

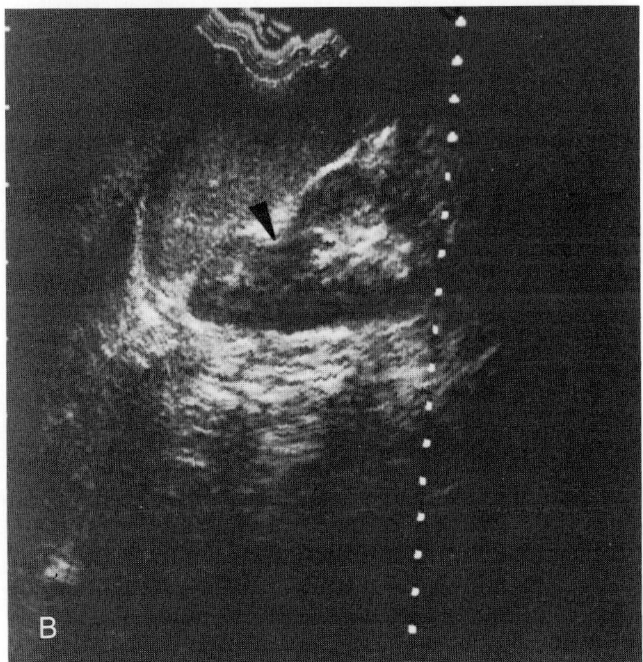

FIG. 4.14. A 17-year-old quadriplegic girl with *E. coli* septicemia. (A) Coronal scan of the left kidney shows two hypoechoic areas (corresponding to multiple focal bacterial nephritis) (arrows). Diagnostic percutaneous aspiration revealed inflammatory cells only; no pus was obtained. This case emphasized that distinction between focal bacterial nephritis and abscess cannot always be made on initial examination. Needle puncture is easily performed in questionable cases. (B) Coronal scan of the same kidney 4 months after antibiotic therapy alone shows a focal cortical scar in the area of previous nephritis (arrowheads).

Chronic Renal Infection

In chronic atrophic pyelonephritis, ultrasound findings reflect the pathological alterations. A focal loss of parenchyma can be noted. Fibrosis manifested by increased echoes can be demonstrated in the involved area of the cortex and mudulla (Fig. 4.14B). The entire scarring process, if advanced, may be global rather than focal and may produce a small echogenic kidney with an irregular border.[19]

Xanthogranulomatous Pyelonephritis

Ultrasound features of xanthogranulomatous pyelonephritis include a focal (Fig. 4.11A) or diffusely (Fig. 11B) enlarged kidney with a nonhomogenous echo texture usually accompanied by a staghorn calculus. Multiple lucencies in the abnormal disorganized renal parenchyma represent small abscesses.[36]

PROTOCOL FOR DIAGNOSIS OF RENAL INFECTION

All patients suspected of acute renal inflammatory disease should immediately be placed on antibiotic therapy. Failure to respond to medical treatment in 48 hours is an indication for sonographic examination. When a diagnosis of acute renal inflammatory disease is suspected by ultrasound, a follow-up examination is recommended in 5 to 7 days, with continuation of medical therapy. If the second ultrasound examination shows a mass that decreased in size and there is clinical improvement on antibiotic therapy, a diagnosis of focal bacterial nephritis is made. In this situation, aspiration biopsy is not warranted. Where there is diagnostic uncertainty, aspiration biopsy is performed. In all cases when the lesion increases in size or there is evidence of liquefication, diagnostic percutaneous needle aspiration should be performed as the next step. Ultrasound examination may not be possible in patients who have extensive obesity or a large amount of gas which obscures the kidney and retroperitoneum. Computed tomography may be the only modality for diagnosis of lesions in such patients. In doubtful cases, gallium scintigraphy may provide additional information.

CONCLUSIONS

Ultrasound findings in renal inflammatory disease generally depend on the stage, the etiology, and the distribution of the disease in and around the kidney. Neoplasm may be excluded from the differential diagnosis by identifying the progress and resolution of an inflammatory renal disease.

In our experience, pure inflammatory masses (focal nephronia) (Fig. 4.14) tend to be small and wedge-shaped with poorly defined borders. Abscess formation is accompanied by better border definition, an increase in size, greater sonolucency, posterior wall enhancement, and the occasional development of fluid debris levels.[37] Serial ultrasound examinations are essential to follow these changes. Percutaneous needle aspiration provides a specific diagnosis and facilitates the appropriate selection of antibiotics for difficult cases (Fig. 4.14A, B).

The diagnosis of intrarenal infection is based on an understanding and correlation of pathological changes with their corresponding ultrasonographic features. Recognition of this correlation enables the ultrasonographer to make an early accurate diagnosis of kidney infection before the appearance of intrarenal abscesses. The initial examination does not always provide a definitive diagnosis, especially in patients with acute focal nephritis. Clinical correlation and follow-up images are often necessary after the institution of antibiotics to confirm the first diagnostic impression. Rapid sequential changes are the hallmark of these infections. The diagnosis may therefore be confirmed by following the course of illness and the response to therapy. Prompt diagnosis can be made and specific antibiotic therapy instituted on the basis of information obtained by the ultrasound examination. This represents a true advance in medical science because it allows for the early institution of treatment at a time when renal destruction can be minimized. Successful medical treatment without drainage of cortical renal abscesses has been reported.

With early diagnosis and frequent follow-up made possible by ultrasound, this conservative treatment of intrarenal abscess, by antibiotics alone, may become more widespread. Ultrasound enables the physician to follow the course of renal infection to the point of complete resolution without exposing the patient to ionizing radiation or intravenous contrast agents.

REFERENCES

1. Kuligowska E, Newman B, White S, Caldarone A: Interventional ultrasound in detection and treatment of renal inflammatory disease. Radiology 147:2, 1983
2. Hoddick W, Jeffrey RB, Goldberg HI, Federle MP, Laing FC: CT and sonography of severe renal and perirenal infections. AJR 140:517, 1983
3. Morehouse HT, Weiner SN, Hoffman JC: Imaging in inflammatory disease of the kidney. AJR 143:135, 1984
4. Gold RP, McClennan BL, Rottenberg RR: CT appearance of acute inflammatory disease of the renal interstitium. AJR 141:343, 1983
5. Silver TM, Kass EJ, Thornbury JR et al.: The radiological spectrum of acute pyelonephritis in adults and adolescents. Radiology 118:65, 1976
6. Wicks JD, Thornbury JR: Acute renal infections in adults. Radiol Clin North Am 17:245, 1979
7. Rosenfield AT, Taylor KJW, Crade M, DeFraaf CS: Anatomy and pathology of the kidney by gray scale ultrasound. Radiology 128:737, 1978
8. Poporad GA, Kaye D: Urinary tract infections. p. 1,244. In Stein JH (ed): Internal Medicine. 1st Ed. Little, Brown, Boston, 1983
9. O'Grady F (ed): Initiation and ascent of urinary tract infection. In Scientific Foundation of Urology. Vol. 1, p. 177, 1979
10. Milton E: Radiology of the Urinary System. Little, Brown, Boston, 1980
11. Siegel MJ, Glasier CM: Acute focal bacterial nephritis in children:Significance of ureteral reflux. AJR 137:257, 1981
12. Hodson CJ: Reflux nephropathy: A personal historical review. AJR 137:451, 1981

13. Lebowitz RL, Fellows KE, Colodny AH: Renal parenchymal infections in children. Radiol Clin North Am 15:37, 1977

14. Ransley PG, Ridson RA: The renal papilla, intrarenal reflux and chronic pyelonephritis. Reflux Neuropathy Sci Found Urol 7:79, 1976

15. De Wardener HE: The Kidney: An Outline of Normal and Abnormal Structure and Function. 4th Ed. Churchill Livingstone, New York, 1973

16. Alexander L, Ramzi L: Renal Pathophysiology. Oxford University Press, New York, 1976

17. Hoffman EP, Mindelzun RE, Anderson RU: Computed tomography in acute pyelonephritis associated with diabetes. Radiology 135:691, 1980

18. Subramanyam BR, Raghavendra BN, Bosniak MA et al.: Sonography of pyonephrosis: A prospective study. AJR 140:991, 1983

19. Kay CJ, Rosenfield AT, Taylor KJW, Rosenberg MA: Ultrasonic characteristics of chronic atrophic pyelonephritis. AJR 132:47, 1979

20. Van Kirk OW, Go RT, Wedel VJ: Sonographic features of xanthogranulomatous pyelonephritis. AJR 134:1035, 1980

21. Sty JR, Starshak RJ: Sonography of pediatric urinary tract abnormalities. In Seminars in Ultrasound. Vol. 2. Grune & Stratton, New York, 1981

22. Bosniak MA, Ambos MA, Lefleur RS: Angiography of renal infection. p. 1175. Abrams HL (ed): Angiography. Vol 2. Little, Brown, Boston, 1983

23. Adler J, Greweldinger J, Conradi H: Gallium-67 scans in renal tumors. Urol Radiol 3:27, 1981

24. Hurwitz SR, Kessler WO, Alazraki NP: Gallium-67 imaging to localize urinary-tract infections. Br J Radiol 49:156, 1976

25. Filly RA: Detection of abdominal abscesses: A combined approach employing ultrasonography, computed tomography and gallium-67 scanning. J Assoc Can Radiol 30:202, 1979

26. Moss AA, Gamsu G, Genant HK: Computed Tomography of the Body. W.B. Saunders, Philadelphia, 1983

27. Berger PE, Munschauer RW, Kuhn JP: Computed tomography and ultrasound of renal and perirenal diseases in infants and children. Pediatr Radiol 9:91, 1980

28. Parienty RA, Pradel J, Picard JD et al.: Visibility and thickening of the renal fascia on computed tomograms. Radiology 139:119, 1981

29. Rosenfield AT, Siegel NJ: Renal parenchymal disease: Histopathologic-sonographic correlation. AJR 137:793, 1981

30. Edell SL, Bonavita JA: The sonographic appearance of acute pyelonephritis. Radiology 132:683, 1979

31. Lee JKT, McClennan BL, Melson GL, Stanley RJ: Acute focal bacterial nephritis: Emphasis on gray scale sonography and computed tomography. AJR 135:87, 1980

32. Rosenfield AT, Glickman MG, Taylor KJW: Acute focal bacterial nephritis (acute lobar nephronia). Radiology 132:553, 1979

33. Conrad MR, Bregman R, Kilman WJ et al.: Ultrasonic recognition of parenchymal gas. AJR 132:395, 1979

34. Coleman BG, Arger PH, Mulhern CB Jr. et al.: Pyonephrosis:Sonography in the diagnosis and management. AJR 137:939, 1981

35. Yoder IC, Pfister RC, Lindfors KK, Newhouse JH:Pyonephrosis: Imaging and intervention. AJR 141:735, 1983

36. Boutros GA, Athey PA: Ultrasonic Demonstration of Xanthogranulomatous Pyelonephritis. J.C.U. Vol. 6, p. 427. John Wiley, New York, 1978

37. Funston MR, Fisher KS, van Blerk JP, Bortz JH: Acute focal bacterial nephritis or renal abscess? A sonographic diagnosis. Br J Urol 54:461, 1982

5 Interventional Ultrasound

R. BROOKE JEFFREY, JR.
EWA KULIGOWSKA

The development of high-resolution real-time sonography has greatly facilitated the performance of many percutaneous interventional procedures of the genitourinary tract. In many instances ultrasound-guided techniques are effective and rewarding alternatives to surgery that lessen morbidity, length of hospitalization, and cost to the patient. This chapter will review some of the more important ultrasound-related interventional procedures in the genitourinary system and stress their basic technique and clinical applications.

ULTRASOUND-GUIDED PERCUTANEOUS NEPHROSTOMY

Percutaneous nephrostomy is an increasingly important technique for the treatment of a wide variety of benign and malignant disorders of the genitourinary tract.[1-5] The ability to rapidly and effectively drain the renal pelvis and collecting system with minimal morbidity represents a major therapeutic advance in urology. In addition to the management of obstructive uropathy, percutaneous nephrostomy has important applications for the removal of renal and ureteral calculi and the treatment of ureteral fistulae.[4,5] Ultrasound used in conjunction with fluoroscopy may be of considerable value in guiding percutaneous nephrostomy by decreasing the time of the procedure and number of attempts at puncturing the renal collecting system.[1]

INDICATIONS, TECHNIQUE, AND COMPLICATIONS

There are a growing number of indications for percutaneous nephrostomy.[1] The main indications for sonographically guided percutaneous nephrostomy include management of obstructive uropathy and pyonephrosis.[6-9] In patients with normal renal function and renal obstruction, percutaneous nephrostomy can be performed directly under fluoroscopic control following the intravenous

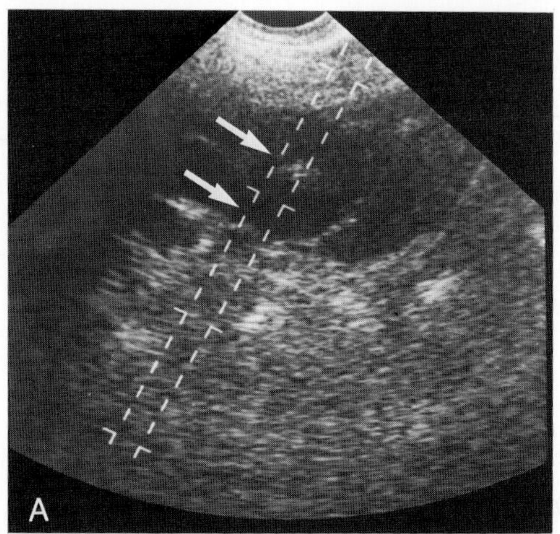

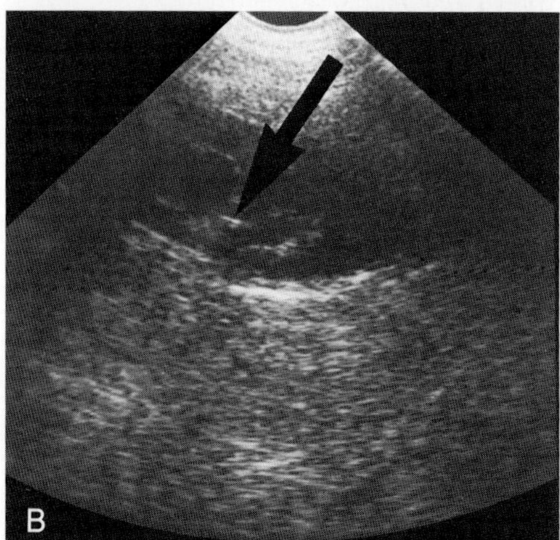

FIG. 5.1. Technique of ultrasound-guided percutaneous nephrostomy. (A) Demonstrates longitudinal scan of dilated collecting system. Parallel lines indicate path of needle aiming for middle calyx (arrows). (B) Same patient demonstrates bright echo from needle within dilated collecting system (arrow). (C) Is another example of visualizing needle tip in markedly dilated collecting system (arrow) (Figure continues).

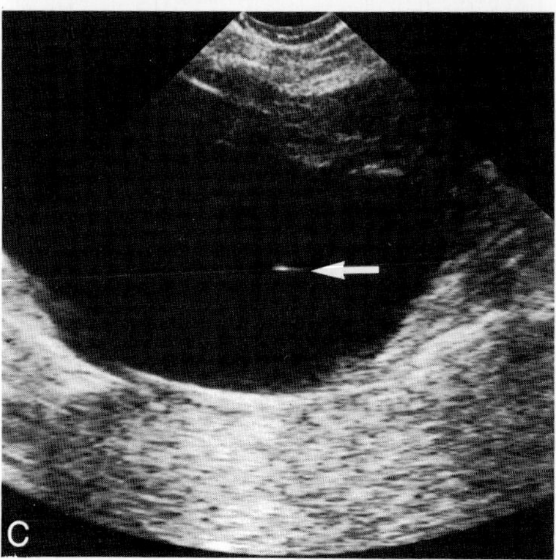

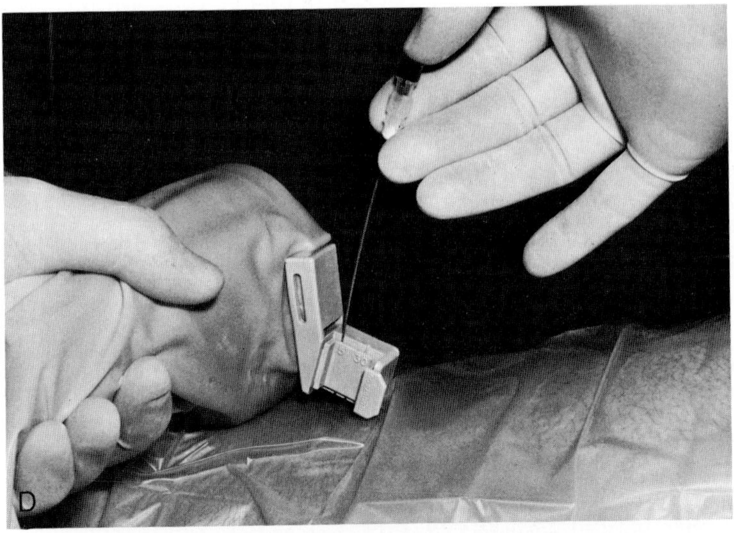

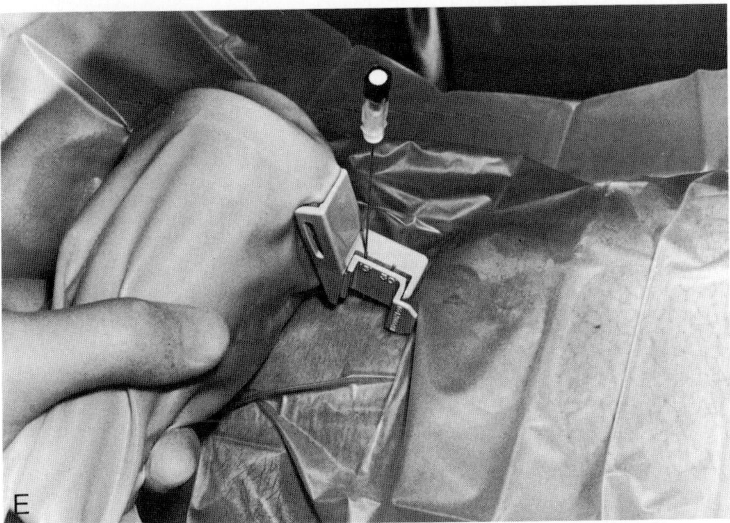

FIG. 5.1. (Continued). (D) and (E) demonstrate use of sidearm adapter for guided puncture. While holding transducer steady needle is inserted under continuous sonographic monitoring.

administration of urographic contrast. However, many patients with severe renal obstruction have significantly delayed contrast excretion; thus, visualization of the renal collecting system in this setting may be quite difficult with excretory urography. Sonographic visualization of a dilated renal collecting system is independent of renal function and avoids the small but measurable nephrotoxicity of urographic contrast.

In the past, blind antegrade pyelography with a skinny needle was performed in patients with obstruction and poor renal function to first opacify the renal collecting system. The collecting system is then punctured under direct fluoroscopic control. However, blind antegrade pyelography may be hazardous in patients with pyonephrosis, as it may be very difficult to effectively decompress an infected system through a skinny needle. Contrast injection into a pus-filled renal collecting system may induce severe bacteremia.

Ultrasound-guided percutaneous nephrostomy obviates the need to perform blind antegrade pyelography. It is also well documented that with ultrasound guidance fewer attempts are required to puncture the renal collecting system than with fluoroscopically guided procedures.[10] Although comparison studies have documented no difference in the morbidity of ultrasound versus fluoroscopic guidance,[10] sonography has several distinct advantages: (1) it is less time consuming as fewer attempts at puncture are required, (2) it does not involve injection of contrast media either intravenously or directly into the collecting system by antegrade pyelography, and (3) it allows small-gauge needles to be inserted initially into the collecting system that have the theoretical advantage of decreasing renal parenchymal hemorrhage. Newer side-arm attachments and real-time guidance systems have greatly improved the continuous visualization of the needle as it punctures the renal collecting system (Fig. 5.1).

The optimal method for performing sonographically guided percutaneous nephrostomy is in combination with fluoroscopy. The puncture of the renal collecting system is guided by sonography, and all subsequent catheter and guidewire manipulation is monitored by fluoroscopy. Although percutaneous nephrostomy can be performed entirely under sonographic guidance, it is often very difficult to visualize the exact position of guidewires and catheters. In desperately ill patients who cannot be transported to the interventional suite, sonography may be used to perform percutaneous nephrostomy at the bedside. However, in general, placement of guidewire and catheters within the renal collecting system is best determined by fluoroscopic control. We prefer to use portable real-time sonography directly in the interventional suite so that the sonographic guidance can be readily combined with fluoroscopy.

Patient preparation for percutaneous nephrostomy is minimal. As with other invasive procedures, coagulation studies should be normal to avoid significant renal hemorrhage. In patients with suspected pyonephrosis, broad-spectrum antibiotics should be given intravenously prior to the procedure. In adults, nephrostomy is performed entirely under local anesthesia with mild sedation. In small children, general anesthesia may be required.

Percutaneous nephrostomy is best performed in the prone or prone oblique position. Generally, a lower pole or middle calyx is punctured in the midcoronal plane of the kidney. The puncture site is below the twelfth rib in the posterior axillary line. This posterior lateral approach avoids traversing the colon, liver, spleen, or pleura. Puncture of the kidney in the relatively avascular midcoronal plane also decreases the degree of bleeding associated with nephrostomy. Addi-

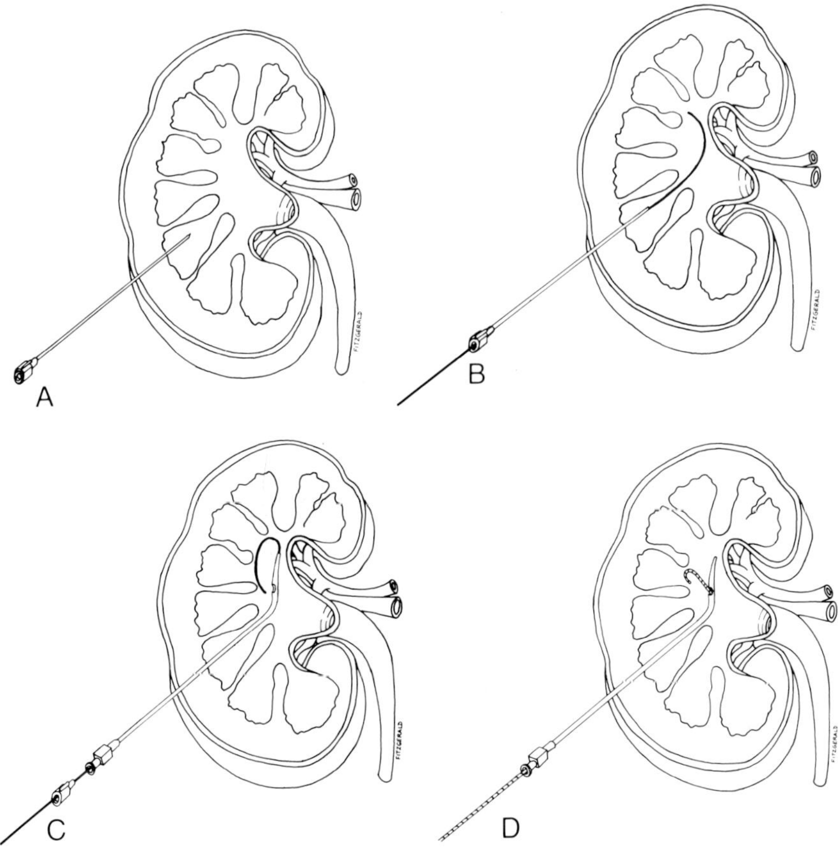

FIG. 5.2. Schematic representation of percutaneous nephrostomy. Initial puncture of collecting system performed with 21-gauge Cope needle (A). Next 0.18-guidewire is inserted in through the needle and coiled in the collecting system (B). Dilator (6.3-F) tapered to 4F inserted over guidewire with inner stiffening cannula (C). Guidewire, 0.18 then removed and heavy-duty 0.38-guidewire inserted through side port of dilator (D). This guidewire readily permits dilatation of the tract and final drainage catheter insertion.

tionally, it avoids the larger paraspinous muscles and is more comfortable for the patient than a direct posterior approach.

Although a variety of needles may be used for sonographically guided puncture of the renal collecting system, we often prefer to use a 21-gauge Cope needle (Cook, Bloomington, Indiana) (Fig. 5.2). The relatively small size of the needle produces less bleeding and a 0.18 guidewire can then be directly inserted through the needle after aspirating urine from the collecting system. A dilator can then be passed that allows insertion of a heavy-duty 0.38 guidewire into the renal collecting system. Larger dilators can then be readily inserted before advancing the final drainage catheter. In postoperative patients with perirenal scarring or in obese patients, a larger-caliber needle (such as a 5F-needle sheath) may be required to penetrate the perirenal tissues without deflecting the needle tip. In general, a pigtail or Cope-loop configuration catheter is used for initial nephrostomy drainage, ranging from 8 to 12 French. The catheter is then secured by suturing it to the plastic disc of an ileostomy stomadhesive.

As with fluoroscopically guided percutaneous nephrostomy, major complications are uncommon but include hemorrhage, bacteremia, pneumothorax, urine extravasation, and urocutaneous fistula.[11] Transient hematuria and flank discomfort are the most common minor complications. If the hematuria fails to clear promptly or increases significantly, angiography may be required to exclude a bleeding pseudoaneurysm.[11]

SONOGRAPHY IN THE DIAGNOSIS AND MANAGEMENT OF PYONEPHROSIS

Pyonephrosis is the presence of pus within an obstructed collecting system. It represents a true urological emergency requiring prompt drainage and relief of obstruction. In the past, nephrectomy was often performed for pyonephrosis. Percutaneous nephrostomy offers an effective and rewarding alternative to surgery with minimal morbidity and patient invasion. Further it has the potential to relieve urosepsis and preserve renal function.[3,7]

Sonography should be performed early in the course of patients with significant urosepsis to exclude the presence of pyonephrosis or a sizable perirenal or renal abscess. In uncomplicated hydronephrosis, the renal collecting system is often anechoic. However, patients with pyonephrosis often demonstrate coarse intraluminal echoes or fluid debris within the collecting system levels[12] (Fig. 5.3). Rarely, gas-forming organisms within the collecting system result in acoustic shadowing from emphysematous pyonephrosis. On occasion it may be necessary to perform a diagnostic needle aspiration of a dilated renal collecting system to absolutely exclude pyonephrosis. This is because a small percentage of patients may have few internal echoes within the renal collecting system associated with pyonephrosis.[3] The risk of a diagnostic needle aspiration under sonographic guidance is far less than missing the diagnosis of pyonephrosis.

As previously noted, antegrade pyelography may be hazardous in patients with pyonephrosis and carries a significant risk of bacteremia. Sonography is therefore the method of choice in guiding the initial puncture and decompression of an infected collecting system. It is also very important to make as few attempts at puncturing the renal collecting system as possible in order not to leak pus out of the renal pelvis and convert a pyonephrosis into a perirenal abscess. If renal radioisotope scans demonstrate some renal function, ultrasound-guided percutaneous nephrostomy may result in significant improvement of renal function.[1]

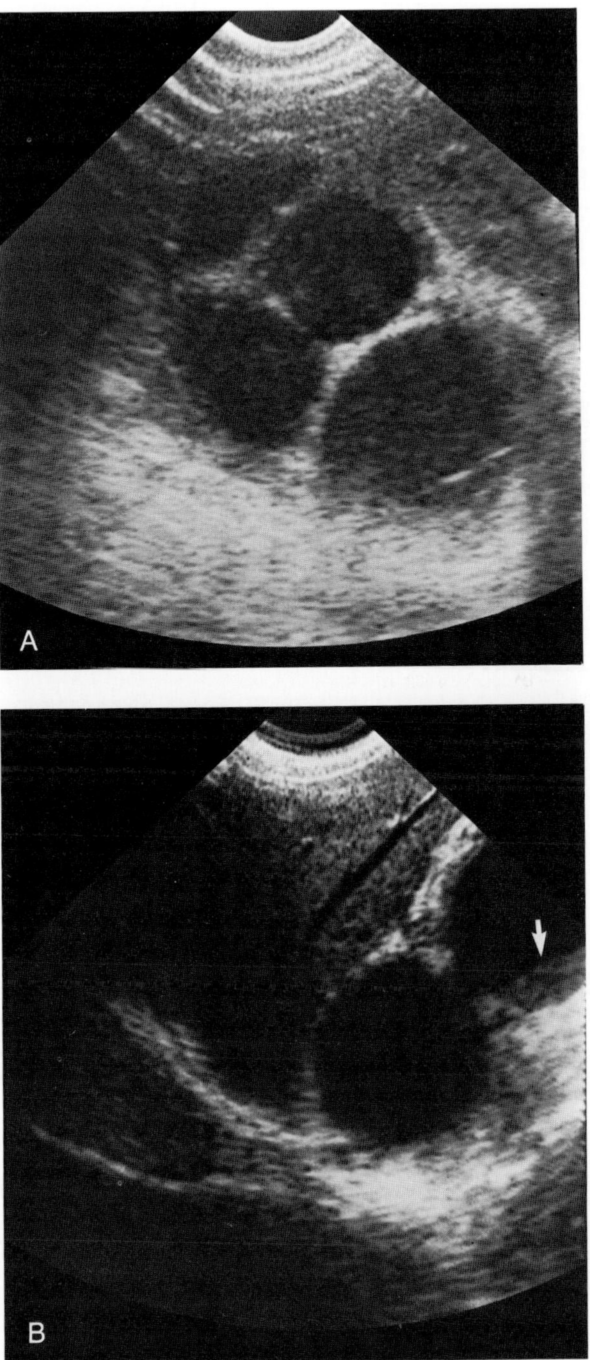

FIG. 5.3. Sonographic spectrum in pyonephrosis. (A) Coarse intraluminal echoes dispersed throughout collecting system. (B) Demonstrates fluid debris level (arrow) (Figure continues).

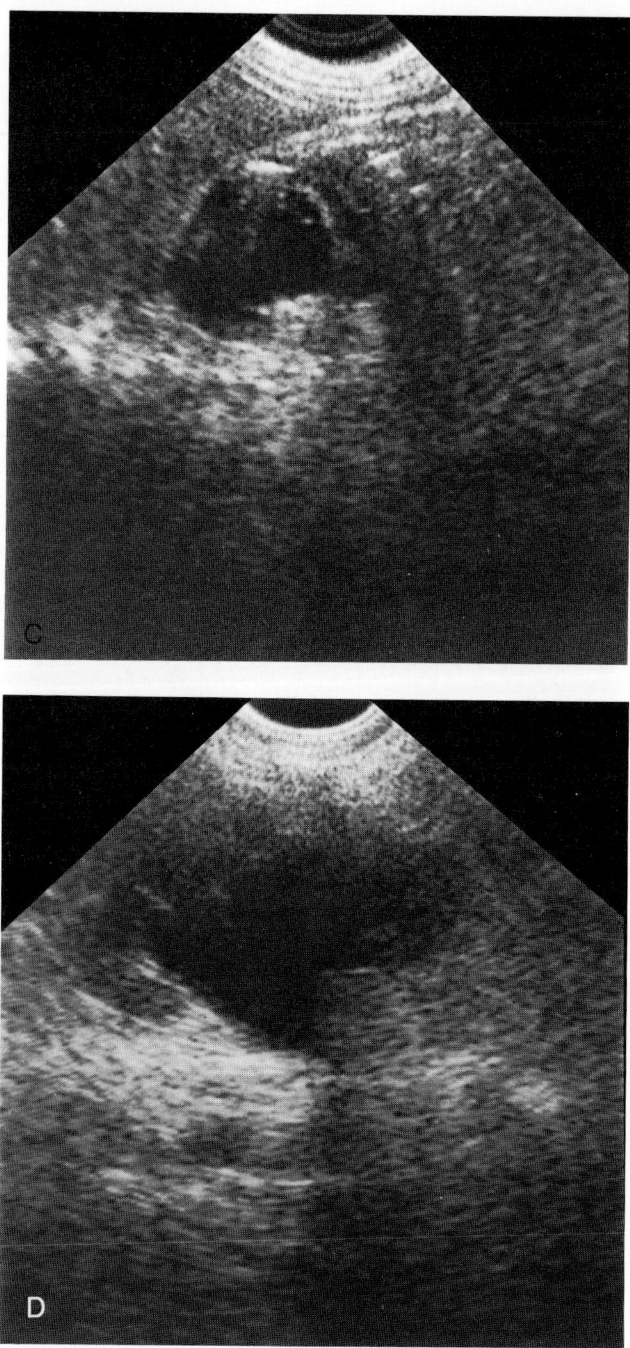

FIG. 5.3. (Continued). (C) Exhibits extensive acoustic shadowing from gas-forming organisms in collecting system. (D) Shows relatively anechoic collecting system with proven pyonephrosis (Figure continues).

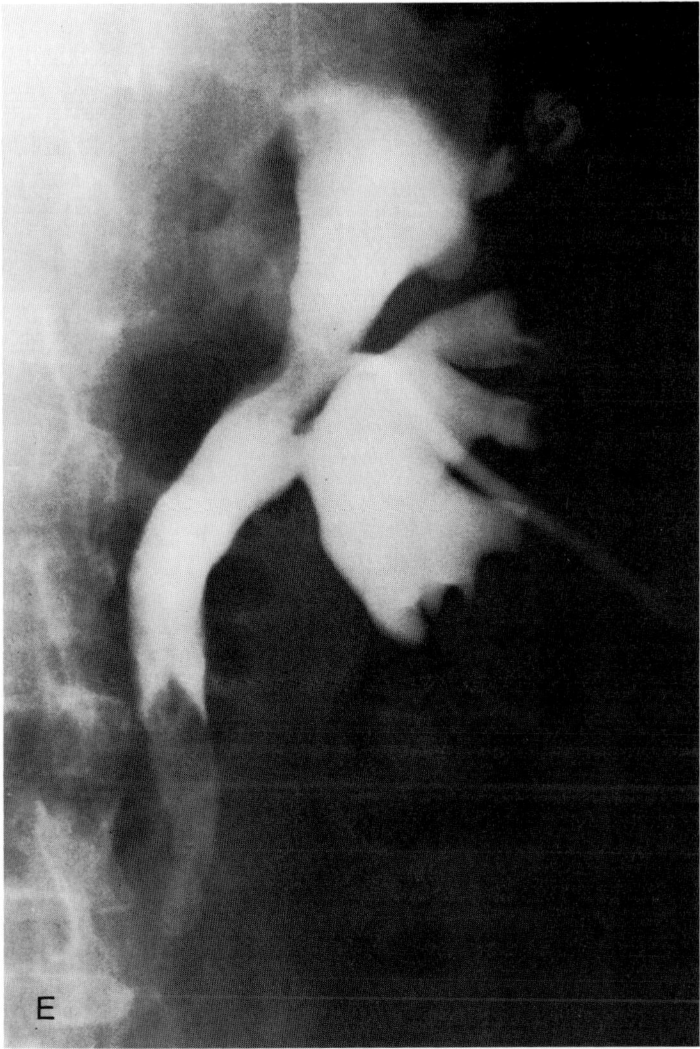

FIG. 5.3. (Continued). (E) Nephrostogram following sonographically guided percutaneous nephrostomy of patient. Note obstructing calculus in proximal ureter.

PERCUTANEOUS DRAINAGE OF RENAL ABSCESSES

The diagnosis and treatment of renal and perirenal abscesses continue to be a serious clinical problem because of their considerable morbidity.[14] Early diagnosis and treatment of renal abscess are essential for effective clinical management. Since the advent of ultrasound and computed tomography, the approach to the diagnosis and treatment of renal and perirenal abscesses has changed significantly. In the past, many of these lesions were recognized late in their

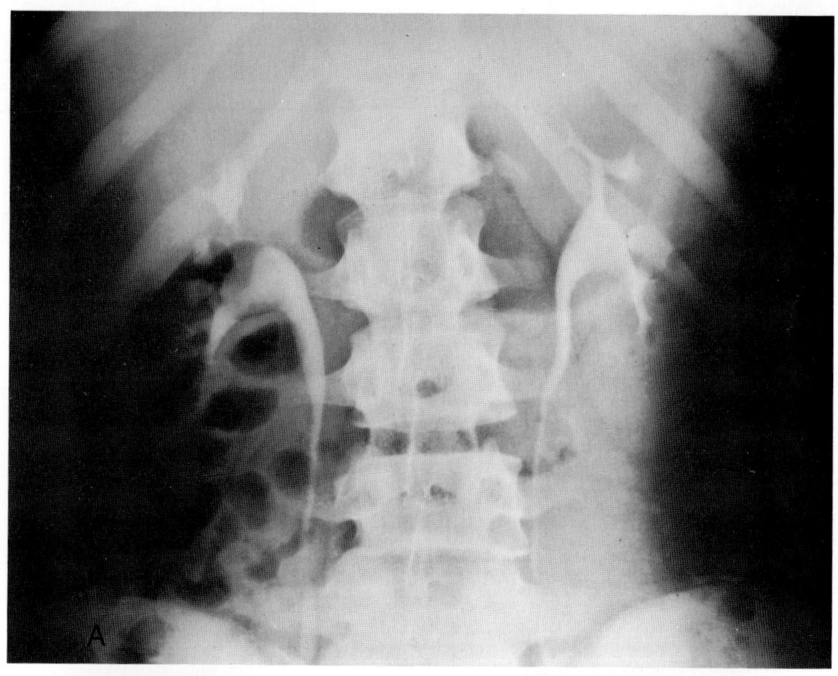

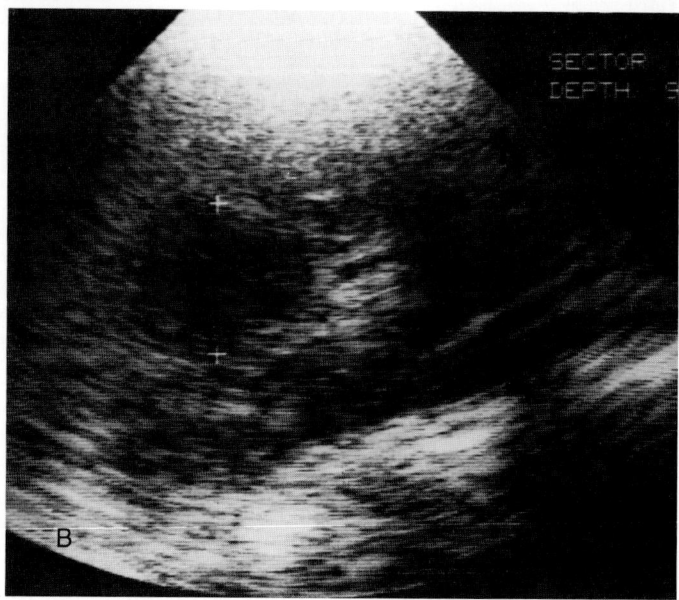

FIG. 5.4.   Ten-year-old girl with high fever and *E. coli* sepsis. (A) Excretory urography is normal. (B) Coronal scan of the left kidney delineates a small intrarenal lesion (Figure continues).

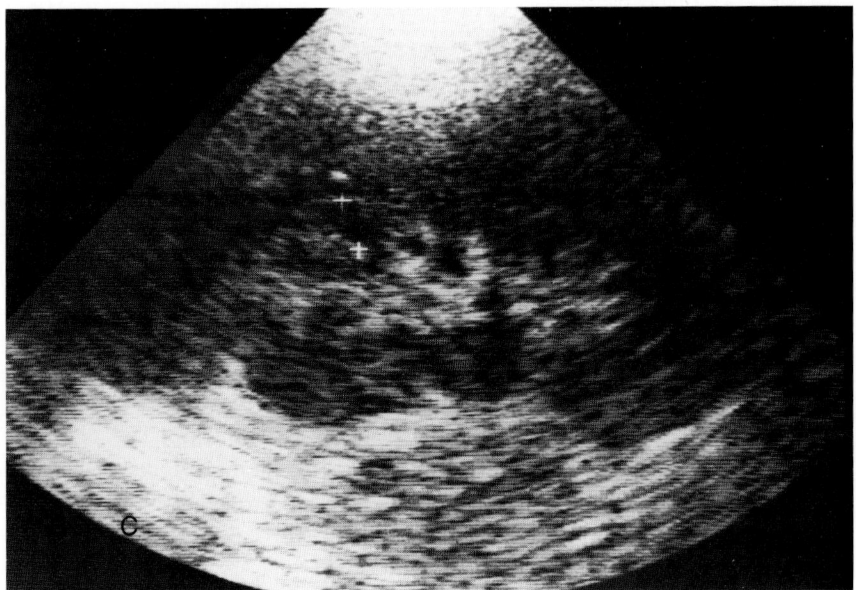

FIG. 5.4. (Continued).   (C) Sonogram of this kidney following complete evacuation of the abscess with 20-gauge needle.

clinical course, and treatment necessitated nephrectomy. Some renal abscesses were only discovered at autopsy.

Early diagnosis and prompt, effective treatment are possible for this condition today.[15,16] Our experience at Boston University with over 500 percutaneous drainage procedures of abscesses includes 54 renal abscesses, 9 of which had perinephric extension. There were no deaths or recurrences in this group of patients treated for renal abscess.

Indications

In patients with urosepsis and the demonstration of a renal mass by either ultrasound or other imaging modalities, a diagnostic puncture should be performed utilizing a 22-gauge needle (Fig. 5.4).[15,16] If diagnostic puncture confirms an abscess, percutaneous drainage should be the next step. Coagulation studies must be performed prior to the procedure, including a platelet count, prothrombin, and partial thromboplastin time. Broad-spectrum antibiotics should be administered intravenously prior to the procedure.

Techniques of Abscess Drainage Under Ultrasound Guidance

Renal and retroperitoneal abscesses should be drained extraperitoneally via the flank to avoid contamination of the peritoneum.[15,16] Patients are placed in the right or left prone oblique position for this procedure as for percutaneous

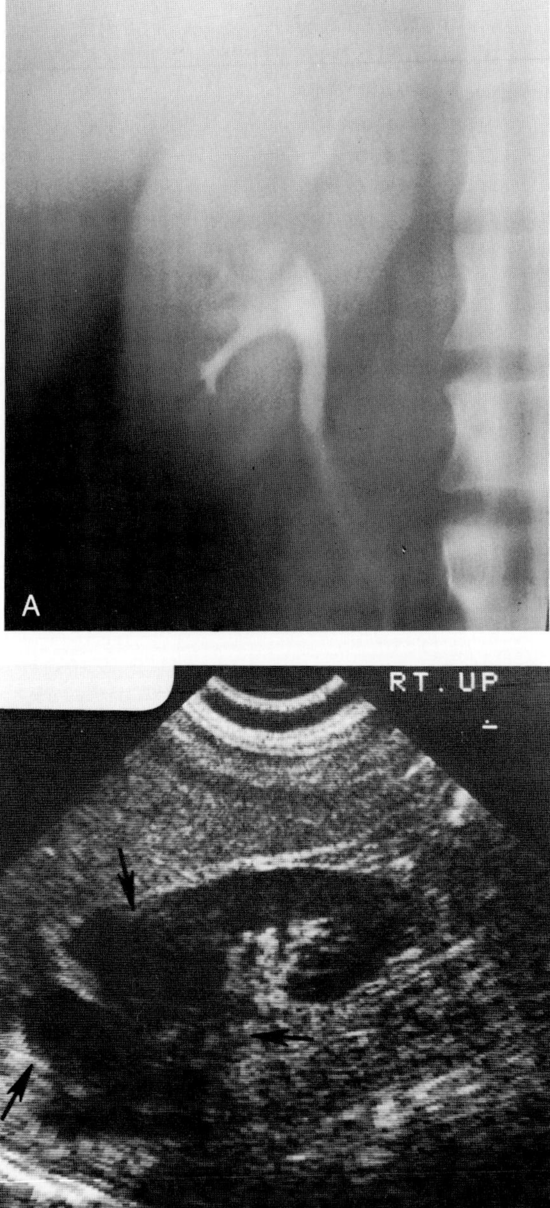

FIG. 5.5.   Thirty-eight-year old man with low-grade fever and back pain for 3 months. (A) Excretory urography suggests a mass in the upper pole of the right kidney. (B) Longitudinal sonogram of the right kidney reveals a hypoechoic mass with extension to perirenal space (arrows) (Figure continues).

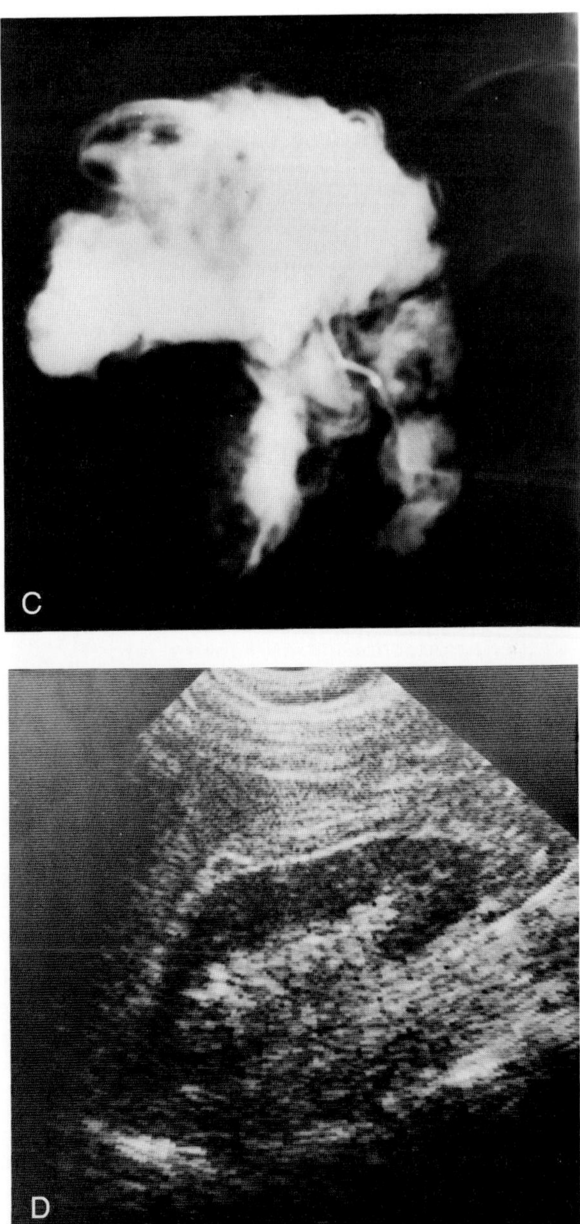

FIG. 5.5. (Continued).   (C) Three hundred cc of thick, purulent material was drained utilizing a 12-French pigtail catheter. Instillation of water-soluble contrast into the cavity shows irregularity of the wall of abscess and extension to the perirenal space. (D) Follow-up scan 14 days later shows complete resolution of the abscess.

nephrostomy. The shortest distance between the skin and the lesion is chosen for the puncture route. The entry site and depth from the skin surface to the lesion are determined during meticulous ultrasound examination performed in two perpendicular planes. After routine preparation, surgical draping and local anesthesia with lidocaine (Xylocaine), a small skin incision is made. The incision is then widened by blunt dissection. Puncture with a 22-gauge needle is made to the appropriate depth determined from the scan. The needle is directed into the central region of the abscess under continuous ultrasound monitoring using real-time sonography. A small amount of pus is aspirated from the abscess cavity and analyzed for bacteria and cells. If the specimen is too thick to be aspirated by a 22-gauge needle, a second puncture utilizing a 20-gauge needle should be performed in the same manner (Fig. 5.4).

Percutaneous drainage is performed only when purulent material has been aspirated during the diagnostic puncture. The drainage catheter is inserted using either a modified Seldinger or a trochar technique.[15,16] The choice of technique for the placement of the catheter is determined by the location and size of the abnormality. For drainage of small and deeply located, less accessible abscesses, a pigtail catheter is inserted. To drain large, easily accessible abscesses, a trochar is usually used.

Small or deeply located abscesses are best drained via modified angiographic Seldinger technique. This technique involves an initial puncture with a 22-gauge needle and the introduction of a guidewire into the fluid. The tract is dilated by passing angiographic dilators over the initial guidewire. This wire is then exchanged for a larger, stiffer guidewire which is advanced and coiled within the cavity.

The tract can then be dilated to accommodate the appropriate pigtail catheter using several vessel dilators over the guidewire (Fig. 5.5). This entire procedure may be carried out under combined ultrasound or CT and fluoroscopic guidance. The method is very effective; however, it requires angiographic expertise to control guidewire manipulation and catheter exchange.[17] There are several commercially available prepackaged drainage catheter sets which are very convenient and contain all of the necessary equipment. The most widely used kits are the percutaneous nephrostomy set, Cook-Cope type loop and the Van Sonnenberg sump kit.[18]

The second technique is the trochar stylet method which is used to drain superficial collections with no intervening bowel or other organs (Fig. 5.6).[15-19] This technique offers several significant advantages. The time required to perform the trochar technique is significantly shorter. It eliminates the need for guidewires, sequential dilatation of the tract, and fluoroscopic manipulation for proper placement. The entire drainage can be performed in a single step. No fluoroscopy is needed, and it can also be performed at the bedside.[17]

There are several excellent trochar catheter sets which are commercially available for draining abnormal fluid collections. The argyle Ingram Trocar Catheter and Cystocath Suprapubic Drainage System which were originally intended for suprapubic percutaneous cystostomy is well suited for draining large retroperitoneal abscesses.[15,16] For smaller collections we recently have used the Sacks

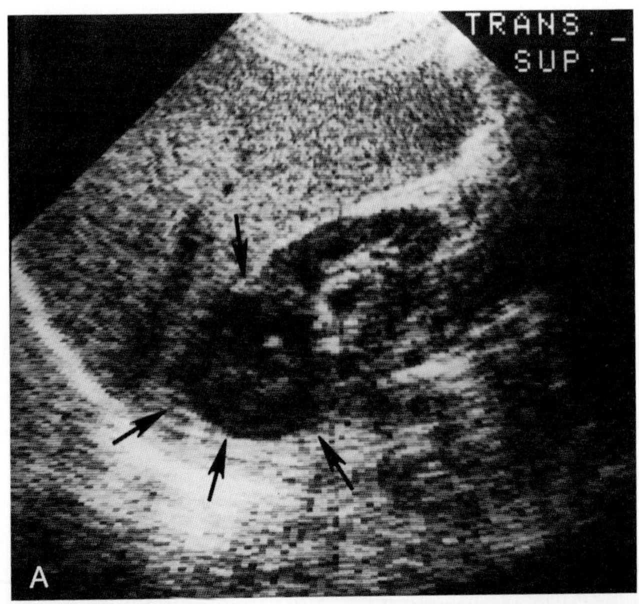

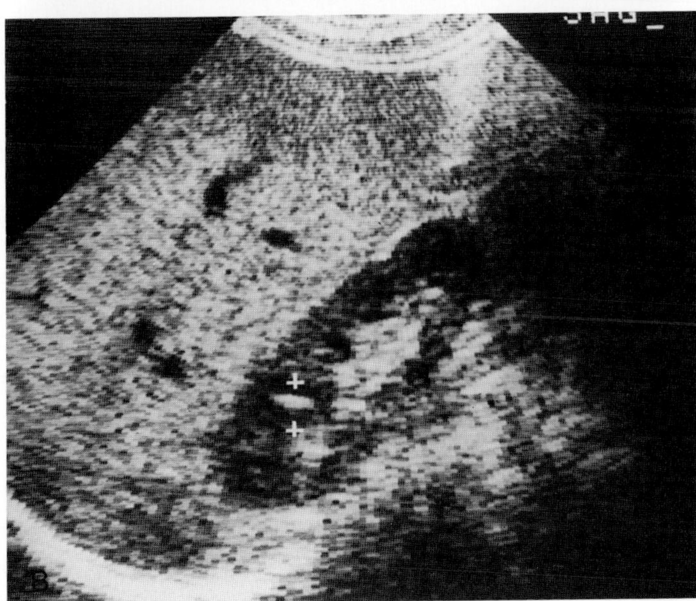

FIG. 5.6. Fifty-year-old man with back pain and elevated white blood cell count. (A) An abscess was discovered on a longitudinal sonogram of the right kidney (arrows). (B) After 7 days of drainage a sonogram reveals complete healing and no reaccumulation of fluid after clamping the catheter (crosshairs).

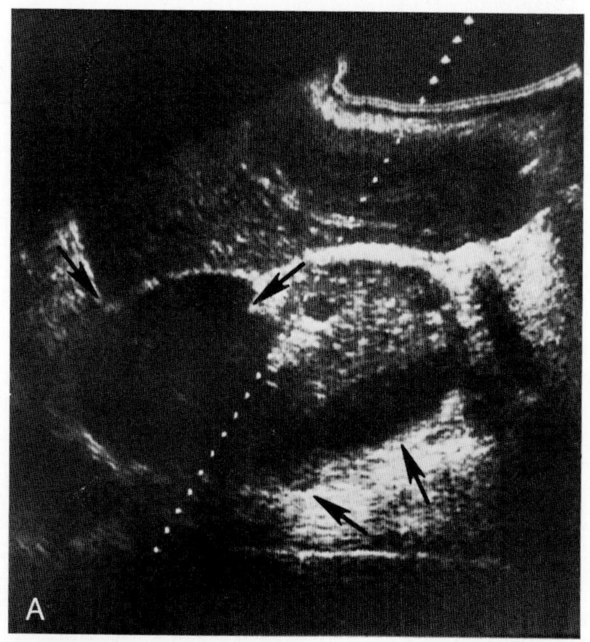

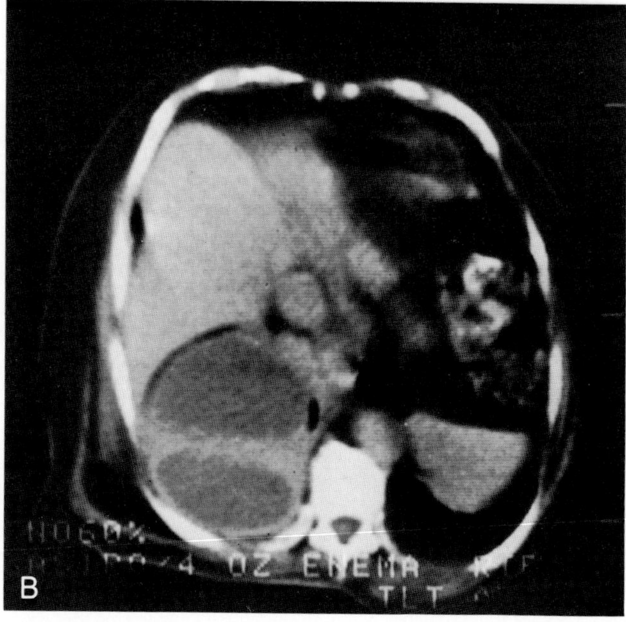

FIG. 5.7. Seventy-one-year-old woman with hypertension, fever and, elevated white blood cell count. (A) Longitudinal sonogram of the right kidney shows two large anechoic masses (arrows) representing abscesses. (B) CT scan reveals two distinct abscesses in the kidney (Figure continues).

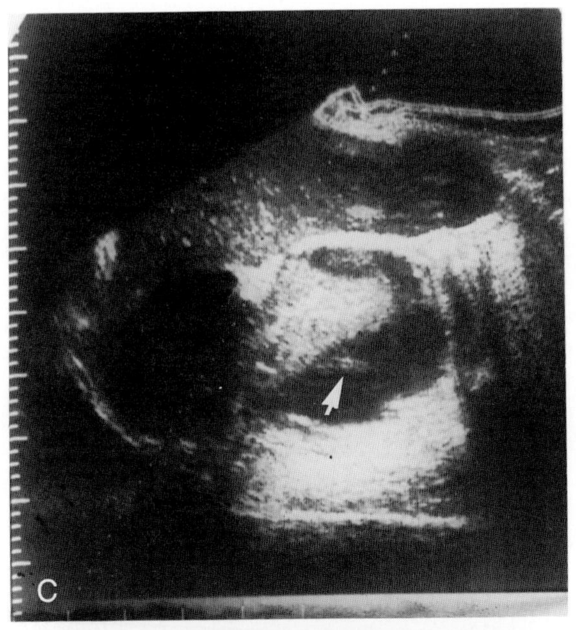

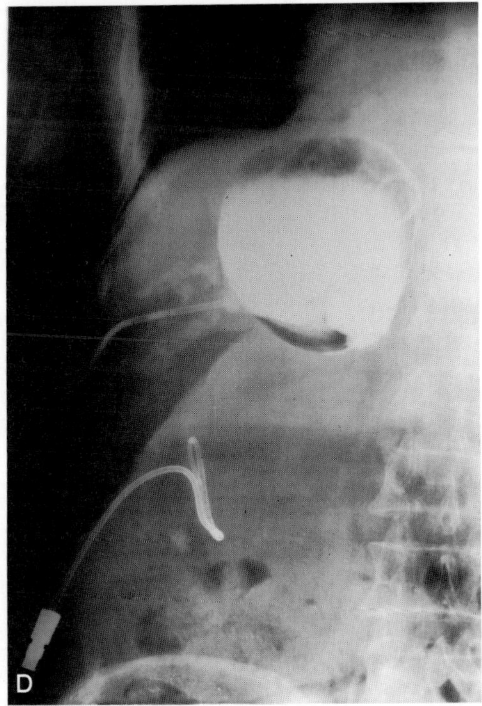

FIG. 5.7. (Continued).   (C) Drainage was accomplished by placement of two 7.5-French pigtail catheters (arrow). (D) Instillation of water-soluble contrast into the cephalad mass fails to demonstrate a connection between the two abscesses.

needle catheter system with extremely good results.[17] This catheter is a modified pigtail with sideholes on the inner aspect of the distal curve.

A variety of drainage catheters are used which range in size from 5.5 to 14 (French). These catheters differ in internal diameter as well as in the number of holes along the catheter. The choice of catheter depends upon the viscosity of the aspirate and location of abscesses.[15,16,18,19]

Once the catheter is placed in the cavity using an appropriate technique, and a free flow of purulent material is obtained, the remaining abscess contents should be completely evacuated by manual syringe suction, and the volume should be recorded. Complete evacuation should be confirmed on a subsequent ultrasound scan. The abscess cavity is then lavaged with copious amounts of sterile saline until the effluent is clear and contains no purulent material. Water-soluble contrast material is then injected through the catheter into the cavity in an amount not exceeding one-tenth of the volume of the initial drainage. Roentgenograms of the abdomen are then obtained in several different positions (decubitus, supine, erect, and/or cross lateral) to determine the size, shape, and possible extension of the abscess to other organs or structures[15,18] (Figs. 5.5C, 5.6C, 5.8D). Finally, the catheter is fixed in place with adhesive tape, attached to the tubing, and connected to a drainage bag which provides a closed-gravity drainage system. The catheter is left in place from 7 to 21 days.

Catheter Management

Drainage catheters require special attention. The catheter must be irrigated with 5 to 10 cc of sterile saline on a regular basis every 8 hours during the first 4 days and then daily until day 7. Additional aspiration and lavage with sterile saline is only performed later when ultrasound examination reveals residual fluid collections. Irrigation decreases the viscosity of the cavity contents, promotes flow, and maintains catheter patency. Portable ultrasound examination is performed daily to monitor the treatment during the first few days and later biweekly. The interventional ultrasound team must be responsible for the total management of catheter drainage in order to assure complete resolution and healing of the abscess.

When drainage stops and sonography or CT confirm the complete resolution of the abscess, the catheter should be clamped for 2 days before the final withdrawal. The catheter can then be totally withdrawn if there is no reaccumulation of abnormal fluid (Fig. 5.7).

All patients should receive intravenous antibiotic therapy while the drainage catheter is in place. Fever usually subsides within 24 to 48 hours. The white blood count also returns to normal usually within 1 week.[15,16]

Contraindications

There are no absolute contraindications for percutaneous drainage of renal abscesses, except for an uncorrectable bleeding disorder.[15,16,18,19] Most coagulopathies can be corrected to allow abscess drainage. It is theoretically possible

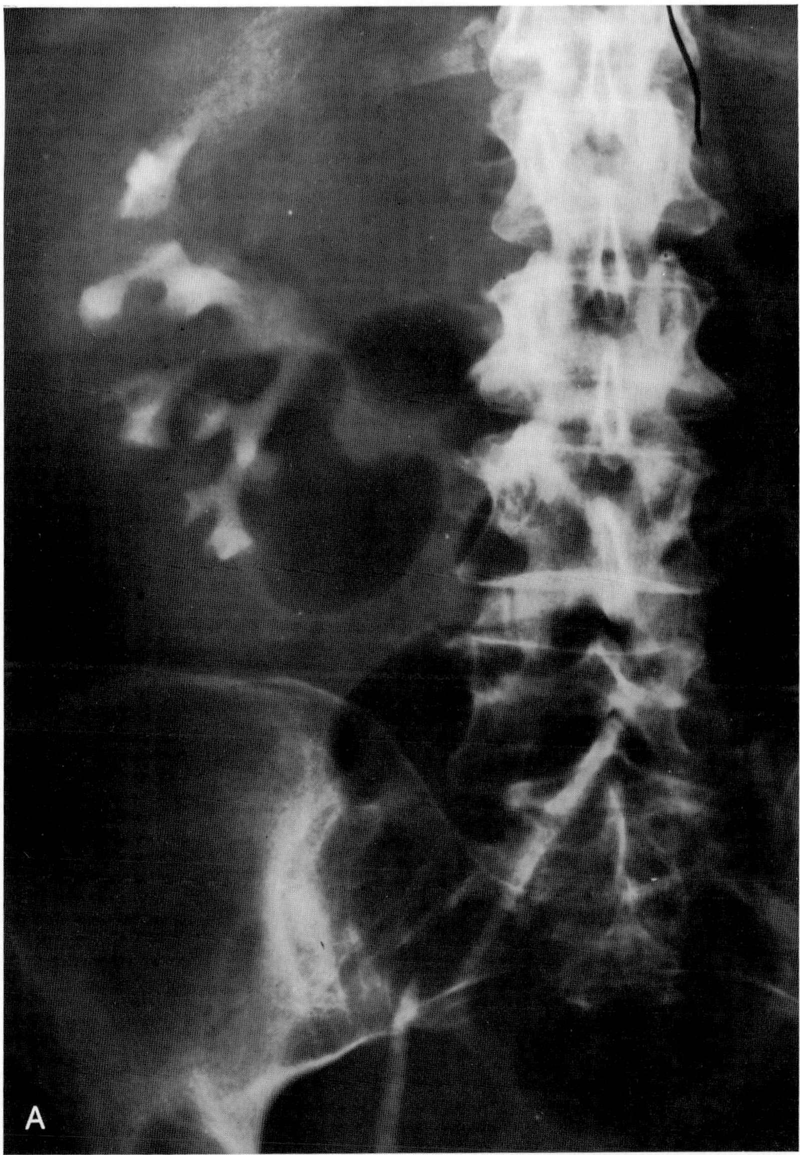

FIG. 5.8. Elderly woman with flank pain and fever 3 weeks after trauma. (A) Excretory urography revealed a right paraspinal mass producing displacement of kidney and proximal ureter (Figure continues).

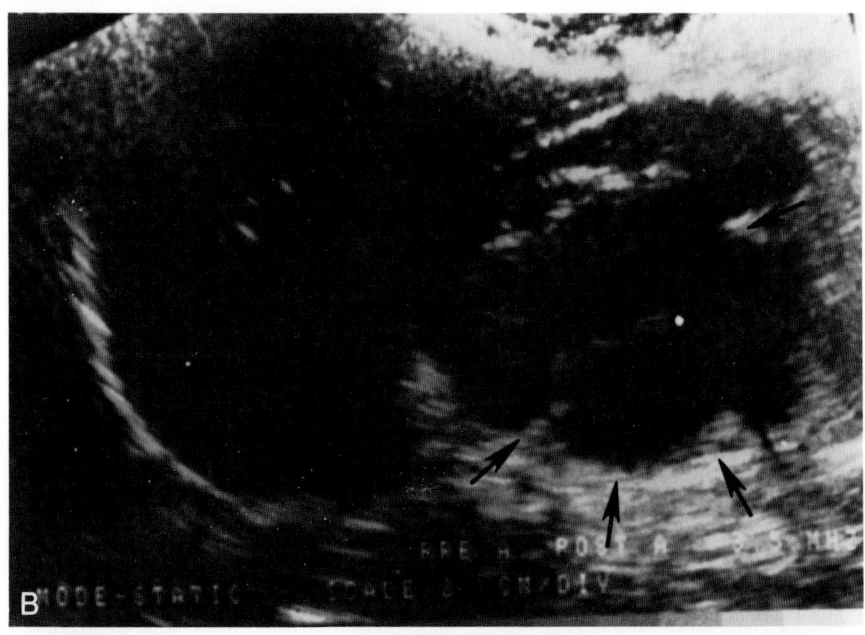

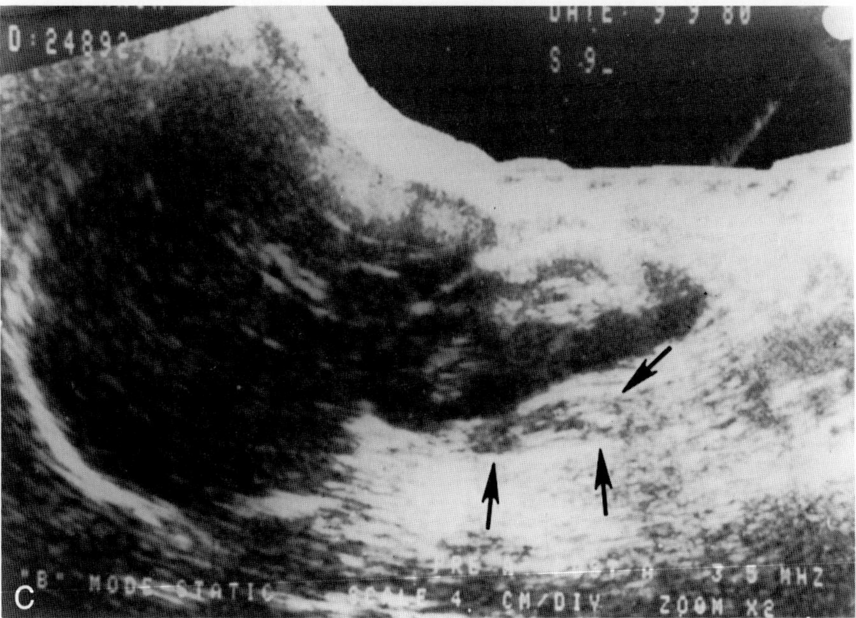

FIG. 5.8. (Continued). (B) Longitudinal scan of right kidney shows anechoic mass occupying the posterior aspect of the kidney with extension to psoas muscle (arrows) which elevates the right kidney. Pus (400 cc) was drained by placement of a 12-French trochar catheter under ultrasonic guidance. (C) Follow-up scan 18 days later shows complete resolution of the abscess. Note the psoas muscle (arrows).

132

that no safe route for percutaneous drainage may be identified without traversing bowel or other organs. In our experience during the past 6 years, however, this situation has never occurred. A retroperitoneal approach in the lateral right or left semidecubitus position has always obviated this problem. Septations and multiloculated abscesses are not a contraindication to percutaneous drainage. The septa between abscesses usually rupture during adequate drainage and lavage procedures. If there is a truly multiloculated abscess, multiple catheters will be required for drainage[15] (Fig. 5.8).

GENERAL CONSIDERATIONS

Percutaneous catheter drainage in combination with antibiotics provides definitive therapy for intrarenal abscess, even with perinephric extension (Figs. 5.5, 5.7, 5.8). Responses are usually so dramatic that we believe this to be the treatment of choice for intrarenal abscesses (Figs. 5.5–5.8). Multiple abscesses pose a difficult problem for the clinician and surgeon. The relatively blind surgical approach for finding and draining deep or small lesions creates significant trauma to surrounding normal renal tissue and often necessitates nephrectomy. This can be completely avoided by using ultrasound to place catheters into each abscess cavity. In our experience, complete and successful drainage has been accomplished by placing as many as four catheters into a multiloculated intrarenal and perirenal lesion.

The initial drainage and lavaging of an abscess cavity are clearly the most important parts of a percutaneous drainage procedure. Complete healing of abscesses has been noted in instances where it has not been possible to maintain catheters in the abscess cavity for more than a short period of time following the initial drainage and lavage procedure.

Many patients with renal infection are poor surgical candidates with multisystem disease. The low morbidity of this interventional ultrasound technique is of obvious benefit to these patients. Sonography affords precise location of an abscess for aspiration, biopsy, and drainage. Recent advances in real-time technology have also contributed to the increased safety and higher accuracy of percutaneous placement of diagnostic needles and drainage catheters. The complete image of the needle or trochar can be monitored in the target lesion during the entire process of placement.[15] Safe percutaneous procedures make it possible to avoid major surgery.[13,14,18,19]

In rare instances, sonographic examination may not be possible in patients who have extreme obesity or large collections of gas which obscure the kidney and retroperitoneum. Computed tomography may be the only modality for diagnosing lesions and guiding drainage procedures in such patients.[16,18,19] Ultrasound remains the modality of choice because it requires a significantly shorter period of time for the procedure; it is cheaper and eliminates radiation exposure.[15]

ACKNOWLEDGMENTS

We greatly thank Louise Koike for secretarial assistance and Ms. Gala Fitzgerald for technical assistance and illustrations.

REFERENCES

1. Lang EK, Price ET: Redefinitions of indications for percutaneous nephrostomy. Radiology 147:419, 1983

2. Pfister RC, Newhouse JH: Interventional percutaneous pyeloureteral techniques. II. Percutaneous nephrostomy and other procedures. Radiol Clin North Am 17:351, 1979

3. Barbaric ZL, Davis RS, Frank IN, Linke CA, Lipchik EO, Cockett ATK: Percutaneous nephropyelostomy in the management of acute pyohydronephrosis. Radiology 118:567, 1976

4. Lang EK: Diagnosis and management of ureteral fistulas by percutaneous nephrostomy and antegrade stent catheter. Radiology 138:311

5. Dretler SP, Pfister RC, Newhouse JH: Renal stone dissolution via percutaneous nephrostomy. N Engl J Med 300:341, 1979

6. Bacon RL, Lee JKT, McClennan BL, Nelson GL: Percutaneous nephrostomy using real-time sonographic guidance. AJR 126:1018, 1981

7. Yoder IC, Pfister RC, Lindfors KK, Newhouse JK: Pyonephrosis:Imaging and intervention. AJR 141:735, 1983

8. Pederson JF, Douglas FC, Kristensen JK, Holm HH, Hancke S, Jensen F: Ultrasonically-guided percutaneous nephrostomy. Radiology 119:429, 1976

9. Burnett KR, Handler SJ, Conroy RM, Khonsaro F, Nelson C: Percutaneous nephrostomy utilizing B-mode and real-time ultrasound guidance:The lateral approach and puncture facilitation with furosemide. J Clin Ultrasound 10:252, 1982

10. Zegel HG, Pollack HM, Banner MP, Goldberg BB, Arger PH, Mulhern C, Kurtz A, Dubbins P, Coleman B, Koolpe H: Percutaneous nephrostomy: Comparison of sonographic and fluoroscopic guidance. AJR 137:925, 1981

11. Gavant MC, Gold RE, Church JC: Delayed rupture of renal pseudoaneurysm: Complication of percutaneous nephrostomy. AJR 138:948, 1982

12. Subramanyam, Raghavendra BN, Bosniak MA, Lefleur RS, Rosen RJ, Horii SC: Sonography of pyonephrosis: A prospective study. AJR 140:991, 1983

13. Jeffrey RB, Laing FC, Wing VW: Sensitivity of sonography in pyonephrosis, AJR (in press)

14. Altemeire WA, Alexander JW: Retroperitoneal abscess. Arch Surg 83:512, 1961

15. Kuligowska E, Newman B, White, SJ, Caldarone A: Interventional ultrasound in detection and treatment of renal inflammatory disease. Radiology 147:521, 1983

16. Gerzof SG, Gale ME: Computed tomograph and ultrasonography for diagnosis and treatment of renal and retroperitoneal abscesses. Urol Clin North Am 9:185, 1982

17. Sacks BA, Palestrant A, Vine H, Ellison H, Hann L, Ackerman B: Catheter/needle assembly for drainage of fluid collections. AJR 137:418, 1981

18. Papanicolaou N, Butch RJ, Mueller PR: Percutaneous abscess drainage. Semin Ultrasound 4(2):117, 1983

19. Sones PJ: Percutaneous drainage of abdominal abscesses. AJR 142:35, 1984

6 Renal Masses

NEAL JOSEPH
HARVEY L. NEIMAN
ROBERT L. VOGELZANG

Traditionally, the imaging diagnosis of renal masses has been made by excretory urography performed for clinical findings suggestive of a renal tumor or for other unrelated reasons such as renal colic. More recently, ultrasound and computed body tomography (CT) have proven to be extremely sensitive techniques for detection and characterization of renal masses. Ultrasound, in particular, has been shown to be a rapid, safe, and accurate, noninvasive method in which distinctive sonographic characteristics often allow for differentiation of a mass into a cystic or solid space occupying lesion. This chapter discusses ultrasound diagnosis of renal masses, as well as addressing its role with respect to other imaging techniques namely CT and/or magnetic resonance (MRI).

CYSTIC RENAL MASSES

Simple Renal Cyst

The most commonly encountered renal mass lesion is the simple cyst. It is estimated that simple renal cysts occur in at least 50 percent of people over the age of 50.[1] The etiology is unknown, and there is no heritable tendency. These lesions have an epithelial lining and, while they generally arise in the renal cortex, they may be located anywhere in the kidney. Simple cysts rarely cause symptoms, although peripelvic cysts may occasionally obstruct portions of the collecting system and become clinically apparent. Hematuria is another rare complication of simple cysts.

The criteria for sonographic diagnosis of a simple renal cyst include: (1) rounded or ovoid lesion, (2) anechoic (no internal echoes), (3) all the walls are sharply defined, (4) acoustic enhancement beyond the posterior wall, and (5) narrow bands of shadowing lateral to the acoustic enhancement. This lateral shadows sign is related to refraction of the sound beam along the curved surface

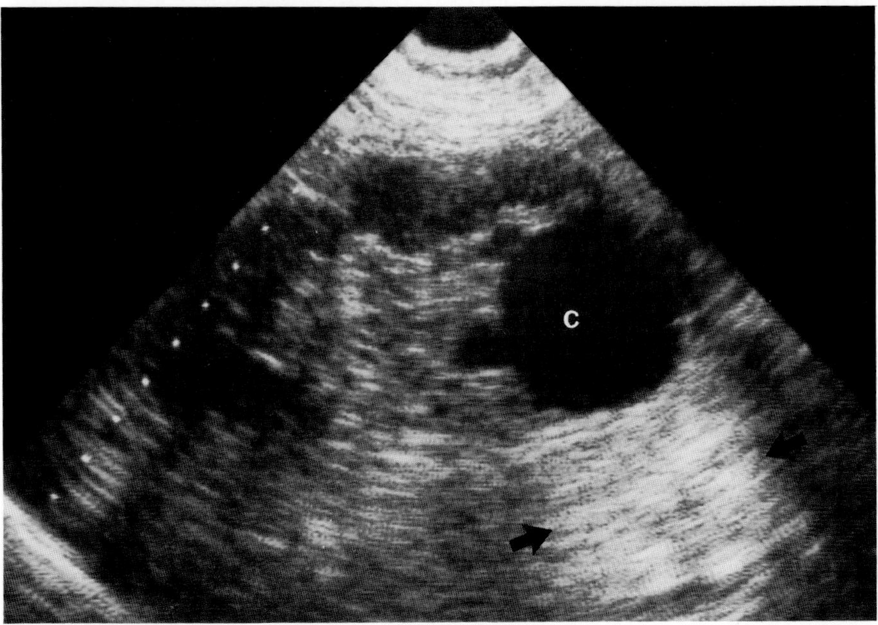

FIG. 6.1.   Anechoic lower pole mass fulfills all criteria for a simple renal cyst (c). Note prominent posterior acoustic enhancement. (arrows)

of a mass in which there is a change in acoustic velocity from the adjacent tissue[2-4] (Fig. 6.1). The ability to apply these criteria depends on several factors. Occasionally, reverberation echoes are seen at the anterior aspect of a cystic lesion and should not be mistaken for abnormal internal echoes. Renal cysts 2 cm or greater in diameter are usually easy to delineate sonographically. When the lesion is less than 2 cm in diameter, there is often a lack of clearly defined acoustic enhancement. Cysts smaller than the diameter of the sound beam will appear as complex structures due to the inclusion of adjacent echoes, the so-called partial volume artifact. In order to clearly delineate a lesion, it is therefore imperative that the lesion be placed within the focal zone of the transducer where the beam width is narrowest.[5,6] With high-frequency transducers in the range of 5 MHz, cysts as small as 5 mm in size may be correctly delineated. When all the sonographic criteria are fulfilled, the diagnosis of a simple renal cyst can be made with an accuracy of between 92 and 100 percent[7-9] It is important to emphasize that all the criteria should be fulfilled strictly in order to make a definite diagnosis. If a cyst does not meet all the criteria, it should be considered suspicious and further studies, such as computed tomography (CT), performed.

CT has proved to be a valuable tool for separating benign cysts from neoplasm with an accuracy said to be between 95 percent and approaching 100 percent.[10,11] The characteristics of a simple cyst on CT are (1) homogeneous attenuation values of water density, (2) an indiscernible wall, (3) lack of enhancement

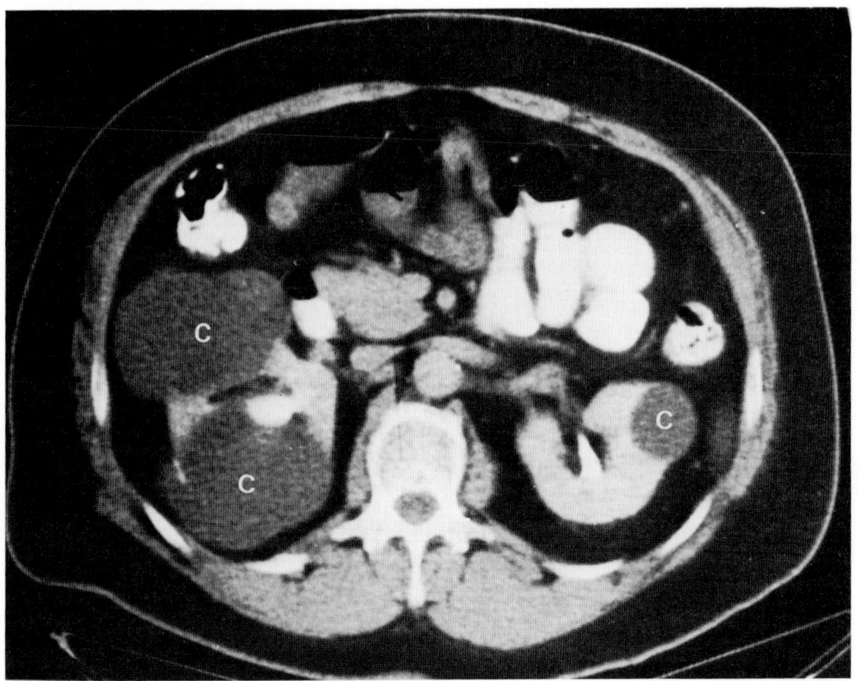

FIG. 6.2. Two right renal masses and one left renal mass (c) fulfill the CT criteria for simple renal cysts.

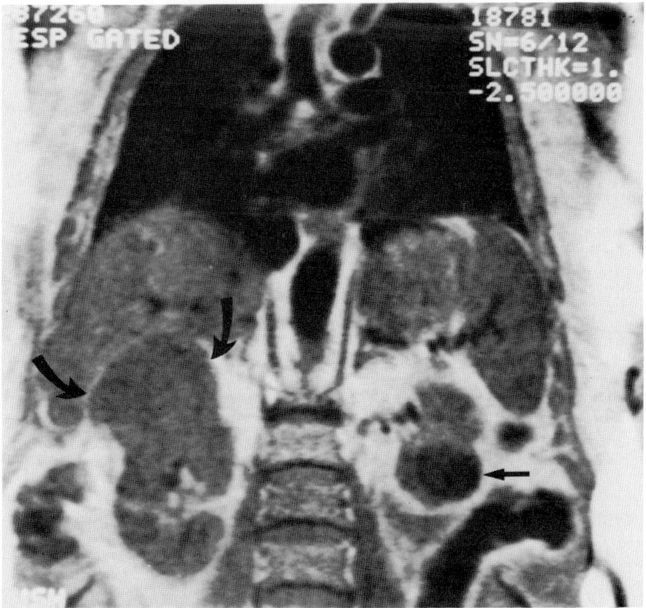

FIG. 6.3. Coronal image obtained using partial saturation sequence demonstrates low-intensity signal of a simple cyst of the lower pole of the left kidney (straight arrow). A renal cell carcinoma of the upper pole of the right kidney (curved arrows) is isointense with normal renal parenchyma.

following intravenous contrast infusion, and (4) smooth interface with renal parenchyma[11] (Fig. 6.2).

Early experience suggests that magnetic resonance imaging (MRI) can accurately differentiate simple renal cysts from the remaining renal mass lesions. Cystic lesions are generally low in signal on partial saturation sequences reflecting the long T-1 time[12] (Fig. 6.3).

Atypical Cysts

Atypical cysts can demonstrate mixed echogenicity. Some cysts are divided by fibrous septae which have no pathological significance.[13] The septa appear sonographically as groups of linear, internal echoes which may suggest liquified solid mass. Simple renal cysts that become infected present a complex pattern of internal echoes from inflammatory debris and thickened walls[14] (Fig. 6.4). Approximately 6 percent of renal cysts undergo hemorrhage.[15] Blood clots may form and appear within the mass as a complex group of echoes. As a result of prior hemorrhage or infection, mural calcifications occur in 1 to 2 percent of all simple renal cysts.[13] The calcification within the wall of the cyst often attenuates the insonating beam and makes accurate diagnosis difficult.

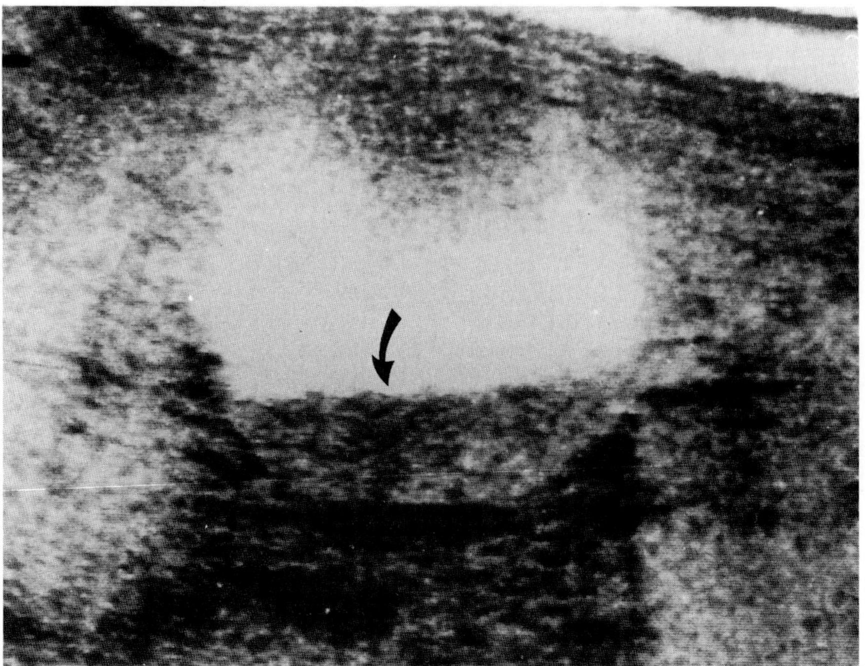

FIG. 6.4.   Layering of debris (arrow) in dependent portion of an infected simple cyst.

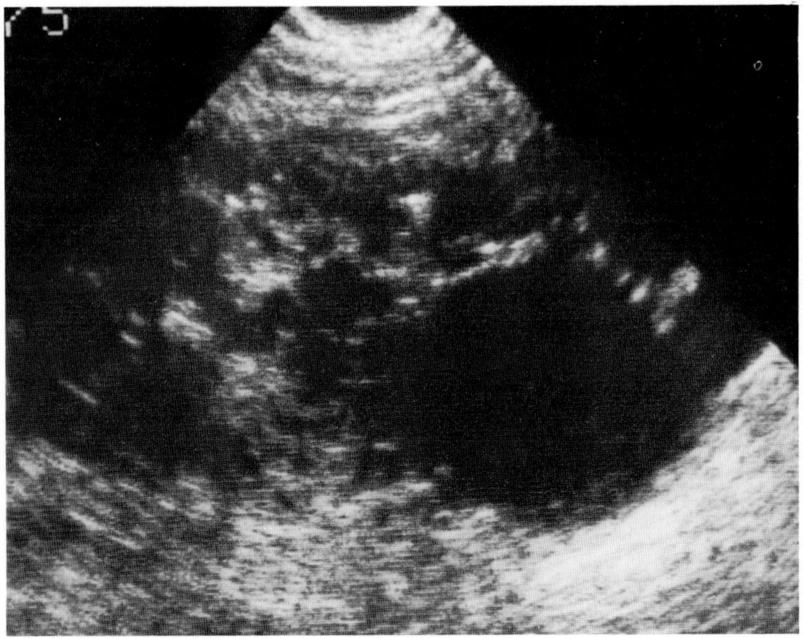

FIG. 6.5. Longitudinal scan of the left kidney demonstrates multiple cystic masses of various sizes with an irregular renal contour in a patient with adult polycystic kidney disease.

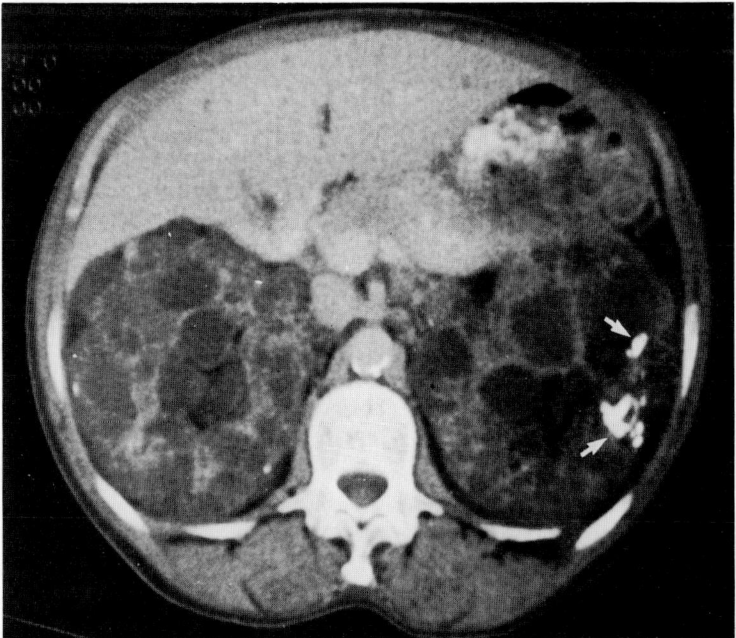

FIG. 6.6. Note massively enlarged kidney containing multiple cystic masses and focal areas of calcification (arrows) in a patient with adult polycystic kidney disease.

Adult Polycystic Kidney Disease (APKD)

The adult form of polycystic kidney disease is inherited as an autosomal dominant trait with high penetrance. In most patients, the disease becomes clinically manifest during or after the fourth decade of life. Sonography demonstrates kidneys with irregular margins and multiple anechoic structures of varying sizes randomly distributed throughout the parenchyma[16,17] (Fig. 6.5). At the beginning of the disease, the extent of involvement of the two kidneys may vary greatly. However, as the renal failure progresses, renal size, number, and size of the cysts become symmetrical. Associated abnormalities such as hepatic and pancreatic cysts can also be demonstrated, with an incidence of about 33 and 9 percent, respectively. Ultrasound is an ideal method for following these patients, and has also been advocated as a method of screening family members.

Occasionally, it may be difficult to distinguish between polycystic renal disease and bilateral multiple simple cysts. An elderly patient with multiple cysts and no evidence of renal failure or family history of APKD is unlikely to have polycystic disease. Occasionally, the differential diagnosis of polycystic renal disease versus advanced hydronephrosis can be difficult, but scans in different planes (especially coronal views) can solve the problem.

CT is also extremely successful in evaluating patients with known or suspected APKD (Fig. 6.6). The cysts vary markedly in size and attenuation value. Some cysts have attenuation measurements higher than water density, which reflects the varying characteristics of fluid cysts in patients with APKD. Cysts are usually noted throughout the entire kidney, and other organ involvement can be evaluated.

Pediatric Cystic Diseases

Multicystic dysplastic kidney (MDK) is a pediatric disease and is the most common cause of an abdominal mass in the newborn. The pathogenesis of MDK is atresia of the ureter or pelvis during the metanephric stage of development. Renal sonography demonstrates multiple cysts that vary in size and have a random distribution[16] (Fig. 6.7). This pattern is similar to that of adult polycystic disease. The normal central echo pattern of the renal pelvis is generally absent. Sonography can be used to examine the contralateral kidney, which has been found to have approximately a 30 percent incidence of anomalies. These include ureteropelvic junction obstruction, horseshoe kidney, and MDK.[18] The differential diagnosis of MDK includes hydronephrosis which demonstrates confluent central cystic spaces of a more uniform size (Fig. 6.8) and perhaps a cystic form of Wilms' tumor.

Infantile polycystic disease is inherited as an autosomal recessive trait and presents in the neonate as bilateral abdominal masses. The large kidneys contain ectatic renal tubules 1 to 2 mm in diameter. Although the ectatic tubules are too small to be resolved sonographically, the interfaces provided by the walls

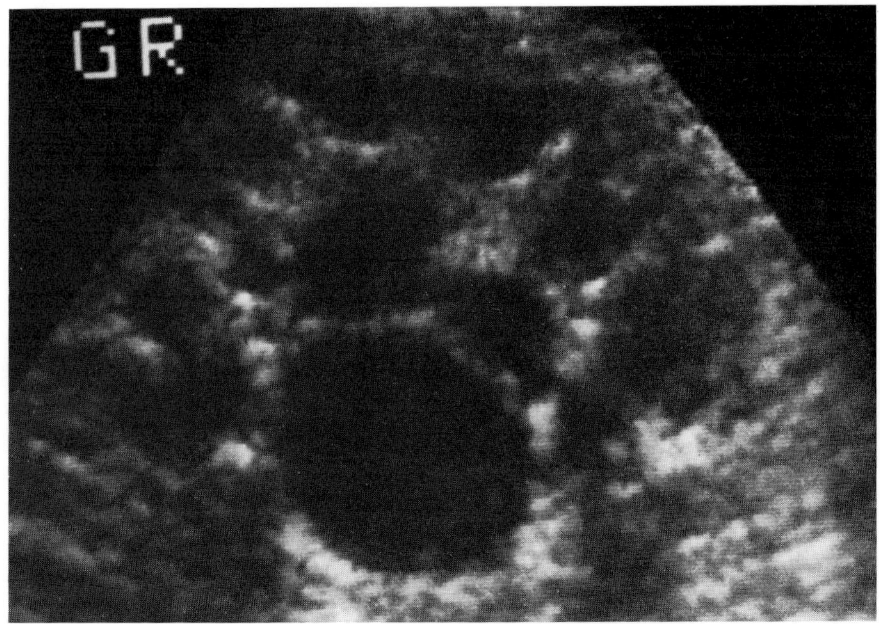

FIG. 6.7. Multiple cystic masses replacing renal parenchyma in a neonate with multi-cystic dysplastic kidney. The largest cyst is centrally located but no communication between them is seen.

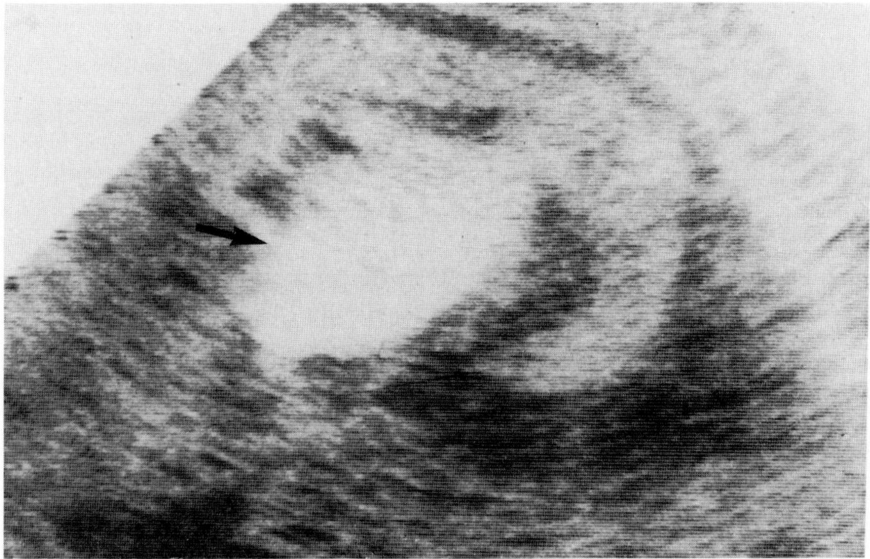

FIG. 6.8. Confluent central cystic space (arrow) of hydronephrosis is contrasted with peripheral cystic masses of multicystic dysplastic kidney.

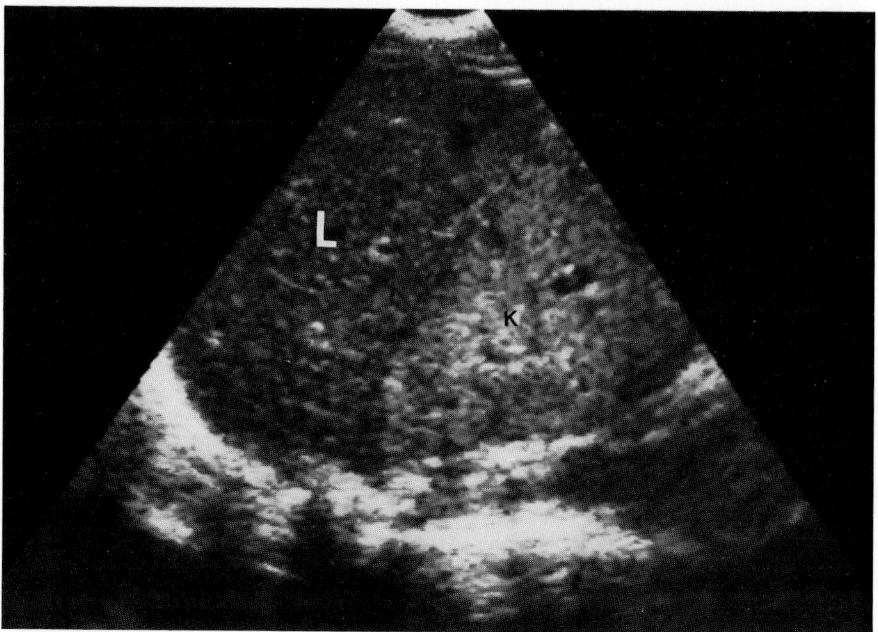

FIG. 6.9.   Large echogenic right kidney (K) with loss of the normally distinct corticol medullary junction in this neonate with infantile polycystic kidney disease. The left kidney was similar in appearance (L = liver).

of the tubules cause increased parenchymal echogenicity. Therefore, the usual sonographic appearance of infantile polycystic disease is bilateral renal enlargement with diffusely echogenic parenchyma and loss of the normal corticomedullary differentiation[16,19] (Fig. 6.9).

Multilocular Renal Cyst

Multilocular renal cyst is a rare nonheriditary disease that is limited to one area of the kidney. The involved cystic part of the kidney is bulky, well encapsulated, and contains multiple noncommunicating cysts that are sharply demarcated from the surrounding normal tissue. Although this uncommon entity is of uncertain etiology, it generally behaves in a benign nature.[16] Of the reported cases, about half occurred in young children and half in adults.[20] This entity has a distinctive sonographic appearance consisting of multiple fluid-filled masses, separated by highly echogenic septations. The remainder of the kidney is normal[20,21] (Fig. 6.10).

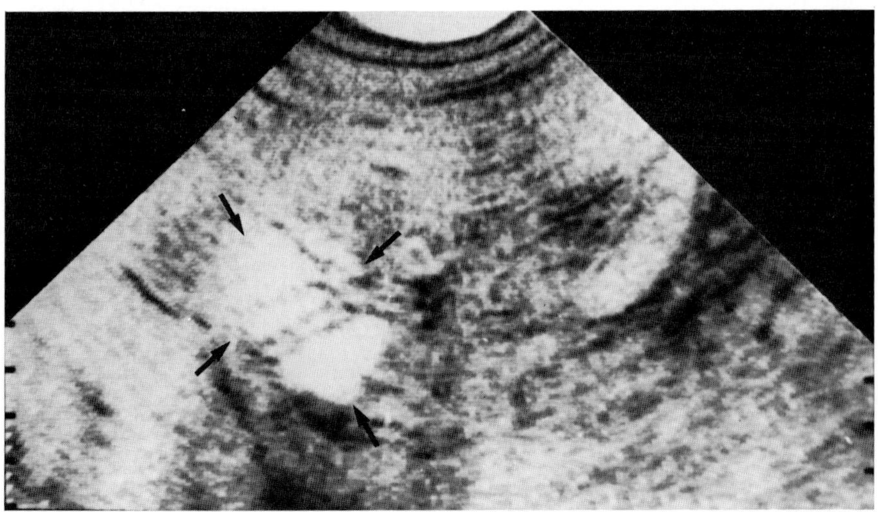

FIG. 6.10. Focal upper pole mass (arrows) of the right kidney consisting of multiple cystic spaces separated by echogenic septations. Pathologically proven multilocular renal cyst. (Case courtesy of David Rochester, M.D., Evanston Hospital, Evanston, Illinois.)

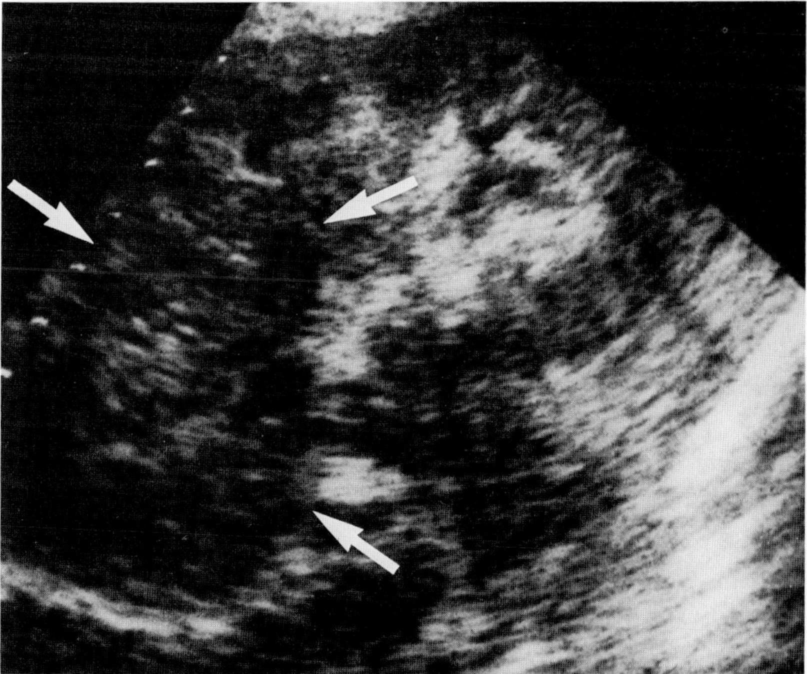

FIG. 6.11. Large mass of the upper pole of the left kidney (arrows) which proved to be a renal cell carcinoma.

Vascular Cystic Mass

Saccular aneurysms are the most common form of renal artery aneurysm. They always occur at the bifurcation of the renal artery into the intralobar branches. They are often calcified and are associated with arteriosclerosis. If not calcified, they may sonographically appear similar to a simple renal cyst.[13] Posttraumatic renal artery aneurysms may also be identified sonographically and present as an anechoic sharply marginated mass. Arteriovenous malformations may also appear as multiloculated cystic masses and can be associated with a large renal vein and inferior vena cava.[13]

SOLID AND COMPLEX RENAL MASSES

Renal Cell Carcinoma

Renal cell carcinomas are the most common solid renal mass, accounting for over 90 percent of the primary malignant neoplasms of the kidney. These neoplasms may be hypoechoic, hyperechoic, or isoechoic with the normal renal parenchyma.[22,23] (Fig. 6.11). The appearance of the lesion may vary from an encapsulated sharply marginated mass with a smooth outline to an irregularly marginated mass with infiltration of the surrounding tissues.[22,23] Occasionally, acoustic enhancement may be noted distal to a neoplasm because of extensive tumor necrosis or hemorrhage. Up to 40 percent of the lesions may demonstrate cystic components, due to areas of hemorrhage, necrosis, or tumor vascularity.[23] A correlation between the tumor echogenicity and vascularity as demonstrated by angiography has been noted,[24] but others have not supported this relationship.[22] The detection of a renal cell carcinoma necessitates a significant workup in an attempt for correct preoperative staging. Emphasis must be placed on visualization of the contralateral kidney, liver for metastatic disease, retroperitoneum for periaortic lymphadenopathy, and ipsilateral renal vein and inferior vena cava for tumor extension[25] (Fig. 6.12).

CT is also reliable in determining the presence of renal malignancy. Renal carcinomas are recognized when the following criteria are utilized: (1) attenuation value greater than that of water density and often heterogeneous; (2) definite contrast enhancement, usually less than that of normal renal parenchyma; (3) an unsharp interface with the normal renal parenchyma; and (4) secondary characteristics may be noted, such as extension into the perinephric space.[26] CT has proven to be extremely valuable in staging renal cell carcinomas with a complete workup involving evaluation of the liver contralateral kidney, renal vein, inferior vena cava (IVC), and retroperitoneal lymph node groups (Fig. 6.13). CT can now replace angiography in this regard.

MRI is sensitive in identifying renal lesions of a variety of types, and the variations in signal intensity appear helpful in characterizing these lesions.[12] Renal carcinoma has shown a spectrum of intensities ranging from hypointense to hyperintense on spin echo images[27] and has shown high-signal intensity

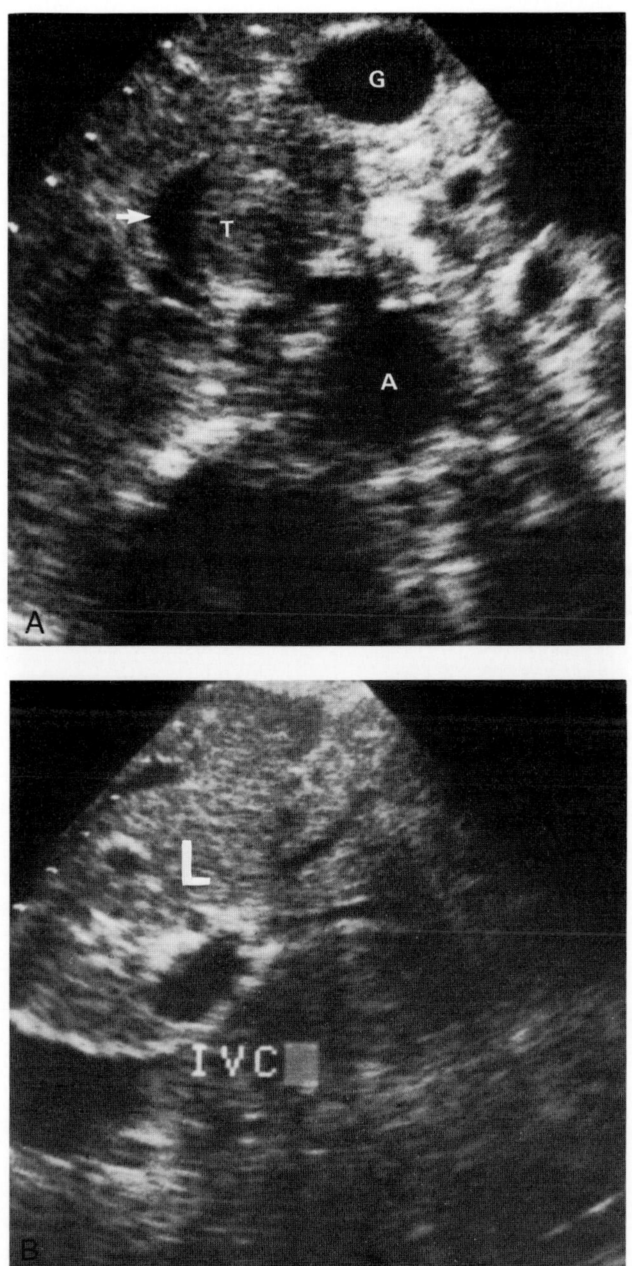

FIG. 6.12. (A) Transverse scan demonstrates extension of tumor thrombus (T) into the IVC (arrow). A = aorta, G = gallbladder. (B) Longitudinal scan in same patient also demonstrates thrombus in the IVC. The liver (L) is seen anterior to the IVC.

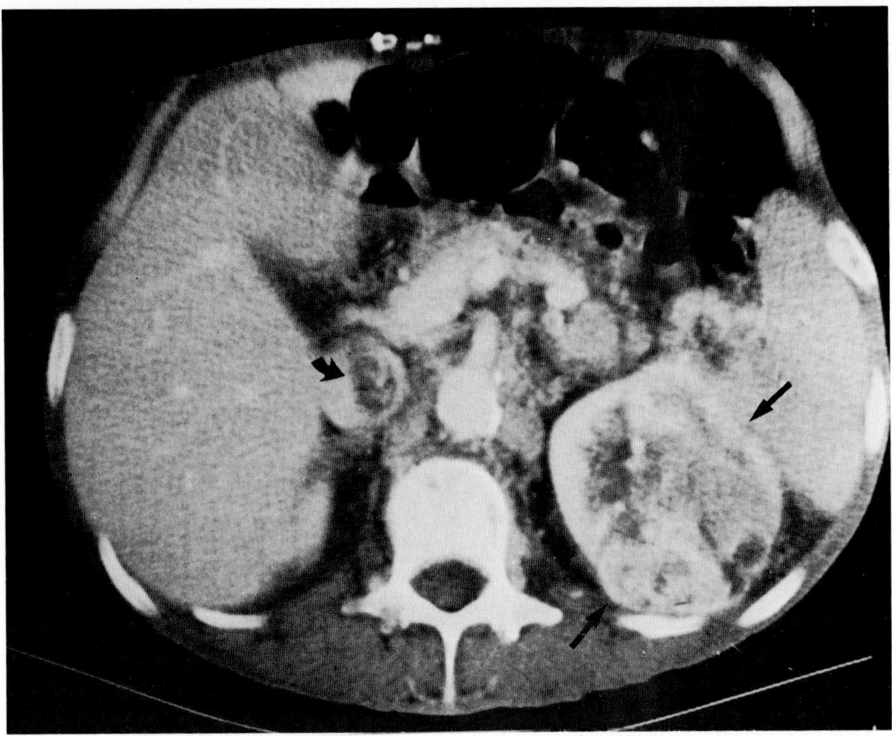

FIG. 6.13. Heterogeneous, enhancing mass with ill-defined margins (straight arrows) represents a left renal cell carcinoma. Note invasion of the IVC by the tumor (curved arrow).

on partial saturation scans[12] (Fig. 6.14). Tumor invasion into the intrarenal veins and inferior vena cava may be diagnosed on MRI,[12,27] and MRI has been able to accurately stage carcinomas.

Lymphoma

Involvement of the kidney by lymphoma is common in end-stage disease, although it is usually clinically silent. Lymphoma may present as multiple focal lesions, diffuse infiltration, or a solitary mass. The sonographic pattern has been said to be characteristic with the mass being hypoechoic with respect to adjacent renal parenchyma.[28] This, however, is true only in those forms of lymphoma in which there is marked homogeneity of the lesion such as lymphocyte predominant varieties. Those forms with multiple cellular components or a large fibrous tissue component may have varying degrees of echogenicity[29] (Fig. 6.15). The central echo complex remains intact in the majority of patients with lymphomatous masses.

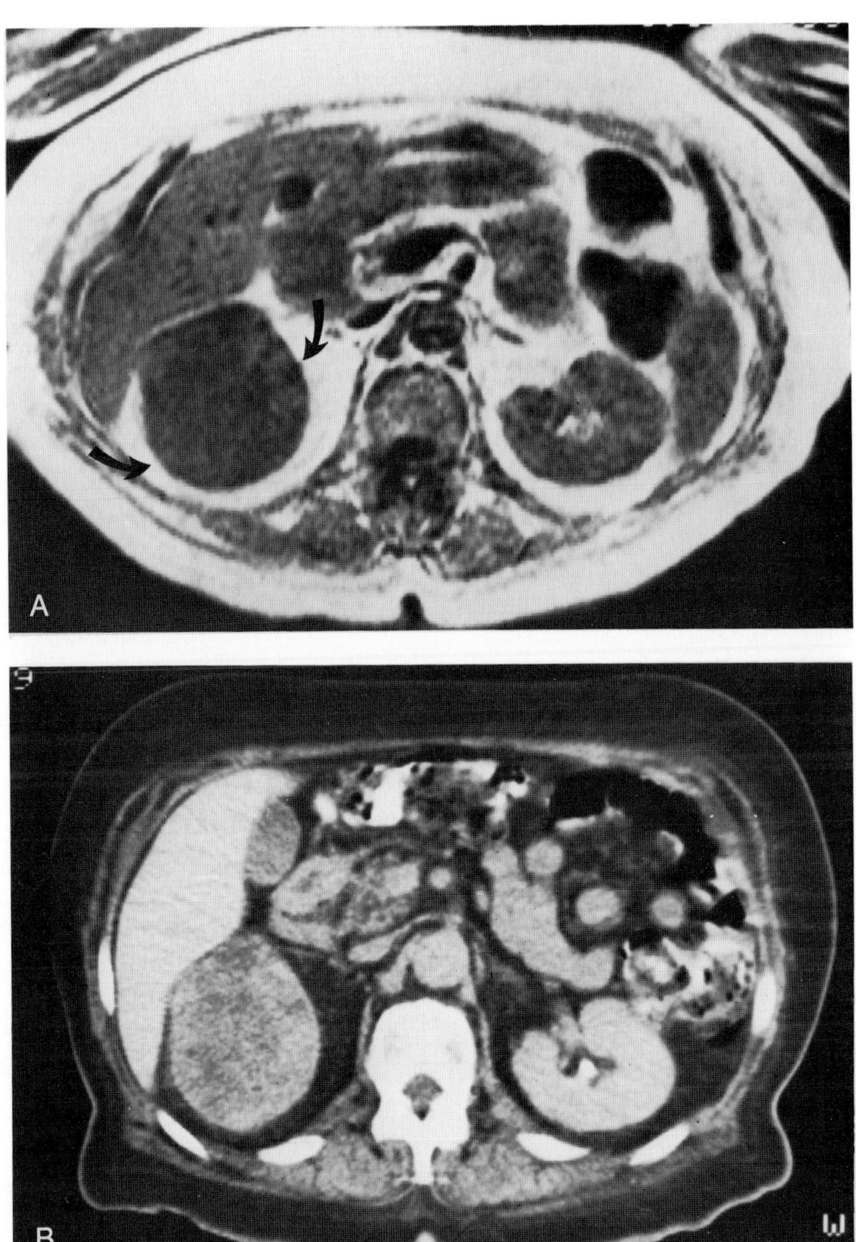

FIG. 6.14.   (A) Axial MRI image of the same patient demonstrates a right renal cell carcinoma (arrows). (B) Corresponding postcontrast enhanced CT image. (Case courtesy of Terence Matalon, M.D., Rush-Presbyterian-St. Luke's Medical Center, Chicago, Illinois.)

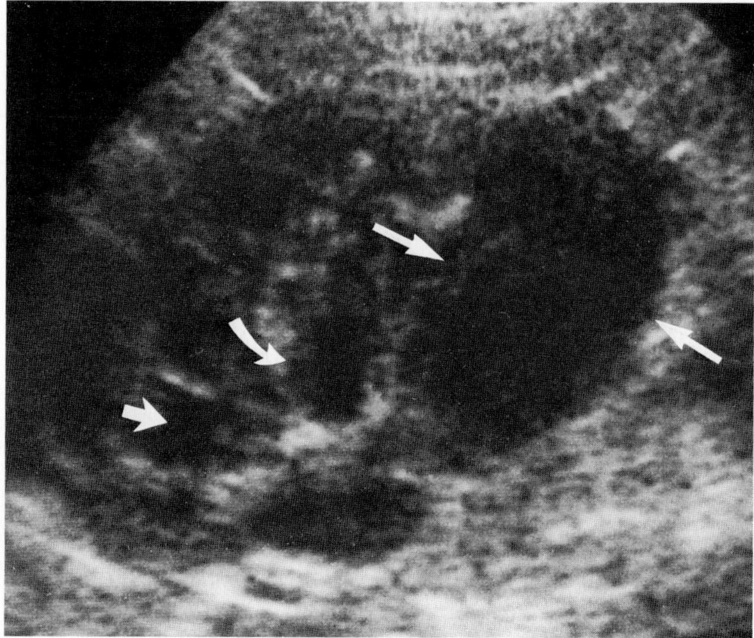

FIG. 6.15. Longitudinal scan of the left kidney in a patient with lymphoma demonstrates multiple focal hypoechoic masses (arrows).

Transitional Cell Carcinoma

Transitional cell carcinoma shows separation of the central portion of the kidney and if identified shows separation of the central complex of echoes. The lesion has been reported to contain low-level echoes[23,28] and can be confused with blood clot or sloughed papilla. Serial studies may allow for distinction of tumor from clot as the latter may change in shape and echogenicity with time. It may not, however, adequately demonstrate a small transitional carcinoma with hemorrhage in which the bulk of the mass is blood clot. Although transitional cell carcinoma can be confused with nonopaque renal pelvic calculi on excretory urography, the latter can be differentiated from other lesions by sonographic demonstration of the stone and its acoustic shadowing. Occasionally, transitional cell carcinoma presents as a bulky mass similar in appearance to renal cell carcinoma.

Metastatic Renal Tumors

Renal metastases rarely cause symptoms leading to antemortem diagnosis, but are frequently noted at autopsy in patients dying of malignant disease. Lung and breast tumors are the main source of renal metastases. There is no specific pattern to differentiate these lesions from other solid masses and may present as hypoechoic to hyperechoic patterns.[13]

Renal Adenoma

Renal adenomas are the benign counterpart of renal cell carcinoma. The existence of this lesion is controversial as many pathologists believe that it actually represents a low-grade malignancy. This school of thought holds that a lesion greater than 3 cm, in spite of the cellular pattern, is by definition malignant. The lesion may be discovered incidentally at surgery or autopsy and is usually quite small, less than 1 cm. Oncocytomas, large vascular adenomas, cannot be distinguished sonographically from typical renal cell carcinomas[23,30] (Fig. 6.16).

Angiomyolipoma

An angiomyolipoma is a hamartoma composed of smooth muscle, blood vessels, and fat in varying portions. Angiomyolipomas occur in two distinct clinical forms: (1) a unilateral solitary mass, usually noted in middle-aged females,

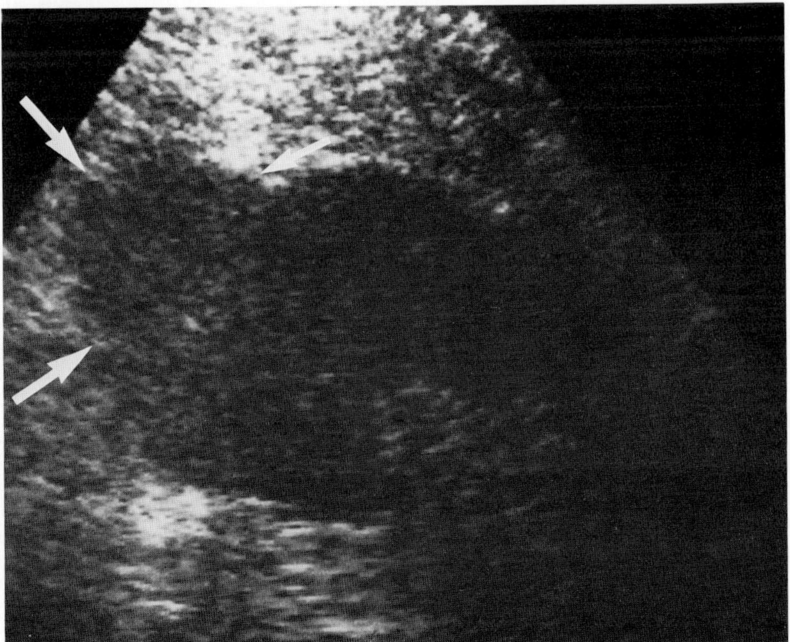

FIG. 6.16.   Note isoechoic mass of upper pole of left kidney (arrows). This oncocytoma cannot be distinguished sonographically from a renal cell carcinoma.

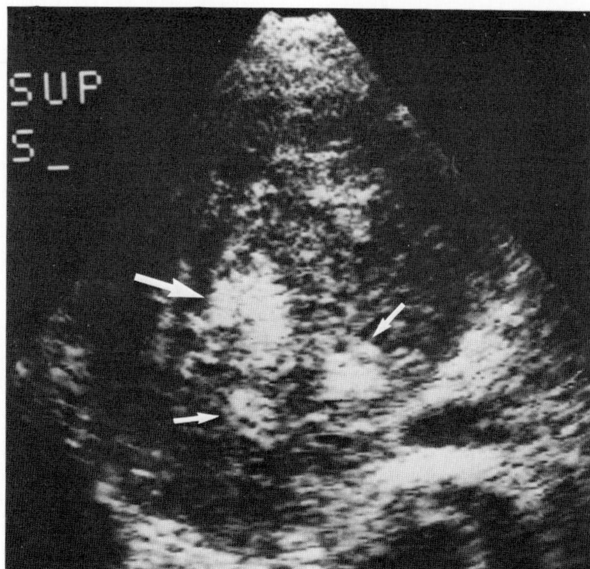

FIG. 6.17. Multiple focal, highly echogenic masses (arrows) are characteristic of angiomyolipomas in a patient with tuberous sclerosis.

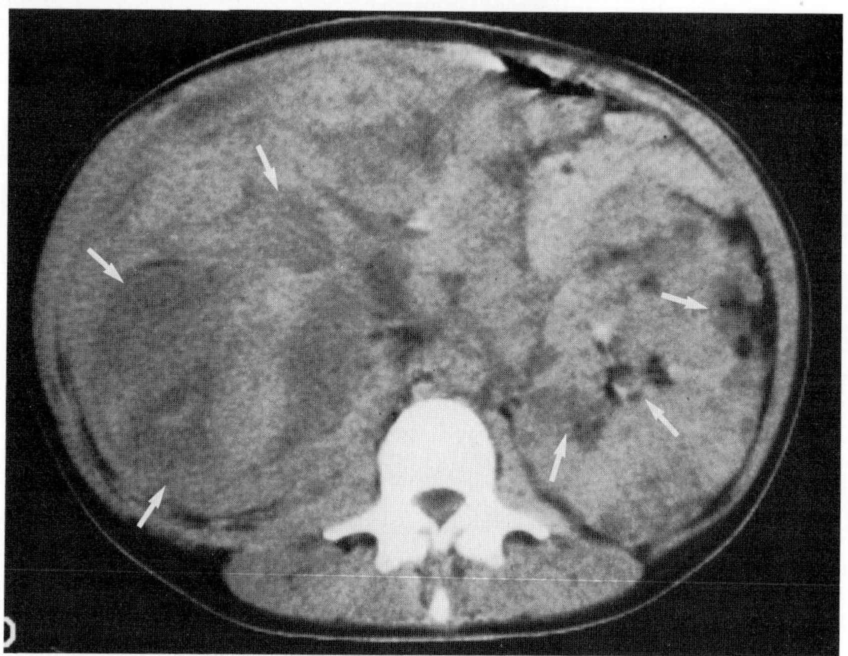

FIG. 6.18. Multiple bilateral renal masses containing fat density (arrow) represent angiomylipomas in a patient with tuberous sclerosis.

and (2) multiple bilateral masses usually, but not always, in patients with tuberous sclerosis. Ultrasound presents a fairly characteristic pattern of a focal, highly echogenic intrarenal mass[31,32] (Fig. 6.17). Several possibilities have been suggested for this appearance, including a rather inhomogeneous tissue architecture and the numerous blood vessels within the tumor, but it is most likely related to the high-fat content.[23,32] Although the mass has a somewhat specific sonographic appearance, it is not pathognomonic, as true lipomas and renal cell carcinoma may occasionally simulate the appearance.[22,33] The ultrasonographic diagnosis of angiomyolipoma can be confirmed by CT. In most cases, enough fat is present within the tumor to allow a specific CT diagnosis[34] (Fig. 6.18).

Wilms' Tumor and Other Pediatric Masses

Wilms' tumor is the most common solid renal tumor in the pediatric age group over 1 year of age. The incidence peaks at 3 years and is unusual past 8 years of age. Most Wilms' tumors are echo-producing lesions, although anechoic spaces within the mass which presumably represent hemorrhage and/or liquification necrosis are often seen[13] (Fig. 6.19). It is essential to evaluate the contralateral kidney with diligence, as the incidence of bilateral Wilms' tumors is 5 percent.[35]

If a solid renal mass occurs in the newborn, the diagnosis is usually benign mesoblastic nephroma.[36] The sonographic pattern appears to be extremely variable, running the entire gamut of echogenicity (Fig. 6.20). Nephroblastomatosis presents as multiple solid or complex masses seen bilaterally on ultrasound.[19] Nephroblastomatosis has been reported to progress to Wilms' tumor.[37]

Inflammatory Masses

A solid renal mass identified by sonography may also be caused by an acute focal infection without liquification. This has been termed "acute focal bacterial nephritis" or "acute lobar nephronia."[38] Ultrasound demonstrates focal irregular hypoechoic masses with an ill-defined posterior wall and no distal acoustic enhancement[38,39] (Fig. 6.21). Although lobar nephronia may resemble a renal cell carcinoma sonographically, clinical findings are usually helpful in establishing the diagnosis. Follow-up examination after appropriate antibiotic therapy shows resolution of the inflammatory change.

Focal bacterial nephritis (lobar nephronia) is to be differentiated from abscess formation. A renal abscess presents as an irregular mass with few internal echoes (the degree of echogenicity depending on the amount of debris), a well-defined distal wall, and acoustic enhancement—features consistent with a fluid-filled mass[39] (Fig. 6.22). Gas, when present within the abscess cavity, significantly alters the sonographic appearance.[40] The sonographic findings of xanthogranulomatous pyelonephritis are nonspecific but may be suggestive.

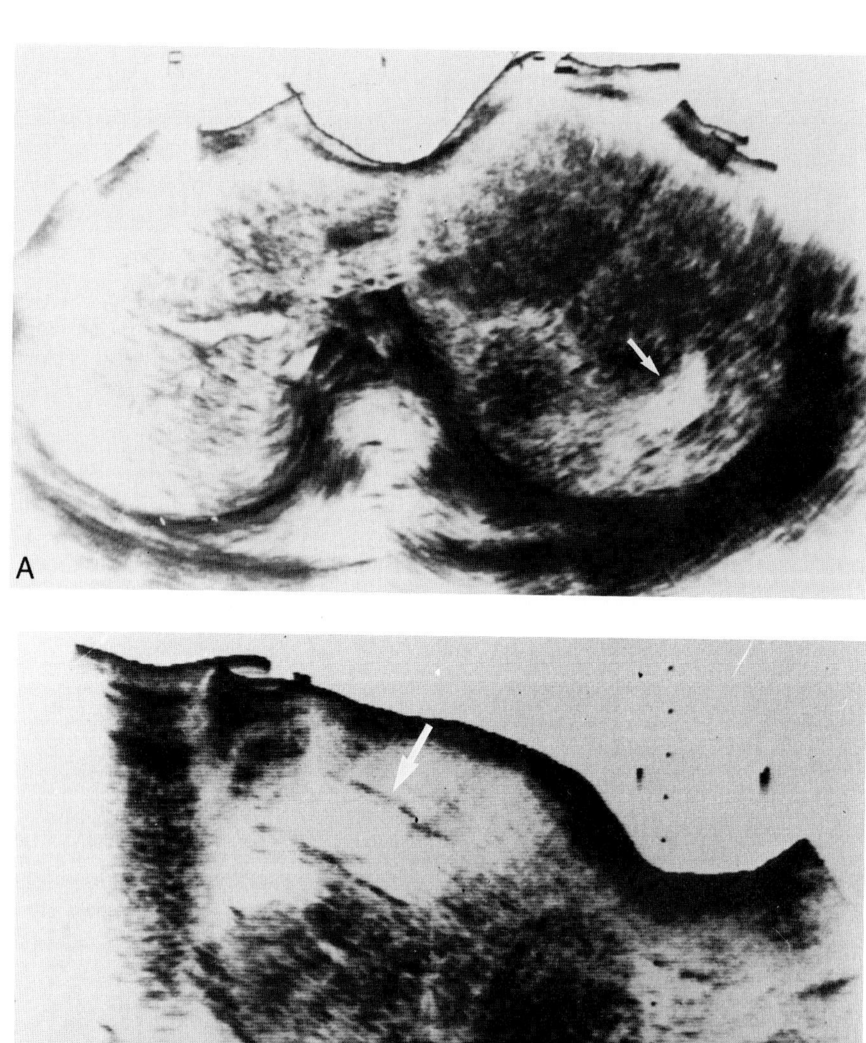

FIG. 6.19. Transverse (A) and longitudinal (B) scan of a large left-sided echogenic mass in a patient with Wilms' tumor. Note cystic spaces (arrows).

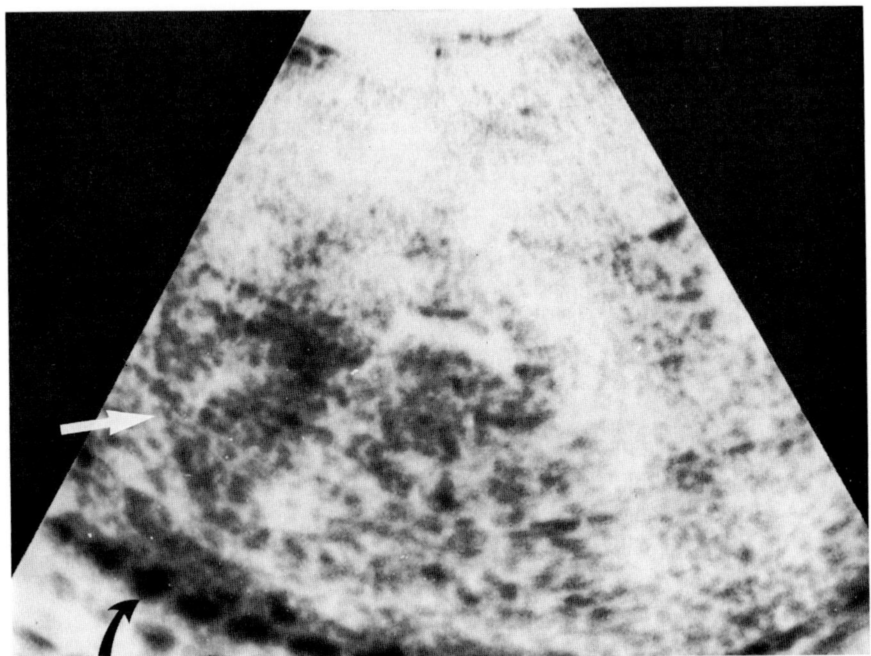

FIG. 6.20. Neonate with large mass of mixed echogenicity filling the left side of the abdomen on a longitudinal scan (straight arrow). Note central anechoic region. The appearance of this mesoblastic nephroma is similar to that of a Wilms' tumor. Curved arrow = spine. (Case courtesy of David Rochester, M.D., Evanston Hospital, Evanston, Illinois.)

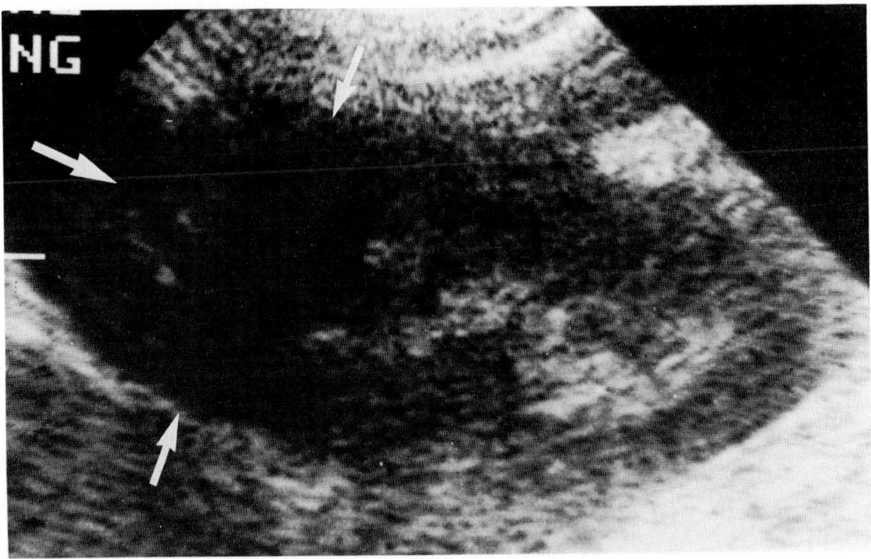

FIG. 6.21. Irregular, hypoechoic, upper pole mass (arrows) proven to be a lobar nephronia. Follow-up study following appropriate therapy demonstrated resolution of the mass.

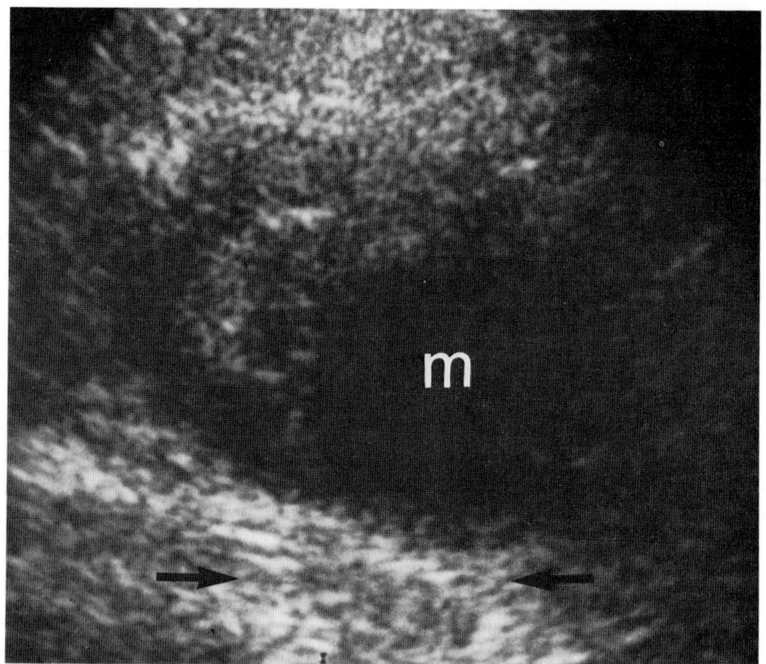

FIG. 6.22.   A renal abscess presenting as a hypoechoic mass (M) on a transverse scan of the left kidney. Posterior acoustic enhancement (arrows) aids in differentiating this abscess from a lobar nephronia.

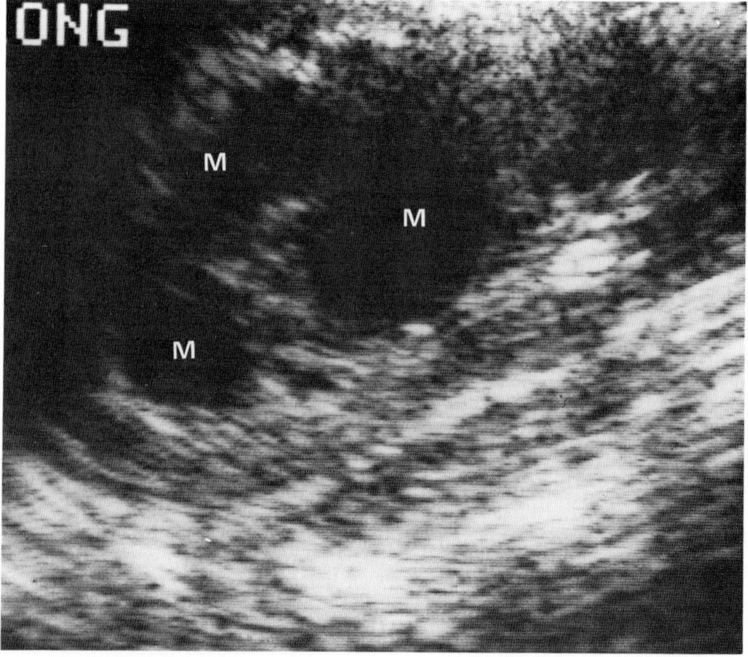

FIG. 6.23.   Longitudinal scan of the left kidney demonstrates multiple anechoic masses (m) representing small abscesses in a patient with xanthogranulomatous pyelonephritis.

There is often diffuse enlargement of a kidney which contains multiple anechoic areas representing small abscesses (Fig. 6.23). Renal calculi may be seen as strongly echogenic foci associated with acoustic shadowing. Other areas of increased echogenicity, frequently bandlike hyperechoic areas, are secondary to fat deposition.[41]

CT can also aid in the diagnosis of inflammatory masses, and is often able to distinguish medically treatable, acute focal bacterial nephritis from a frank abscess requiring drainage. CT and/or ultrasound can also serve to localize the abscess in those cases requiring percutaneous drainage. Acute focal bacterial nephritis can have one of several appearances including: (1) a focal mass without definable walls; (2) wedge-shaped areas corresponding to the renal lobule that are isodense with normal renal parenchyma and exhibit varying degrees of enhancement after intravenous contrast administration; and (3) patchy striated pattern to the CT nephrogram after contrast enhancement[42] (Fig. 6.24). An abscess, on the other hand, is often well defined, of lower density than the normal renal parenchyma, and may have a thick irregular wall which exhibits variable degrees of contrast enhancement but without central enhancement[42] (Fig. 6.25). Chronic infection in an obstructed kidney may lead to xanthogranu-lomatous pylonephritis, which has the following CT appearance: (1) a calculus in the renal pelvis or collecting system; (2) absence of contrast material excretion in the involved kidney or a focal area involvement; (3) multiple nonenhancing rounded areas within the medullary space having higher attenuation than urine, arranged in a hydronephrotic pattern; (4) discrete solid mass; and (5) areas of fat[41] (Fig. 6.26).

Renal Hematoma

Renal hematomas may result from a variety of causes and are divided into two main groups, spontaneous and posttraumatic. Spontaneous hematomas usually occur due to a bleeding diathesis, and may be associated with renal infarcts or tumors including arteriovenous malformations. The sonographic appearance of a renal hematoma depends on its age and can range from an anechoic to a hypoechoic lesion.[13] As the hematoma organizes, it develops internal echoes and sonographically is indistinguishable from a neoplasm (Fig. 6.27).

Pseudotumors

Renal pseudotumors are localized, enlarged areas of normal renal tissue which produce a false impression of a renal mass on an imaging technique. The most common pseudotumors are dromedary humps, fetal lobulations, and a column of Bertin. Ultrasonography can be used to determine the solid or cystic character of the lesion, but is sometimes unable to distinguish a pseudotumor from a solid neoplasm (Fig. 6.28). Additional studies may be necessary for definitive evaluation.

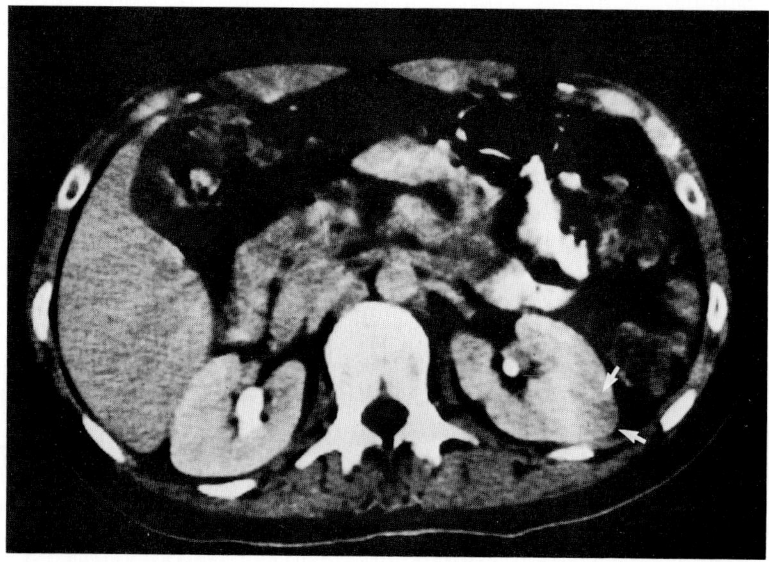

FIG. 6.24. Wedge-shaped area of relatively decreased contrast enhancement (arrows) represents labor nephronia.

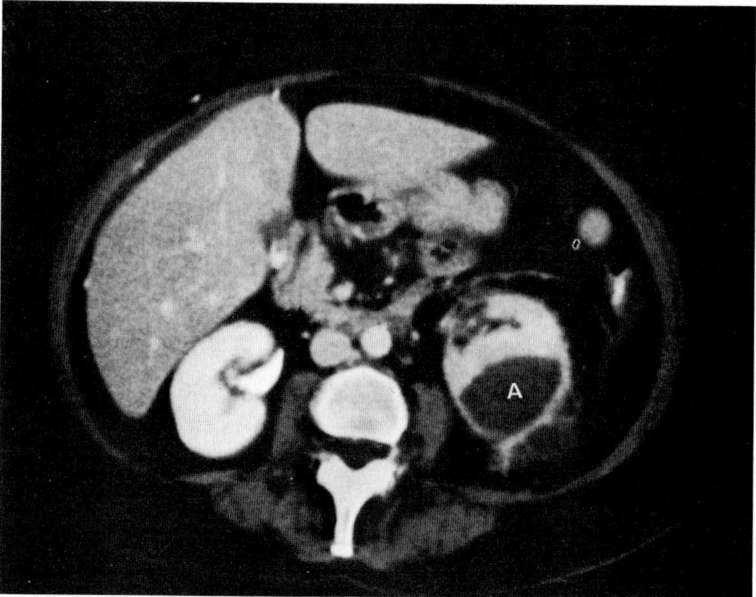

FIG. 6.25. Well-defined left renal mass (A) with a thick, enhancing wall and a nonenhancing center is typical of a renal abscess.

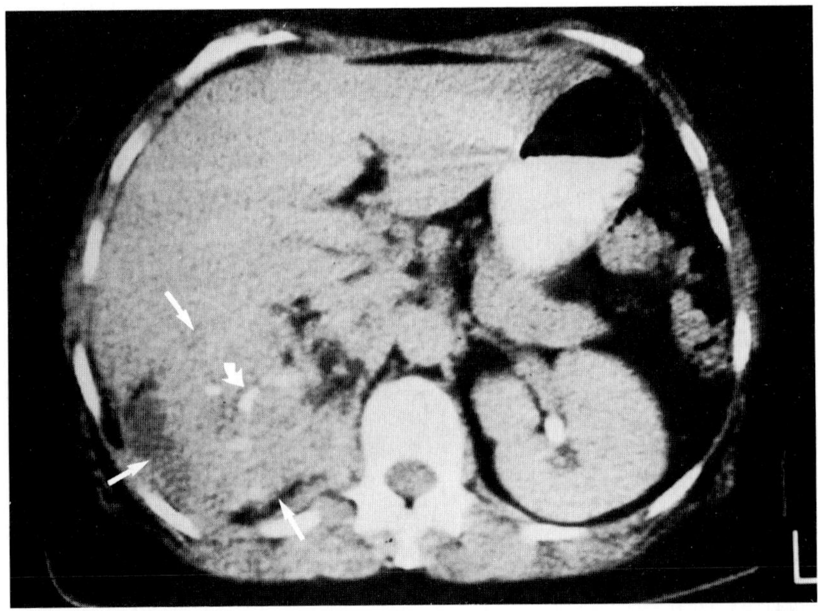

FIG. 6.26. A right-sided renal mass (straight arrows), a calculus in the right renal pelvis (curved arrow), and absence of contrast excretion on the right side are findings consistent with the diagnosis of xanthogranulomatous pyelonephritis.

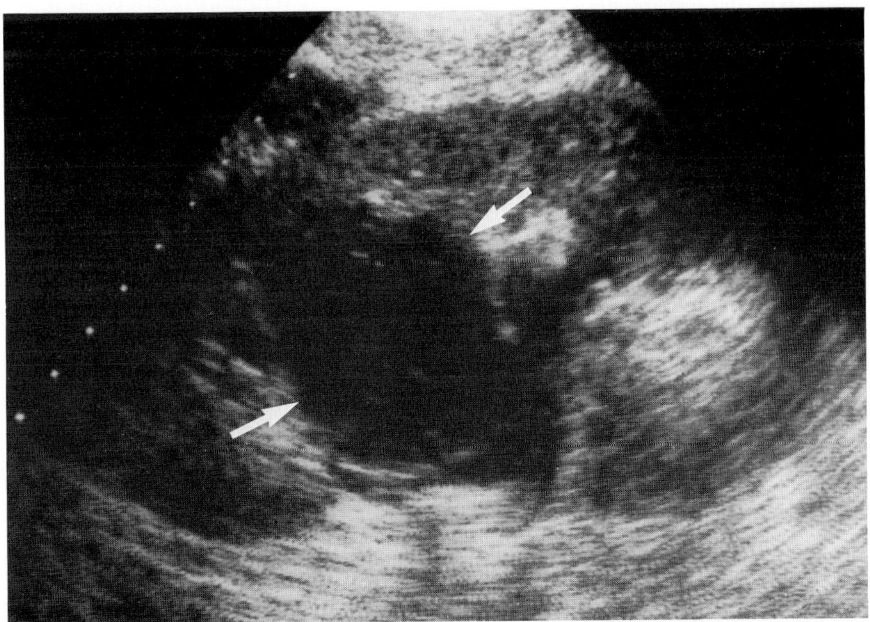

FIG. 6.27. Cystic mass (arrows) with internal echoes in a patient with a subacute renal hematoma.

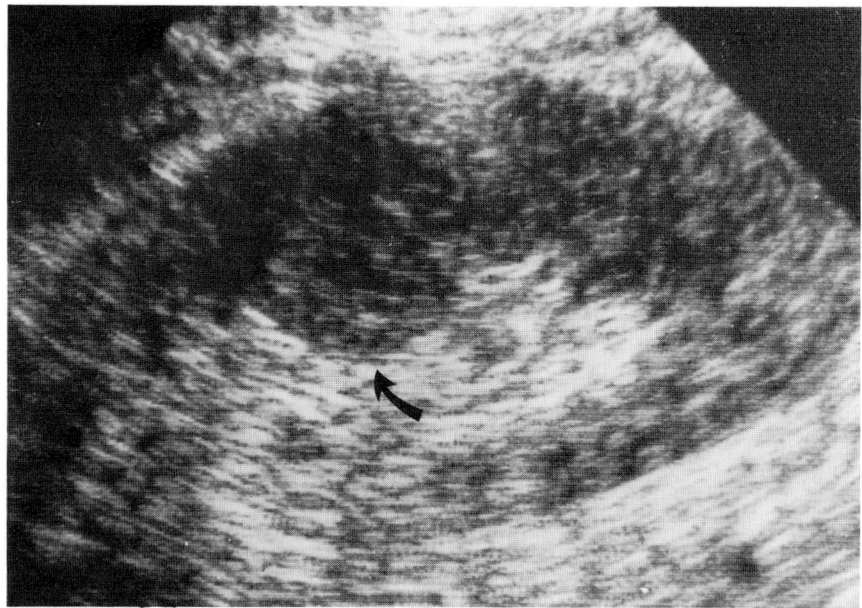

FIG. 6.28.   Solid mass (arrow) representing a column of Bertin cannot be distinguished from a renal neoplasm.

RADIOLOGICAL APPROACH TO RENAL MASSES

Renal mass evaluation is currently in a state of flux as the use of various imaging techniques has changed. Although a renal mass was traditionally identified on excretory urography, patients are now more frequently seen with ultrasound or computed tomography as the initial imaging modality.

Ultrasound remains a cost-effective way to triage renal masses. If ultrasound establishes a definitive diagnosis of cyst, it is not necessary to proceed further. However, if ultrasound does not confirm the presence of a mass, if the ultrasound is unsatisfactory for technical reasons, or a complex or solid mass is present, then it is advisable to proceed with CT. (An exception occurs when a solid mass is expected to represent a column of Bertin. In this situation, a radionuclide scan is indicated rather than CT.) Once CT is performed, the etiology of the mass can usually be determined to represent a simple cyst, a malignancy, or an inflammatory process, particularly in those cases where ultrasound was equivocal. Approximately 8 percent of masses detected by CT will remain indeterminate.[43] In these cases, if the mass is suggestive of a cyst but has features that still place it in the indeterminate category, or the mass has complex CT features which are not typical of either a cyst or malignancy, skinny needle aspiration biopsy is recommended. A mass which is indeterminate by CT is generally also indeterminate by angiography. Newer-generation ultrasound and CT equipment has relegated angiography to being used in those cases where: (1) an indeterminate mass lesion is identified for which renal-sparing surgery is contemplated; (2) when identification of the vascular supply of a large mass prior to nephrectomy is important to the urologist; (3) where the status of the venous drainage is uncertain and renal venography may be of value; and (4) where embolotherapy is contemplated.

REFERENCES

1. Lauks SP Jr, McLachlan MSF: Aging and simple cysts of the kidney. Br J Radiol 54:12, 1981

2. Filly R, Sommet R, Minton M: Characterization of biologic fluid by ultrasound and computed tomography. Radiology 134:167, 1980

3. Sommers FG, Filly RA, Minlon MJ: Acoustic shadowing due to reflective and refractive effects. Am J Roentgenol 132:973, 1979

4. Bree RL, Silver TM: Differential diagnosis of hypoechoic and anechoic masses with gray scale sonography: New observations. J Clin Ultrasound 7:249, 1979

5. Jaffe CC, Taylor KJW: The clinical impact of ultrasonic beam focusing patterns. Radiology 131:469, 1979

6. Jaffe CC, Rosenfield AT, Sommer G, Taylor KJW: Technical factors influencing the imaging of small anechoic cysts by B-scan ultrasound. Radiology 135:429, 1980

7. Chan SL, Cooperberg P, McLaughlin MG, Ewart B: Grey-scale ultrasonography: A refined tool for differentiating renal mass lesions. Can Med Assoc J 122:321, 1980

8. Behan M, Wixson D, Pitts WR Jr, Kazam E: Sonographic evaluation of renal masses: Correlations with angiography. Urol Radiol 1:137, 1980

9. Pollack HM, Banner MP, Arger PH, Peters J, Mulhern CB Jr, Coleman BG: The accuracy of gray-scale renal ultrasonography in differentiating cystic neoplasms from benign cysts. Radiology 143:741, 1982

10. Sagel SS, Stanley RJ, Levitt RG, Geisse G: Computed tomography of the kidney. Radiology 124:359, 1977

11. McClennan BL, Stanley RJ, Melson GL, Levitt RG, Sagel SS: CT of the renal cyst: Is cyst aspiration necessary? AJR 133:671, 1979

12. Choyke PL, Kressel HY, Pollack HM, Arger PM, Azel L, Mamourian AC: Focal renal masses: Magnetic resonance imaging. Radiology 152:471, 1984

13. Pollack HM, Banner MP, Arger PH, Goldberg BB, Mulhern CB: Comparison of computed tomography and ultrasound in the diagnosis of renal masses. In Resenfield AT (ed): Genitourinary Ultrasonography—Clinics in Diagnostic Ultrasound 2. Churchill Livingstone, New York, 1979

14. Kyung JC, Maklad N, Curran J, Ting YM: Angiographic and ultrasonographic findings in infected simple cysts of the kidney. Am J Roentgenol 127:1015, 1976

15. Jackman RJ, Stevens GM: Benign hemorrhagic renal cysts. Radiology 110:7013, 1974

16. Grossman H, Rosenberg ER, Bowie JD, Ram P, Merten DF: Sonographic diagnosis of renal cystic diseases. AJR 140:81, 1983

17. Lawson TL, McClennan BL, Shirkhoda A: Adult polycystic kidney disease: Ultrasonographic and computed tomographic appearance. J Clin Ultrasound 6:297, 1978

18. Greene LF, Feinzaig W, Dahlin DC: Multicystic dysplasia of the kidney: With special reference to the contralateral kidney. J Urol 105:482, 1971

19. Rosenberg ER: Ultrasonographic evaluation of the kidney. CRC Crit Rev Diag Imaging 17:239, 1982

20. Banner MP, Pollock HM, Chatten J, Witzleben C: Multilocular renal cysts. AJR 136:239, 1980

21. Wood BP, MUurahainen N, Anderson VM, Ettinger LJ: Multicystic nephroblastoma: Ultrasound diagnosis (with a pathologic-anatomic commentary). Pediatr Radiol 12:43, 1982

22. Coleman BG, Arger PH, Mulhern CB, Pollack HM, Banner MP, Arenson RL: Gray-scale sonographic spectrum of hypernephromas. Radiology 137:757, 1980

23. Charboneau JW, Hattery RR, Ernst EC III, James EM, Williamson B Jr, Hartman GW: Spectrum of sonographic findings in 125 renal masses other than benign simple cyst. AJR 140:87, 1983

24. Ladwig SH, Jackson D, Older RA, Morgan CL: Ultrasonic, angiographic, and pathologic correlation of noncystic-appearing renal masses. Urology 17:204, 1981

25. Green B, Goldstein H, Weaver R: Abdominal pansonography in evaluation of renal cancer. Radiology 132:421, 1979

26. Weyman PJ, McClennan BL, Stanley RJ, Levitt RG, Sagel SS: Comparison of computed tomography and angiography in the evaluation of renal cell carcinoma. Radiology 137:417, 1980

27. Hricak H, Williams RD, Moon KL et al.: Nuclear magnetic resonance imaging of the kidney: Renal masses. Radiology 147:765, 1983

28. Kaude JV, Lacy GD: Ultrasonography in renal lymphoma. J Clin Ultrasound 6:295, 1978

29. Sanders RC: Kidneys. In Goldberg BB (ed): Ultrasound in Cancer—Clinics in Diagnostic Ultrasound 6. Churchill Livingstone, New York, 1981

30. Bonavita JA, Pollack HM, Banner MP: Renal oncocytoma: Further observations and literature review. Urol Radiol 2:220, 1980

31. Scheible W, Ellenbogen PH, Leopold GR, Siao NT: Lipomatous tumors of the kidney and adrenal: Apparent echographic specificity. Radiology 129:153, 1978

32. Lee TG, Henderson SC, Freeny PC, Raskin MM, Benson EP, Pearse HD: Ultrasound findings of renal angiomyolipoma. J Clin Ultrasound 6:150, 1978

33. Hartman DS, Goldman SM, Friedman AC, Davis CJ Jr, Madeweli JE, Sherman JL: Angiomyolipoma: Ultrasonic-pathologic correlation. Radiology 139:451, 1981

34. Totty W, McClennan BL, Melson GL, Patel R: Selective value of computed tomography and ultrasonography in the assessment of renal angiomyolipoma. J Comput Asst Tomogr 5:173, 1981

35. Teele RL: Ultrasonography of the genitourinary tract in children. Radiol Clin North Am 15:109, 1977

36. Stovis TL, Perlmutter AD: Recent advances in pediatric urological ultrasound. J Urol 123:613, 1980

37. Rosenfield NS, Shimkin P, Berdon W, Barwick K, Galssman M, Siegel NJ: Wilms' tumor arising from spontaneously regressing nephroblastomatosis. AJR 135:131, 1980

38. Rosenfield AT, Glickman MG, Taylor KJW, Crade M, Hodson J: Acute focal bacterial nephritis (acute lobar nephronia). Radiology 132:553, 1979

39. Funston MR, Fisher KS, van Blerk PJP, Bortz JH: Acute focal bacterial nephritis or renal abscess? A sonographic diagnosis. J Urol 54:461, 1982

40. Kressel HY, Filly RA: Ultrasonic appearance of gas containing abscess in abdomen. Am J Roentgenol 130:71, 1978

41. Vankirk OC, Cgo RT, Wedel VJ: Sonographic features of xanthogranulomatous pyelonephritis. Am J Roentgenol 134:1035, 1980

42. Wadswirtg DE, McClennan BL, Stanley RJ: CT of the renal mass. Urol Radiol 4:88, 1982

43. Balfe DM, McClennan BL, Stanley RJ, Sagel SS: Evaluation of renal masses considered indeterminate on computed tomography. Radiology 142:421, 1982

7 Ultrasound in Renal Transplantation

HEDVIG HRICAK
WILLIAM K. HODDICK

Over the past 25 years, renal transplantation has evolved into a standard treatment modality for irreversible renal failure. To date, more than 50,000 renal transplants have been performed worldwide, and the procedure continues at an ever-increasing rate.[1] Although the technical aspects of organ perfusion and transplantation have been nearly perfected, the search for effective methods to control the immunological mechanisms responsible for rejection continues. From the moment of implantation, the renal allograft exists and functions in a precarious balance between the rejection reaction, the process by which the organism recognizes and disposes of foreign substances, and survival on immunosuppressive therapy. Advances in transplant immunology have allowed more favorable selection of donor and recipient combinations. Additionally, advances in immunosuppressive therapy have permitted increased allograft survival while simultaneously diminishing the incidence of severe or life-threatening infection. These improvements have led to prolonged allograft survival with 2-year allograft survival rates of 60 to 80 percent recently reported for cadaver grafts, depending on tissue matching.[2]

When the renal function is noted to be deteriorating in an allograft recipient, differential diagnostic possibilities are numerous, including obstruction of the collecting system, renal artery or renal vein occlusion, acute tubular necrosis, renal transplant rejection, infection, and recurrent renal disease. Unfortunately, the clinical setting is seldom specific,[3] and consequently a number of diagnostic studies have been suggested to evaluate acute renal allograft failure. These include radionuclide scintigraphy,[4] dynamic computed tomography (CT) scanning,[5] angiography and digital subtraction angiography,[6] excretory urography[7] pulsed Doppler duplex sonography,[8,9] as well as real-time and articulated arm gray scale ultrasonography.[10,11] All these modalities provide some, but also different, significant information regarding the status of the renal allograft.

With the advent of technologic improvements in both gray scale and real-time ultrasonography over the past decade, the ability of ultrasound to evaluate the renal transplant allograft has gradually become evident. The fact that ultrasonography lacks the potential hazards of ionizing radiation, does not require the parenteral administration of potentially nephrotoxic[12] contrast material, is readily available, relatively inexpensive, independent of allograft function, and noninvasive makes it an invaluable modality in the diagnostic armanemtarium for the evaluation of these patients.

In the past, sonography was primarily used as an indicator of hydronephrosis or perirenal fluid collection. However, the superficial anatomical position of the renal transplant in conjunction with the recent refinements in ultrasound technology has enabled the ultrasonographer to display superb anatomical detail. Although sonography actually depicts gross anatomy, it is affected by the tissue texture and thus gives clues regarding the histopathophysiologic characteristics of an organ.

SCANNING TECHNIQUE

Although the renal allograft may be evaluated with facility throughout the postoperative period with ultrasound, a baseline study in the immediate postoperative period (48 to 72 hours after surgery) is preferable. By observing certain precautions, the small theoretical risk of wound infection secondary to contamination during ultrasonographic imaging can be eliminated. All patients are examined with both real-time and static articulated arm equipment in the supine position. The wider field of view provided by articulated arm scanners allows a more global perspective of the allograft and surrounding structures. Additionally, more accurate measurements of the allograft dimensions are facilitated by articulated arm scanning. Rarely can the entire kidney length be measured with current linear array transducers and mechanical sector real-time devices can significantly distort the allograft dimensions, particularly in the direction perpendicular to the image plane. However, greater scanning agility is provided by modern real-time transducers which makes them helpful, particularly in tracing the course of the dilated ureter to the level of obstruction. Additionally, the ability of real time to detect motion is indispensable in the detection of bowel peristalsis, vascular pulsations and, occasionally, ureteral peristalsis.

Adequate images of the allograft can often be obtained by scanning alongside the surgical incision and angling toward the allograft without removing the sterile dressing. Typically, these images are superior to those obtained from directly over the incision as they are not degraded by artifacts induced by surgical sutures and fibrosis. However, if scanning directly over the wound is imperative, bandages should be removed and sterile acoustic coupling gel applied to the incision and a sterile cover placed over the transducer.

Complete postoperative evaluation of the renal allograft includes scanning the entire renal and perirenal area. The scans should extend from the region of the symphysis pubis to a level above the superior aspect of the allograft.

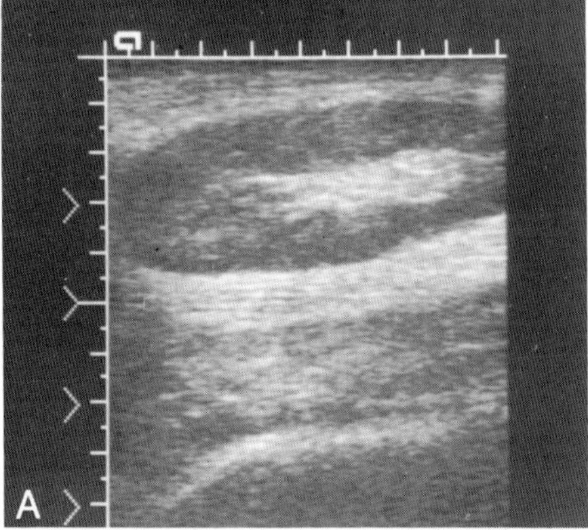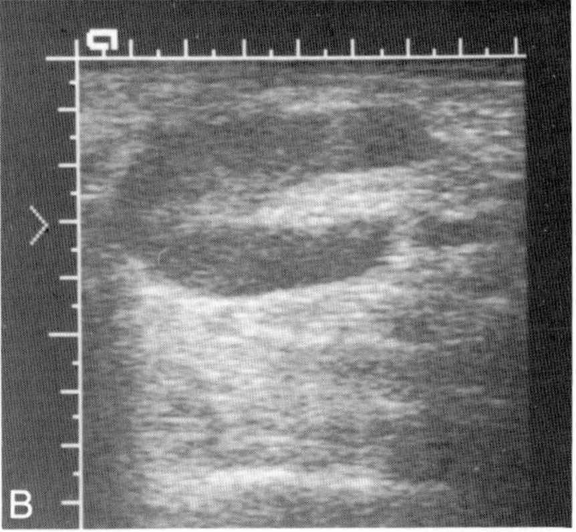

FIG. 7.1.   (A) Longitudinal and (B) transverse ultrasonograms of normal renal allograft. Note the normal elliptical configuration, high-amplitude central sinus fat, and normal renal pyramids.

Optimal scanning of the allograft is along its anatomical coronal plane (Fig. 7.1). This axis permits optimal assessment of renal length and configuration, renal parenchyma, corticomedullary junction, renal collecting system, and the central renal sinus. Angling the transducer at the skin surface and rotating the patient to an oblique position may facilitate the imaging process. Although distention of the urinary bladder provides an excellent acoustic window, over-distention induces an element of hydronephrosis and may lend the illusion of obstructive uropathy. Postvoid images are helpful in this situation.

NORMAL RENAL ALLOGRAFT

The sonographic appearance of the renal allograft is dependent not only upon its inherent anatomy but also on its anatomical relationships within the iliac fossa. Typically, the allograft is transplanted into the recipient's contralateral iliac fossa. Consequently, the kidney is inverted so that the dorsal aspect of the kidney is oriented toward the ventral aspect of the patient. The allograft renal artery and vein are anastomosed end to side to the external iliac artery and internal vein, respectively. Most commonly the allograft ureter is anastomosed with the recipient's bladder by way of a ureteroneocystotomy. Occasionally, and particularly in the past, the recipient's distal ureter was anastomosed with the allograft ureter or renal pelvis. Consequently, the orientation of the renal hilar structure is the converse of the native state. The most anterior structure is the renal pelvis, the most posterior structure is the renal vein, and the renal artery is oriented between these. The kidney is most commonly placed retroperitoneally in an oblique orientation. The allograft can usually be scanned easily without interference from overlying bowel gas. It lies in the iliac fossa anterior to the psoas muscle and iliac veins. The renal hilar structures are medial to the renal parenchyma. The normal allograft is elliptical

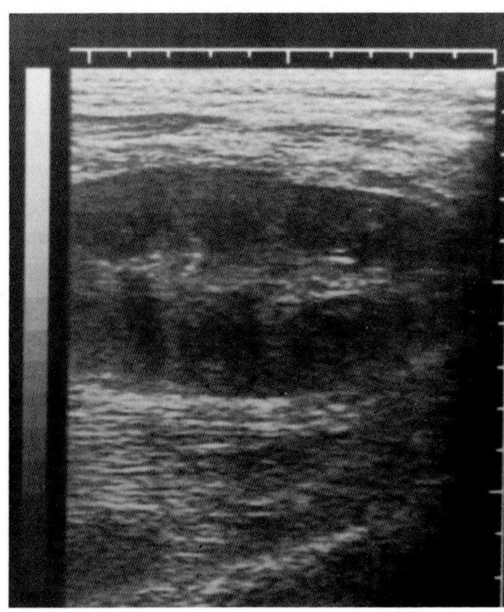

FIG. 7.2. Longitudinal view of normal renal allograft. Note the medullary pyramids are less echogenic than the renal cortex. The renal cortex is less echogenic than the central sinus fat.

in shape. The ratio of the anteroposterior diameter divided by the allograft length is 0.36 to 0.54. A high-amplitude specular reflector surrounding the kidney represents the renal capsule (Glisson's capsule). The intrarenal anatomical structure can also be well-delineated ultrasonographically. The renal parenchyma is divided into the poorly echogenic cortex and the more centrally located hypoechoic centrally located medullary pyramids. The corticomedullary

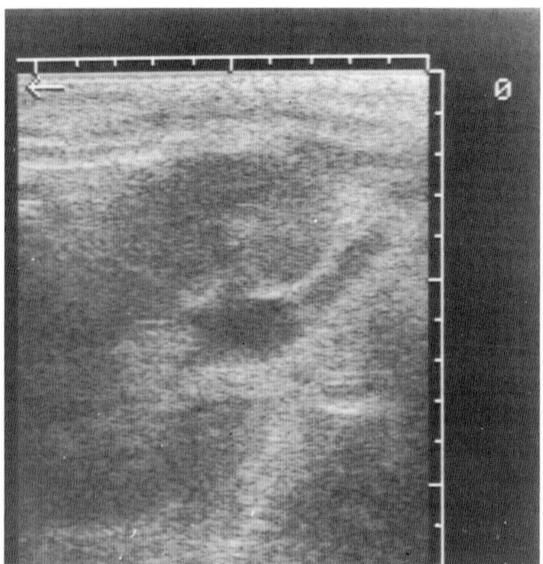

FIG. 7.3. Longitudinal view of renal allograft demonstrating mild dilatation of intrarenal collecting structures and proximal ureter.

junction is normally very distinct. Occasionally high-amplitude specular reflectors in the corticomedullary junction can be identified and are thought to represent arcuate arteries.[13] High-amplitude echoes normally emanate from the central sinus, manifesting the multiple acoustic interfaces present in this region secondary to the multiple lobules and closely packed fat cells separated by fibrous septa and, to a lesser degree, the multiple blood vessels and collecting structures also present in this region[4] (Figs. 7.1, 7.2).[15] The echogenicity of the allograft cortex is greater than that of the medullary pyramids but less than that of the central renal sinus.

Usually, specific identification of the allograft pelvis and proximal ureter can be made. When pylectasis or caliectasis is present, intercommunication with the intrarenal collecting system facilitates identification. Additionally, the pelvis and ureter can be identified anatomically since they lie anterior to the allograft artery and vein. Real-time identification of pulsations within a vessel in the renal hilum identifies the renal artery. Mild dilatation of the intrarenal collecting system is seen frequently, particularly in the immediate postoperative period, and it is considered a normal variant (Fig. 7.3). Although the exact etiology of this phenomenon is uncertain, speculation is possible. Transient edema at the site of the ureteroneocystostomy leading to the temporary low-grade incomplete obstruction of the dilated ureter is a likely cause.[16] Often contributing factors include the prolonged ischemia of the ureter during transplantation and disturbed ureteral innervation secondary to surgery.[17] Regardless of the cause, this temporary dilatation of the collecting system should be considered normal unless it is severe or demonstrates progression on interval scanning.

Following a successful renal transplantation, the renal allograft undergoes normal hypertrophy. The allograft which provided approximately one-half the renal clearance of the donor must solely provide all the renal clearance function for the recipient. Despite hypertrophy, the normal elliptical shape of the allograft is maintained, unless some additional process such as acute tubular necrosis, rejection, or renal vein thrombosis is superimposed.[13] The degree of hypertrophy varies with the age of the donor kidney and is also affected by underlying pathophysiological conditions such as diabetes mellitus.[13] The usual degree of hypertrophy is modest. At the end of the second week following transplantation, the normal allograft hypertrophy has been demonstrated to be between 7 and 25 percent by volume. By the end of the third week, the renal volume has been shown to increase 14 to 34 percent.[16]

RENAL TRANSPLANT PATHOLOGY

Although common in all centers, the incidence of posttransplant renal function is highly variable and depends on many factors relating to the transplant procedure (living related versus cadaver kidney, modality and duration of allograft preservation, operative technique and experience of the transplant team, immunological compatability of the allograft host as well as prophylactic immunosuppresion). The etiological possibilities for allograft failure in the posttransplant period include vascular compromise (arterial or venous), obstruction of the collecting system, infectious processes (viral, bacterial, or fungal), acute rejection, and acute tubular necrosis. Obviously, this is an important differential diagnosis as the appropriate therapeutic regimen must be implemented in order to preserve and maintain allograft function. Unfortunately, the correct diagnosis is rarely clear solely from the clinical setting. Although insufficient data are available to permit generalizations concerning the sonographic appearance of the less common entities, current data indicate that the three most common causes of posttransplant allograft renal failure (acute tubular necrosis, acute rejection, and ureteral obstruction) can be distinguished sonographically.

Acute Tubular Necrosis

Acute tubular necrosis (ATN) is actually a misnomer for renal failure resulting from renal tubular damage. The presence of frank tubular necrosis is rare. ATN is a significant cause of immediate posttransplant renal failure in the posttransplant period with histological evidence of tubular damage identifiable in virtually all renal transplants. However, clinically significant episodes of ATN become manifest in up to 50 percent of cadaver renal transplants. The incidence of ATN is substantially higher in cadaver renal transplants for a variety of reasons. Due to preterminal events in the cadaver donor such as hypotension and disseminated intravascular coagulation, as well as the storage and perfusion of the cadaver allograft prior to transplantation, it is more susceptible to ATN. Clinically, ATN presents with elevated serum creatinine levels. The renal failure may become manifest in the immediate postoperative period, or the urine output may initially be good and progress to oliguria and anuria.

When uncomplicated, ATN is reversible with maintenance of hydration. Therefore, it is important to recognize ATN in distinction from acute rejection which requires alteration in immunosuppressive therapy. Although there are a few isolated reports of the ultrasonographic manifestation of ATN,[14] the majority of reports in both experimental animals[20] and clinical series[16,20,21] indicates there is generally a paucity of ultrasonographic findings in ATN. Typically, the ultrasonographic findings of the allograft undergoing ATN remain unchanged from the baseline study. Therefore, a normal sonogram in a clinical setting of acute renal failure suggests the diagnosis of acute tubular necrosis.

Acute Rejection

The rejection reaction is the universal response to surgical transplantation. Surprisingly, the incidence of rejection episodes is high (up to 93 percent in cadaver kidneys).[22] The early and correct diagnosis of this process must be made in order to avail the patient of the appropriate therapeutic regimen without risking unnecessary side effects. Techniques aimed at reducing the degree of transplant rejection include histocompatibility matching (to minimize the magnitude of the rejection reaction), nonspecific immunosuppression (which renders the host vulnerable to systemic infections), and specific immunosuppression (using monoclonal antibodies and donor-specific transfusions, both relatively new techniques that show great promise).[23]

Acute rejection typically occurs during the first weeks following transplantation. However, due to the current use of immunosuppression, which may delay the rejection process, the exact chronological onset of the process is highly variable.[24] Acute rejection has been reported as early as 5 days or as late as 5 years following transplantation.[25] The histological features of rejection are varied. Acute rejection may histologically be described as primarily vascular or cellular but, in reality, most cases demonstrate elements of both. In cellular rejection, mononuclear cells and edmatous fluid infiltrate the renal interstitium. Vascular rejection is characterized by intimal thickening of arteries and arterioles with associated thrombosis, infarction, and interstitial hemorrhage.[24] Histologically, changes of rejection are present in all renal compartments, including the cortex, medullary, and central sinus fat. During acute rejection, a wide spectrum of sonographic changes occur. These changes are complex and variable.[11,13,18,21,26-32] With the onset of acute rejection, the renal allograft loses its elliptical configuration and becomes more spherical (Fig. 7.4). The allograft increases its size at a rate substantially greater than that associated with compensatory hypertrophy. This alteration in allograft size and configuration is related to the marked interstitial edema and cellular infiltration occurring during acute rejection. A sudden increase in renal volume (20 percent over 5 days or greater than 25 percent over 2 weeks) is typically seen.[18] The anteroposterior diameter/

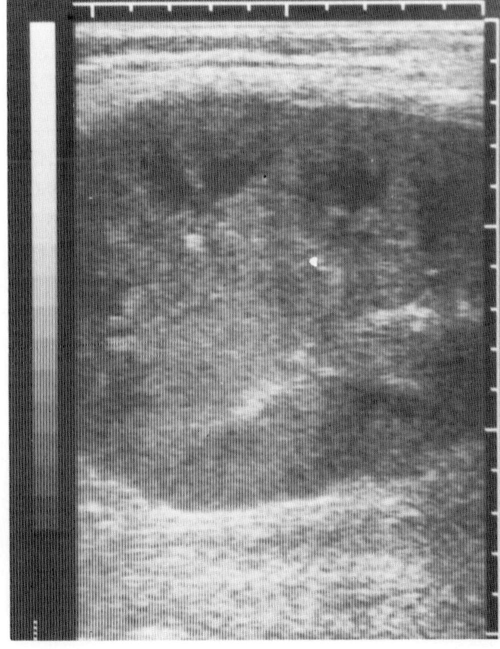

FIG. 7.4.   Longitudinal view of allograft undergoing acute rejection. The configuration is globular, the pyramids are abnormally prominent, and the central sinus fat is diminished.

longitudinal length ratio (AP/L) has been assessed, indicating that in acute rejection the allograft assumed a globular shape with AP/L ratio greater than 0.55 (normal 0.36 to 0.54), with a concomitant increase in allograft thickness with an AP diameter being greater than 5.5 cm.[13] It is important to note that an isolated finding of increased allograft size is not specific for allograft rejection since such processes as renal vein thrombosis and acute pyelonephritis may induce a similar ultrasonographic finding.

Swelling and diminished echogenicity of the renal medullary pyramids have long been recognized as an early sign of acute allograft rejection (Figs. 7.5, 7.6).[18,20,21,33] Histologically, this finding corresponds to the extensive interstitial peritubular edema which involves the medulla in acute rejection.[24] Additionally, the increase in pyramid size is a reflection of the increase in medullary size due to congestion, edema, and hemorrhage in this region. Although this is a highly sensitive and specific finding for acute allograft rejection, one must be cautioned against using this finding in isolation to diagnose acute rejection. The finding of enlarged hypoechogenic medullary pyramids has been noted in both normal adult[29,31] and normal juvenile kidneys,[34] normal kidneys following diuretic therapy,[18] and rarely in allografts undergoing acute tubular necrosis.[29]

Additionally, as the allograft is rejected acutely, the definition between the medullary and cortical portions of the kidney becomes obscured (Fig. 7.6).[18,20,27]

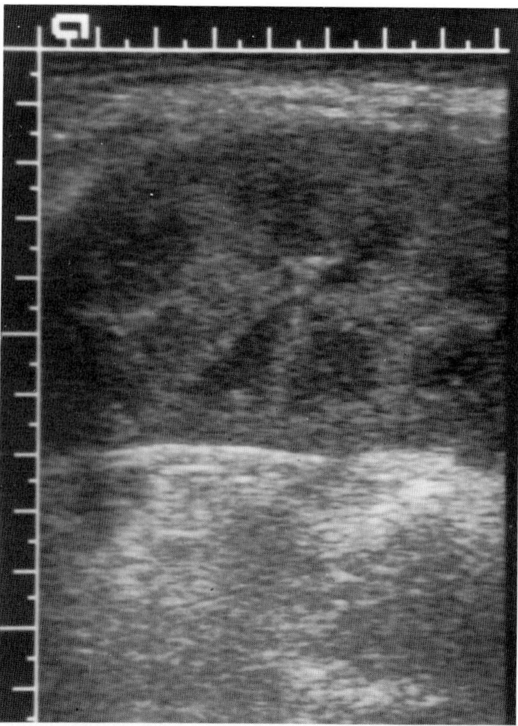

FIG. 7.5. Longitudinal view of allograft undergoing acute rejection. The contour is globular, the medullary pyramids are prominent, and the central sinus fat is diminished.

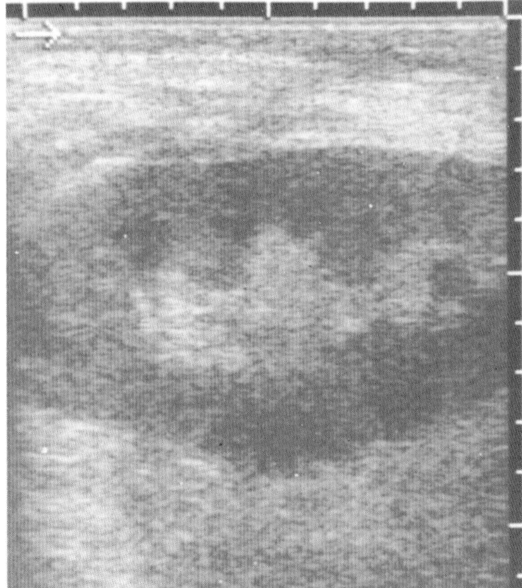

FIG. 7.6. Longitudinal view of allograft demonstrating obscuration of the corticomedullary junction secondary to acute rejection.

Pathological correlation has demonstrated that this is related to the edema and mononuclear cell infiltration which affects the corticomedullary junction early on in the course of acute rejection.

Normally, the central sinus fat in the renal sinus leads to the manifestation of high-amplitude echoes. It is now recognized that the size and echogenicity of the central renal sinus fat is diminished with acute rejection (Fig. 7.7).[11,13] Histologically, the interlobular and intralobular fibrous septa within the renal

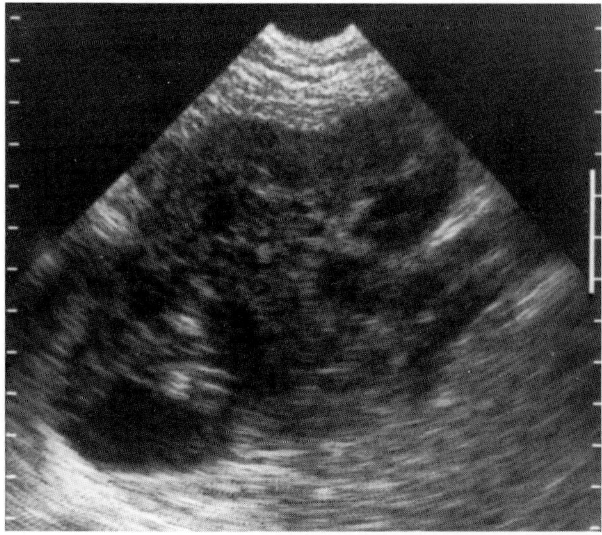

FIG. 7.7. Longitudinal view of renal allograft with virtually no central sinus fat secondary to acute rejection. Focal parenchymal abnormalities are seen as well.

hilum enlarges in size due to edema and infiltrating mononuclear cells. Subsequently, the number and size of the hilar fat cells decrease. The diminished hilar echogenicity is a reflection of a decreased quantity of fat combined with a replacement of fat by edematous infiltrated fibrous septa. Although this finding has been reported in cases of chronic rejection,[21] in the setting of renal failure in the immediate posttransplant period, this appearance of the renal sinus is sensitive and specific in the diagnosis of allograft rejection.

Sonolucencies scattered throughout the allograft parenchyma have been described by numerous observers in acute allograft rejection[18,21,28,29] (Figs. 7.7, 7.8). Pathologically, these focal regions of hypoechogenicity correspond to areas of parenchymal edema, hemorrhage, infection, and necrosis. Although multiple focal sonolucencies are fairly specific for acute rejection, the sensitivity of this finding is somewhat low.[18,28] Rarely, multiple embolic infections or abscesses within the allograft may present with a similar appearance.[31]

The cortical echogenicity has been described as being both increased and diminished in acute transplant rejection.[18,20,27] Histological correlation has demonstrated that the diminished echogenicity is related to parenchymal interstitial edema, and the increased echogenicity is induced by cellular infiltration of the allograft parenchyma. Again, this finding is nonspecific[18] and difficult to interpret secondary to the lack of adjacent reference organs to establish the normal range of echogenicity.

Thickening of the renal pelvis, as well as the infundibulum, has also been seen in allograft rejection[18] (Fig. 7.9).

Limited success in evaluating posttransplant allograft renal failure utilizing duplex Doppler ultrasound has been reported.[9] By calculating a pulsed Doppler index, a relative approximation of renal blood flow can be made. Decreased renal function in view of good renal blood flow correlates more with ATN, whereas diminished function and blood flow correlate more with rejection or vascular compromise. In our experience, this technique is cumbersome and not readily reproducible. Its full utility awaits further evaluation.

In conclusion, rejection is a dynamic process, and different sonographic findings correspond to the stage that the rejection process has reached. To suggest sonographically a diagnosis of acute rejection, at least two of the above described features should be present. Obviously, the ultrasonographic findings should always be correlated with the clinical, laboratory, and radionuclide data.

Obstructive Uropathy

Another cause of acute renal failure in transplant patients is obstruction of the allograft. Ureteral obstruction requiring repeat surgery occurs in 1 to 10 percent of renal transplants.[35] The etiological possibilities leading to obstructive uropathy include intrinsic blockage (blood clot, calculus, fungus ball), stricture formation, and extrinsic pressure from any pelvic mass including periallograft fluid collection.

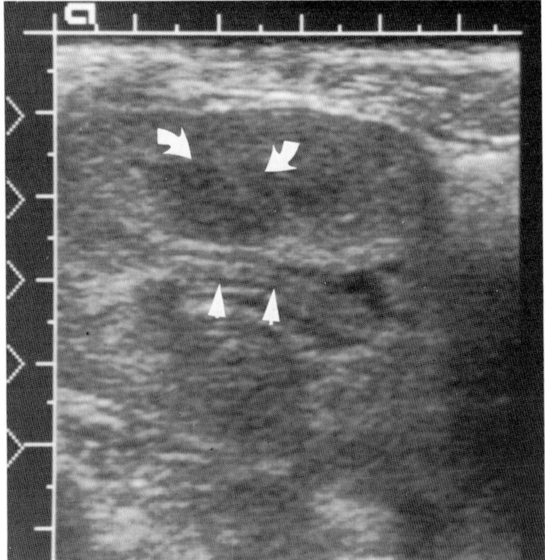

FIG. 7.8. Curved arrows delineate focal parenchymal abnormality secondary to acute allograft rejection. Arrowheads demonstrate ureteral stent in place.

Ultrasound detects dilatation of the intrarenal collecting structures with facility (Fig. 7.10).[36] However, visualization of the entire ureter is unusual as there is no consistent acoustic window along its course.

It is important to note that hydronephrosis and obstruction are not synonymous, and the degree of hydronephrosis does not adequately depict the severity

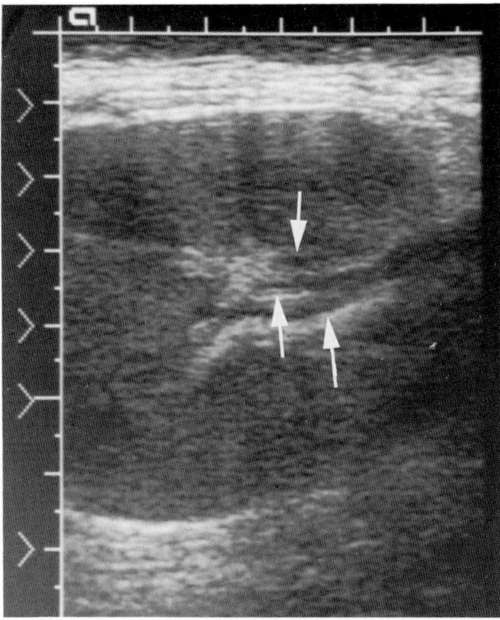

FIG. 7.9. Arrows delineate pelvic and vascular wall thickening secondary to acute allograft rejection.

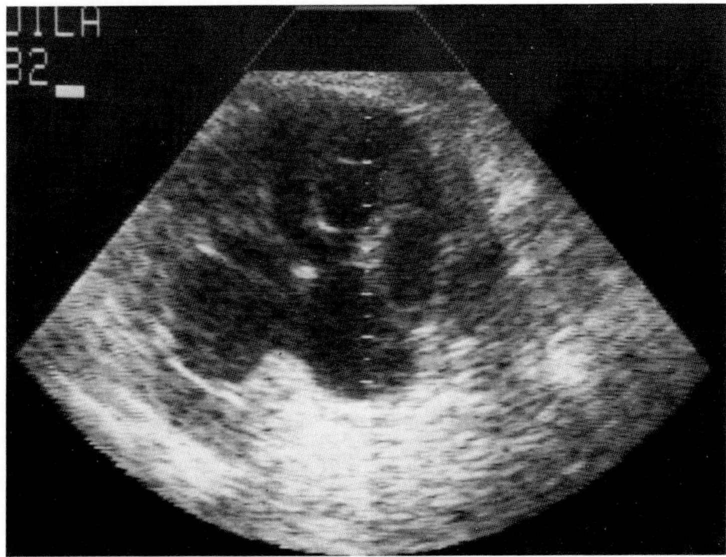

FIG. 7.10. Marked hydronephrosis in renal allograft secondary to ureteral obstruction.

or even the presence of obstruction. The degree of dilatation of the collecting system is a complex product of the amount of urine produced, compliance of the collecting system, and the resistance to flow in the ureter and collecting system. If the allograft is functioning poorly and ureteral compliance is diminished by edema and cellular infiltration, even complete obstruction could result in only modest hydronephrosis and hydroureter. Conversely, as noted earlier, mild dilatation of the collecting structures is quite common, particularly in the immediate posttransplant period as a result of edema at the ureteroneocystostomy site. Additionally, the ureter may be dilated during episodes of both acute and chronic rejection in the absence of any anatomical obstruction.[32] Occasionally, the pressure of a pelvic mass such as a lymphocele or hematoma compressing the ureter can be identified, facilitating the diagnosis of obstruction. However, the accurate diagnosis of obstruction of the urinary tract can only be made in conjunction with a complementary imaging modality such as radionuclide scanning, excretory urography, or retrograde pyelography.

Cyclosporin Toxicity

Cyclosporin A (CsA) is one of a family of fungal metabolites which has proved to be a potent immunosuppressive agent.[37-39] Unfortunately, when CsA is used as an immunosuppressive agent in recipients of renal allografts, deterioration of renal function often develops secondary to CsA nephrotoxicity. This problem is complicated by the fact that allograft biopsy on patients with CsA-induced allograft nephrotoxicity demonstrate no specific pathological marker.[40] Although the ultrasonographic findings of allografts undergoing CsA-induced nephrotoxicity remain to be evaluated in a lare series, preliminary results indicated that the typical appearance of these allografts fall within normal limits without detectable ultrasonographic abnormality (Hricak, unpublished data).

Vascular Compromise

In the postoperative state, the renal allograft is at risk for a number of vascular lesions including renal vein thrombosis, renal arterial occlusion, and segmental arterial occlusion, all of which may present as acute renal failure. The sonographic findings of both venous and arterial vascular compromise are nonspecific, requiring angiography or Doppler ultrasound for a definitive diagnosis. However, the ultrasound findings, in conjunction with clinical, laboratory, and complementary imaging modalities, assist the clinician in arriving at the accurate diagnosis.

Renal Vein Thrombosis

Work with both laboratory animals and allograft patients[18] has demonstrated several sonographic findings in acute renal vein thrombosis. These include immediate renal enlargement, increased cortical thickness, sparsely distributed cortical echoes, diminished echogenicity of the renal cortex, indistinct corticomedullary junction, and hypoechoic regions within the renal parenchyma due to hemorrhage, dilated renal vein, and renal rupture. It is apparent that several of these finding could be confused with the sonographic manifestations of acute allograft rejection, and the definitive diagnosis rests with a complementary imaging modality.

Complete Arterial Occlusion

Only limited reports of the sonographic manifestations of acute renal allograft arterial occlusion are available.[18] These suggest that the findings in this entity are limited, and the allograft may appear unchanged after acute complete arterial occlusion. Animal models have demonstrated only minimal diminution of the allograft echogenicity following acute arterial occlusion.

Segmental Arterial Occlusion

Experimental animals models have demonstrated a sequence of sonographic changes following segmental renal arterial occlusion.[18] Forty-eight hours following segmental arterial occlusion, there are ill-defined anechoic areas corresponding to the region of infarction. The size and configuration of the infarction zone remain unchanged for 5 days. Between 7 and 21 days, there is a decrease in size of the infarction zone, and the region of infarction is more distinct from the adjacent parenchyma. Between 21 and 35 days, the infarction zone continues to diminish in size and increase in its echogenicity.

Peritransplant Fluid Collections

Another frequent complication in recipients of renal allografts is the development of peritransplant fluid collections. Ultrasound has proven of considerable value in the evaluation of these collections. Hematomas, lymphoceles, seromas, urinomas, and abscess all may present in the posttransplant period. The sonographic appearance of each area is largely nonspecific, and the ultimate diagnosis rests with clinical correlation, needle aspiration, or surgical exploration.[41-44]

Abscess

Patients undergoing renal transplantation are at risk for the development of abscess and other infectious processes for a variety of reasons. Longstanding renal failure compromises many body functions and organ systems, including the host defense mechanisms. The host's integumentary boundary is violated during the transplantation procedure, adding to the risk of infection. Perhaps most importantly, the immunosuppression necessary to prevent or mitigate allograft rejection also dramatically lowers the host's ability to combat infection.

Like abscesses in other patients and organ systems, the ultrasonographic appearance of abscesses surrounding the renal transplant is highly variable and dependent on several factors including the degree of liquification of the abscess, the degree of inflammation in surrounding tissues, and the abscence or presence of air within the abscess from gas-forming organisms.[45,46] Typically, the abscess must be at least 1 cm in diameter to be detected ultrasonographically. In liquified collections of pus, the abscess will fulfill the criteria of a cystic lesion, including lack of internal echoes, through sound transmission and posterior wall enhancement. If the abscess is less than fully liquified, the appearance will be heterogeneous with areas of both increased and diminished echogenicity. High-amplitude echoes typically with "dirty" posterior shadowing result when air is present within the abscess cavity.

It is important to keep in mind that immunosuppression will confuse the clinical picture by preventing the patient from mounting a typical response to a septic insult (fever, pain, leukocytosis). Consequently, there should be a low threshold of suspicion for an abscess in these patients, and confirmation of ultrasonographic findings should be obtained via surgery or percutaneous needle aspiration.

Seromas

Seromas are a localized fluid mass caused by the collection of serum in a tissue. They are not uncommon in patients following surgery, particularly those undergoing renal transplantation. They are typically seen in the acute period following surgery. Typically, they are echo-free structures with thin well-defined margins. Again, their appearance is nonspecific and may be mimicked by a number of processes.

Hematoma

When hematomas are demonstrated during the immediate postoperative period, they are most commonly related to the technical aspects of the surgery such as a vascular anastomostic leak. Delayed hematomas may also be seen and are secondary to renal biopsy, hypertensive events, ischemia, or acute rejection. The site of rupture is often along the superior lateral margin of the allograft and results in a superiorily deployed hematoma.

Acutely (before 5 days' duration), the hematoma is quite echogenic secondary to the multiple acoustic interfaces in the organizing clot. Therefore, it is quite difficult to distinguish from the adjacent soft tissues. Often, the only ultrasonographic finding is subtle mass effect necessitating computerized tomographic evaluation to further characterize the mass.[18] A hematoma greater than 5 days of age undergoes liquification and often contains thick septations, making ultrasonographic detection more facile (Fig. 7.11).

Lymphoceles

The surgical procedure involved in renal transplantation by its very nature must result in the disruption of many lymphatic vessels in and around the recipient's transplant bed. These small lymphatics are typically ligated and, if they do not reanastomose spontaneously, a lymphocele or an accumulation of lymph fluid will form around the allograft (Fig. 7.12). Lymphoceles develop in up to 20 percent of transplant recipients. Typically the lymphocele requires 2 to 6 weeks to develop, but episodes of acute rejection may hasten their

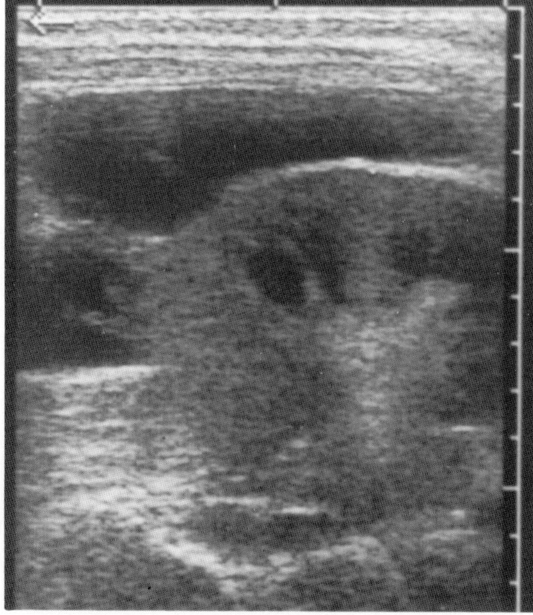

FIG. 7.11. Hematoma along superior aspect of renal allograft. Note the thick septations.

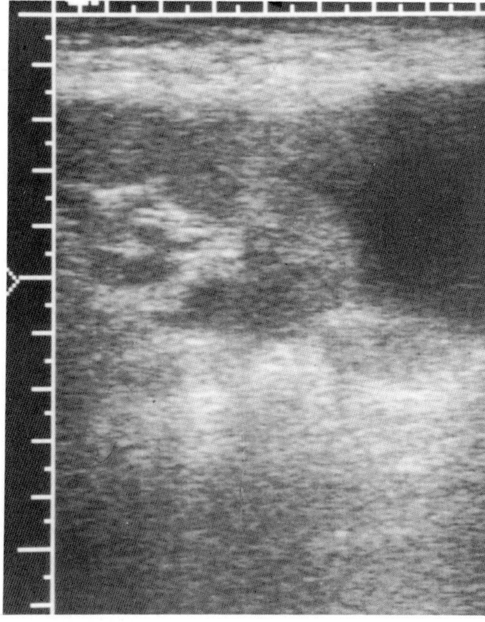

FIG. 7.12. Fluid collections adjacent to the inferior aspect of the allograft represents a lymphocele.

appearance. Lymphoceles may occur anywhere along the extraperitoneal allograft bed, although they are most often seen inferior to the allograft. Usually, they are the largest of the peritransplant fluid collections. After 5 days, stranding or septations often develop within the lymphocele (Fig. 7.13). The location and size of lymphoceles allows them to exert significant pressure on the iliac

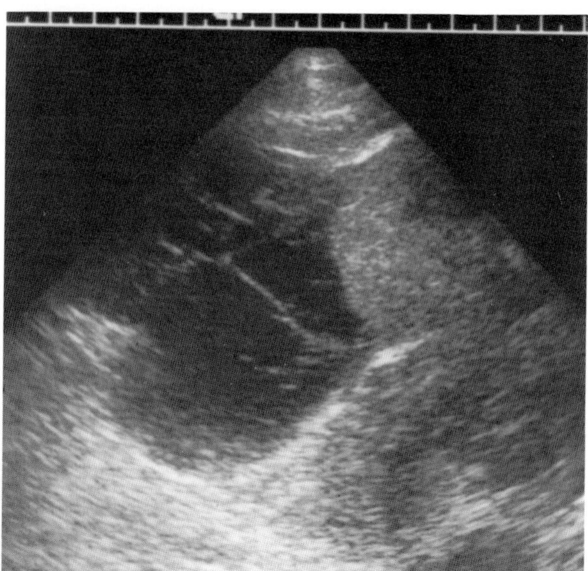

FIG. 7.13. Lymphocele superior to renal allograft containing multiple septations.

vessels, ureter, and bladder, leading to leg edema, obstructive uropathy, and difficulties with control of micturition.[38]

Urinoma

Early diagnosis of urinoma is essential since it may lead to wound sepsis, loss of the allograft or generalized sepsis. Urinomas may occur at any time in the posttransplant period in up to 10 percent of transplant recipients.[19,39]

Urinomas developing during the first week after surgery are usually related to the technical aspects of the procedure, with the site of extravasation at the site of the ureteral anastomosis. Later development of the urinoma is secondary to either renal biopsy, closed allograft injury, obstruction, or urinary fistula.

Sonographically, urinomas have a variable shape but typically are seen adjacent to the lower pole of the allograft. Septations are unusual and, unlike other peritoneal fluid collections, urinomas have a tendency to dissect along tissue planes, necessitating careful sonographic evaluation of the flanks, scrotum, and labia. Again, the appearance of this peritransplant fluid collection is nonspecific, and diagnosis usually requires confirmation by demonstrating urine extravasation by nuclear scintigraphy or excretory urography.

SUMMARY

Ultrasound contributes valuable information in the differential diagnostic dilemma in acute renal transplant failure. However, the ultrasound findings are rarely specific and require careful correlation with clinical and laboratory data as well as complementary imaging modalities.

REFERENCES

1. Health care finance administration: In Contemporary Dialysis, June 1984
2. Morris PJ: Kidney transplantation. Transplant Proc 18:26, 1981
3. Brown EA, Siegel HJ, Finkelstein FO: Symptomless acute renal transplant rejections: Occurrences six months or more after transplantation. JAMA 239:2256, 1978
4. Delmonico FL, McKusick KA, Losimi AB et al.: Differentiation between renal allograft rejection and acute tubular necrosis by renal scan. AJR 128:625, 1977
5. Fuld IL, Metalon TA, Vogelzang RL, Meiman HL, Kowal LE, Hutchins WW, Soper W: Dynamic CT in the evaluation of physiologic status of renal transplants. AJR 142:1157, 1984
6. Hamway S, Novick A, Braun WE et al.: Impaired renal allograft function. Comparative study with angiography and histopathology. J Urol 122:292, 1979
7. Imray TH, Gedgaudas E: Excretory urogrphy in the evaluation of renal transplants. Radiology 95:653, 1970
8. Arima M, Ishibashi M, Usami M et al.: Analysis of the arterial blood flow patterns of normal and allografted kidneys by the directional ultrasonic Doppler technique. J Urol 122:587, 1979
9. Berland LL, Lawson TL, Adams MB, Melrose BL, Foley WD: Evaluation of renal transplants with pulsed Doppler duplex sonography. JUM 215, 1982

10. Bertram RJ Jr, Smith LH, D'Orsi LJ et al.: Evaluation of renal transplants with ultrasound. Radiology 118:405, 1976

11. Hricak H, Romanski RN, Eyler WR: The renal sinus during allograft rejection: Sonographic and histopathologic findings. Radiology 142:693, 1982

12. Light TA, Hill GS: Acute tubular necrosis in a renal transplant recipient: Complication from drip infusion excretory urography. JAMA 232:1267, 1975

13. Heckeman R, Rehwald U, Jakubowski HD, Donhuijsen K: Sonographic criteria for renal allograft rejection. Urol Radiol 4:15, 1982

14. Rosenfield A, Taylor K, Crade M et al.: Anatomy and pathology of the kidney by gray scale ultrasound. Radiology 128:737, 1978

15. Behan M, Karam E: The echogenic characteristics of fatty tissues and tumors. Radiology 129:143, 1978

16. Hricak H, Cruz C, Sandler M, Romanski R, Madrazo B, Levin N, Eyler WR: Sonographic evaluation of the transplanted kidney: A prospective study (abst). Presented at the Radiologic Society of North America, 61st Scientific Assembly and Annual Meeting, Chicago, Ill., 1981

17. Schiff M: Ureter in renal transplantation. Urology 12:256, 1978

18. Hricak H, Cruz C, Eyler WR, Madrazo BL, Sandler MA: Post-transplant renal failure: Differential diagnosis by ultrasound—experimental and clinical obstructions. Med Ultrasound 6:1, 1982

19. Delmonico FL, McKusich KA, Cosin AB, Russel PS: Differentiation between renal allograft rejection and acute tubular necrosis by renal scan. AJR 128:625, 1977

20. Hricak H, Toledo-Perreyra L, Eyler WR et al.: Evaluation of acute post-transplant renal failure by ultrasound. Radiology 133:433, 1979

21. Maklad NF, Wright CH, Rosenthal SJ: Gray-scale ultrasound of renal transplant rejection. Radiology 131:711, 1979

22. Becker JA, Kutcher R: The renal transplant: Rejection and acute tubular necrosis. Semin Roentgenol 13:352, 1978

23. Perloff LJ, Tomaszewski JE, Barka CF: Transplantation biology: Mechanism of rejection and recent advances in immunosuppresion. Hosp Physician 6:42, 1983

24. Olsen S: Pathology of the renal allograft rejection. p. 327. In Chung J, Spango BH, Mostafi KF (eds): Kidney Disease—Present Status. Williams and Wilkins, Baltimore, 1979

25. Brown E, Siegel M, Finkelstein FO: Symptomless acute renal transplant rejection. JAMA 239:2256, 1978

26. Conrad MR, Dickerman R, Love IL, Curry T, Peters P, Hall H, Lerman M, Helderman H: New observations in renal transplants using ultrasound. AJR 131:851, 1978

27. Hillman RJ, Birnholz JL, Busin GJ: Correlation of echographic and histologic findings in suspected renal allograft rejection. Radiology 132:673, 1979

28. Singh A, Conen WH: Renal allograft rejection: Sonography and scintigraphy. AJR 135:73, 1980

29. Frick MP, Feinberg SB, Sibley R, Idstrom ME: Ultrasound in acute renal transplant rejection. Radiology 138:657, 1981

30. Hurkaayi Z, Juray J, Alfoldy F, Perner F, Torak I: Echography of renal transplant patients. Radiology 21:485, 1981

31. Jafri SZ, Kaude JV, Wright PG, Jufri SZ, Kaude JV, Wright PG: Ultrasound findings in renal transplant rejection. Acta Radiol (Diagn) (Stockholm) 22:245, 1981

32. Hricak H, Zammit M, Eyler WR, Farah R: Ureteral peristalsis in the rejecting allograft. Presented at the Association of University Radiologists, 28th Annual Meeting, Tuscon, 1980

33. Fried AM, Woodring JH, Lon FH, Lucas BA, Kryscio RJ: The medullary pyramid index:

An objective assessment of prominence in renal transplantation rejection. Radiology 149:787, 1983

34. Hricak H, Slovin TL, Callen CW, Callen PW, Romanski RN: Neonatal kidneys: Sonographic, anatomic correlation. Radiology 147:699, 1983

35. Palestract AM, DeWolff WL: The pseudostricture of transplant ureteral torsion. Radiology 133:443, 1979

36. Bulchaunes WR, Hill MC, Isokoff MB, Morillo G: The clinical significance of dilatation of the collecting system in the transplanted kidney. J Clin Ultrasound 3:221, 1982

37. Smottid JP: Cyclosporin A Transplantation 32:349, 1981

38. Kostakis AJ, White DJG, Calne RY: Prolongation of rat heart survival by cyclosporin A. IRCS J Med Sci 5:280, 1977

39. Calne RY, White DJG: Cyclosporin A—a powerful immunosuppressant in dogs with renal allografts. IRCS J Med Sci 5:595, 1977

40. Farnsworth A, Hall BM, Kirwan P, Bishop GA, Duggin GC, Goodman B, Harvath J, Johnson J, Ng A, Sheil AGR, Tiller DJ: Pathology in renal transplant patients treated with cyclosporin. Transplantation Proc 15:2852, 1983

41. Silver TM, Campbell D, Wicks JD, Lurber MT, Surace P, Turlett J: Percutaneous plant fluid collection. Radiology 138:145, 1981

42. Brockis JG, Hulbert JC, Patel AS, Golinger D, Hurst P, Saker B, Haywood EF, House AK, Van Merwyk A: The diagnosis and treatment of lymphoceles associated with renal transplantation. Br J Urol 50:307, 1978

43. Yup R, Madrazo B, Oh HK, Dienst SG: Perirenal fluid collection after renal transplantation. Am Surg 47:287, 1981

44. Spigo DG, Tan W, Pavel DG, Moses M, Jonusson O, Capek V: Diagnosis of urine extravasation after renal transplantation. AJR 129:409, 1977

45. Hoddick WK, Jeffrey RB, Goldberg HI, Federle MP, Laing F: CT and ultrasound in the evaluation of severe renal and perirenal infections. AJR 140:517, 1983

46. Schneider M, Becker JA, Striano S, Campos E: Sonographic-radiographic correlation of renal and perirenal infections. AJR 127:1007, 1976

8 Transrectal Sonographic Urodynamics

INDER PERKASH
GERALD W. FRIEDLAND

Neuromuscular dysfunction of the bladder affects nearly 25 million Americans.[1] Of this group, nearly 1.5 million have neuromuscular dysfunction of the bladder due to spinal cord injury, and injuries of this type are occurring at a rate of approximately 10,000 new cases annually.[1] Nearly all of these patients, moreover, are young. They will normally receive relatively large doses of radiation from conventional voiding cystourethrograms, which, in addition to other reasons, might be a problem should they wish to father children in the future. Certainly, the radiation from multiple radiological voiding cystourethrograms does not cause sterility, but the risk of incurring genetic defects in potential children as a result of multiple voiding cystourethrograms is a question that we cannot yet comfortably answer. One of the reasons for the development of the sonographic voiding cystourethrogram is to overcome the effects of radiation in these patients; this chapter discusses how this examination can effectively be used in these patients, as well as its advantages over conventional examinations.

ANATOMY AND PATHOPHYSIOLOGY

The muscular part of the wall of the bladder and of the urethra is made up of two types of muscles, smooth and striated. These muscles are supplied by three separate nerves: the parasympathetic (S2-4), the sympathetic (T11-L2), and the pudendal (S2-4). There is naturally some intermingling both of muscle and of nerve supply, but there are some areas in the bladder and urethra where particular muscles and nerve supplies predominate.

The muscular part of the bladder wall (the detrusor) is made up entirely of smooth muscle. It is supplied by both parasympathetic and sympathetic nerves.

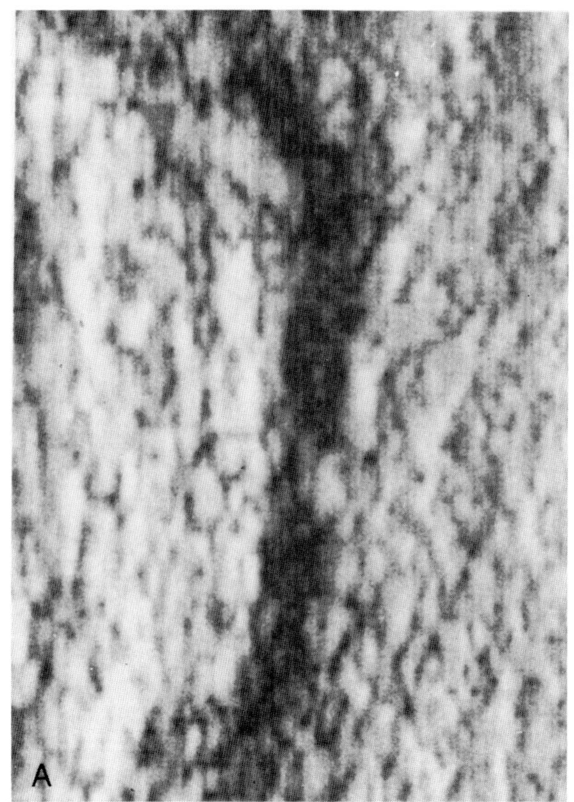

FIG. 8.1. Normal urethral angle in a 27-year-old man. (A) Sonographic voiding cystourethrogram, showing that the normal male urethra kinks posteriorly about 135°. (B) Diagrammatic illustration of part A. (C) Diagram illustrating that, because of the urethral angle, the Credé or Valsalva maneuvers close the bladder neck.

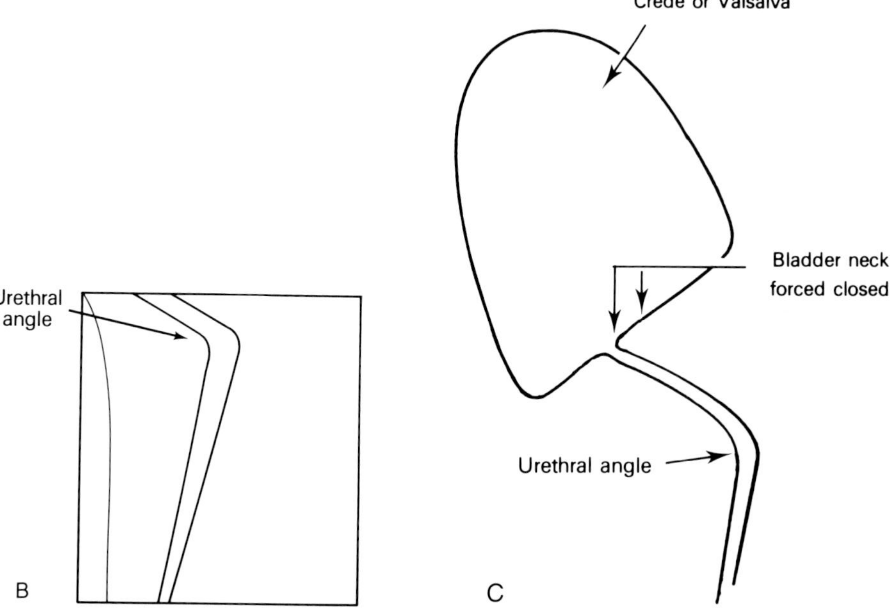

Voiding is mediated via the parasympathetic nerves; as these nerves are stimulated, the detrusor contracts. Bladder filling, on the other hand, is mediated via the sympathetic nerves. When these nerves are stimulated, their nerve endings secrete noradrenalin. The detrusor, which possesses β-adrenergic receptors, relaxes when noradrenalin is present.

Although the muscles surrounding the bladder neck are made up entirely of smooth muscle, in the proximal urethra* smooth muscle only predominates, and the predominant nerve supply is sympathetic. When these nerves are stimulated, their nerve endings secrete noradrenalin, but in this case the relevant muscles, which possess α-adrenergic receptors, contract when noradrenalin is present. Therefore, as the bladder fills, the detrusor relaxes and the bladder neck contracts.

The muscles surrounding the distal half of the urethra are made up predominantly of striated muscle, and are supplied largely by the pudendal nerves.

The male urethra kinks posteriorly at an angle of approximately 135°, dividing the urethra into two equal parts (Fig. 8.1).[3] When the male urethra opens, the anterior wall moves anteriorly and straightens; there is little or no movement of the posterior wall.

When neuromuscular dysfunction occurs, it can affect different parts of the lower urinary tract, including the detrusor, the bladder neck, or the proximal or distal half of the urethra.

In these patients the detrusor may or may not be able to contract. If it can contract, the patient has an upper motor neuron lesion. If it cannot contract, the patient usually has a lower motor neuron lesion, but this inability to contract may also occur in patients with upper motor neuron lesions in whom the bladder was not appropriately managed (and which consequently became chronically overdistended), and in patients with lesions of the sensory nerve roots.

The main functional abnormality that can occur at the bladder neck and urethra involves the inability of their muscles to relax when the patient tries to void. The bladder neck may not relax when the detrusor contracts (detrusor-bladder-neck dyssynergia), a functional abnormality seen in patients with high paraplegia or quadriplegia, or the striated muscles surrounding the distal half of the urethra may not relax when the detrusor contracts (detrusor-sphincter dyssynergia); this can be the result of a lesion anywhere between the pons and the conus.

The result of either functional abnormality, however, is that the patient may find it extremely difficult or impossible to void. Because of the obstruction, the pressure in the bladder will remain chronically high, which may result in detrusor hypertrophy, the formation of saccules and diverticula, and vesicoureteral reflux. Since the urine is chronically infected in such patients, the result may be chronic reflux pyelonephritis or the formation of struvite stones.

It is therefore extremely important to define precisely which functional ab-

---

* In this chapter the term "urethra" refers to the posterior urethra in males and the entire urethra in females.

normality is present in any given patient. We now do this primarily with a combination of transrectal sonography and urodynamic studies, which combination we call transrectal sonographic urodynamics.

TECHNIQUES

The sonographic studies are performed using a Toshiba model SAL 30 machine and a 3.5-MHz linear-array transrectal transducer, model 30A, covered with a water-filled condom and introduced intrarectally, with the window facing anteriorly.[4] During voiding, this unit produces real-time images equivalent to or better than the images obtained during radiological voiding cystourethrograms.

Urodynamic studies consist of a combined electromyogram of the periurethral striated sphincter, a cystometrogram, and a urethral pressure profile.

Our electromyograms (EMGs) are performed as follows: a fine needle is passed through the perineum transcutaneously into the striated muscle surrounding the lower half of the urethra. The electrical activity originating in the striated muscle can then be measured; when the muscle contracts, electrical activity will be present, but when it relaxes, there will be no electrical activity.

When normal people are at rest and the striated muscle contracts enough to prevent incontinence, there is EMG activity. If normal people are asked to contract their perineal muscles, they can easily do so, and EMG activity increases. At the onset of normal voiding, however, the striated muscle relaxes, and EMG activity ceases.

The cystometrogram is simply a recording of bladder pressure, and is useful to show whether the bladder can contract and whether any urethral narrowing visible on ultrasound or a radiological voiding cystourethrogram has any functional significance. The normal bladder pressure during voiding does not rise above 40 cm water in children or above 70 cm water in adults; if pressures are higher, obstruction is present, either at the bladder neck or in the urethra.

The urethral pressure profile is a recording of the pressures in the bladder neck and the urethra. If the pressure in either of these two areas is higher than in the bladder when the patient attempts to void, the attempt will be unsuccessful.

All of the above are displayed on the monitor of a DISA Video Urosystem; a coaxial cable that is usually connected to the television monitor for a radiological voiding cystourethrogram is here attached to the ultrasonographic equipment, enabling the examiner to record the urodynamic studies and the sonographic examination simultaneously on videotape. Subsequent hard copies are obtained using a Polaroid camera.

ROLE OF SONOGRAPHIC URODYNAMICS

Sonographic urodynamics has two important roles to play: it helps establish the correct diagnosis, and it has become important in patient management.

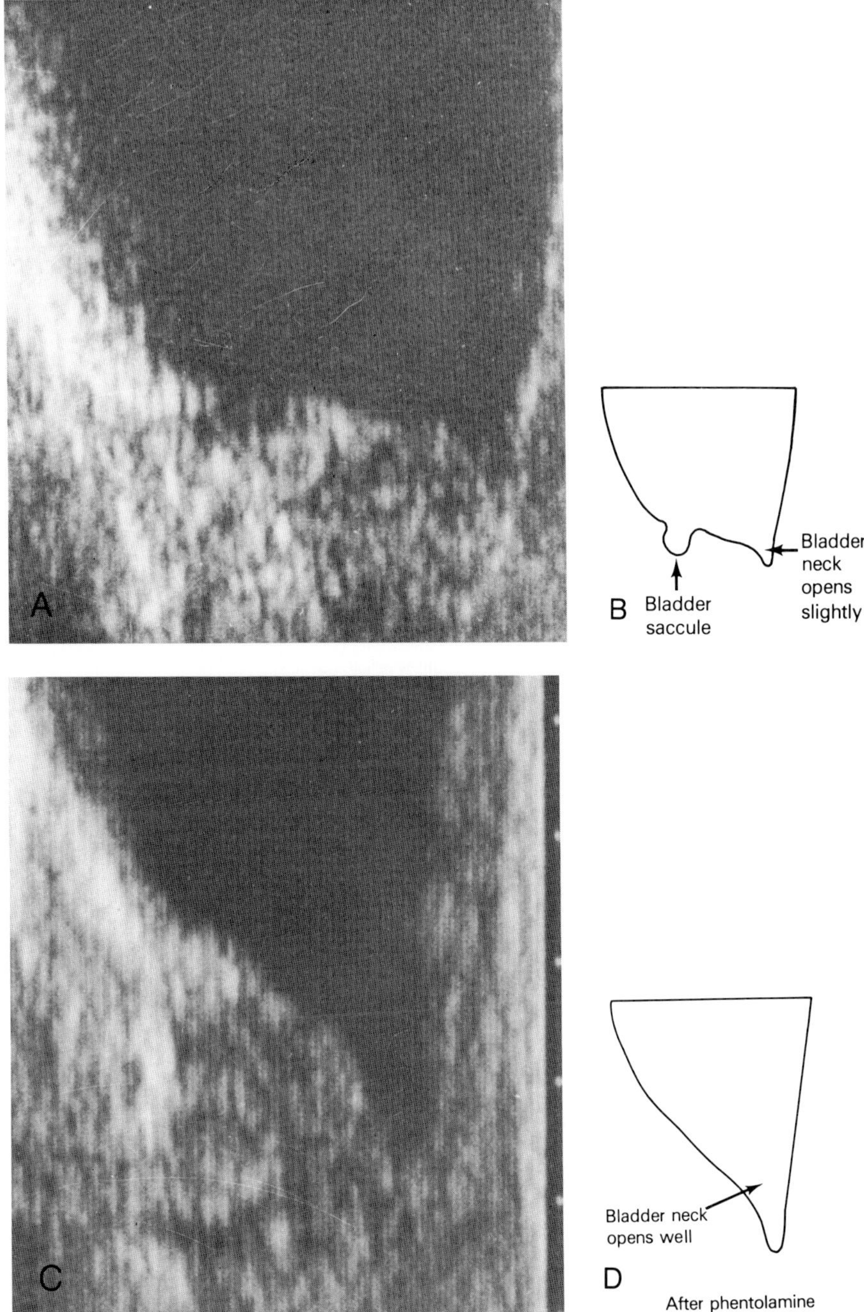

FIG. 8.2.   Detrusor-bladder-neck dyssynergia. (A) Sonographic voiding cystourethrogram shows that the bladder neck fails to relax when the detrusor contracts. (B) Diagrammatic illustration of part A. (C) Sonographic voiding cystourethrogram, performed in the same patient, showing the effect of intravenous phentolamine, and α-adrenergic blocker. (D) Diagrammatic illustration of part C.

Diagnosis

Sonographic urodynamics can provide further information regarding the causes of three common problems in patients with neuromuscular dysfunction: bladder neck obstruction, urethral obstruction, and hyperreflexic bladder. It can also demonstrate the presence of bladder saccules and diverticula, a sign that bladder outlet obstruction has begun to have adverse effects on the urinary tract.

Bladder Neck Obstruction

There are three common causes of bladder neck obstruction in patients with neuromuscular dysfunction: detrusor-bladder-neck dyssynergia,[4] a ledge composed of hypertrophied and atrophied muscle and fibrous tissue that forms posteriorly in the bladder neck as a result of trauma suffered during chronic intermittent catheterization, and benign prostatic hyperplasia. Sonographic urodynamics shows that the bladder neck opens not at all or slightly in patients with detrusor bladder-neck dyssynergia, but when they are given intravenous phentolamine, an α-adrenergic blocker, the bladder neck clearly opens widely (Fig. 8.2).[4]

In addition, about 30 percent patients on chronic intermittent catheterization eventually develop a ledge posteriorly at the bladder neck due to the trauma of intermittent catheterization (Fig. 8.3). This ledge causes difficulty in voiding and considerably complicates catheterization in some patients; this is, however, a new observation, since it is best visualized only on transrectal sonography using a linear-array transducer, which has only recently become available.

Benign prostatic hyperplasia can be readily recognized because it causes a focal or generalized enlargement of the gland; the echo pattern is homogeneous.

Urethral Obstruction

There are three common causes of urethral obstruction in patients with neuromuscular dysfunction, detrusor-sphincter dyssynergia, urethral stricture, and benign prostatic hyperplasia. Sonographic urodynamics reveals a failure of the distal half of the urethra to open adequately in patients with detrusor-sphincter dyssynergia (Fig. 8.4). The sonographic voiding cystourethrogram invariably demonstrates this functional disturbance as well as, or better than, the radiological voiding cystourethrogram (Fig. 8.5).

Sonographic urodynamics can help distinguish between urethral stricture and detrusor-sphincter dyssynergia. Although these can appear almost identical on a voiding cystourethrogram, an EMG will reveal the difference. Electrical activity increases when a patient with detrusor-sphincter dyssynergia tries to void, but ceases in a patient with stricture, since in the latter case the periurethral striated sphincter is relaxed.

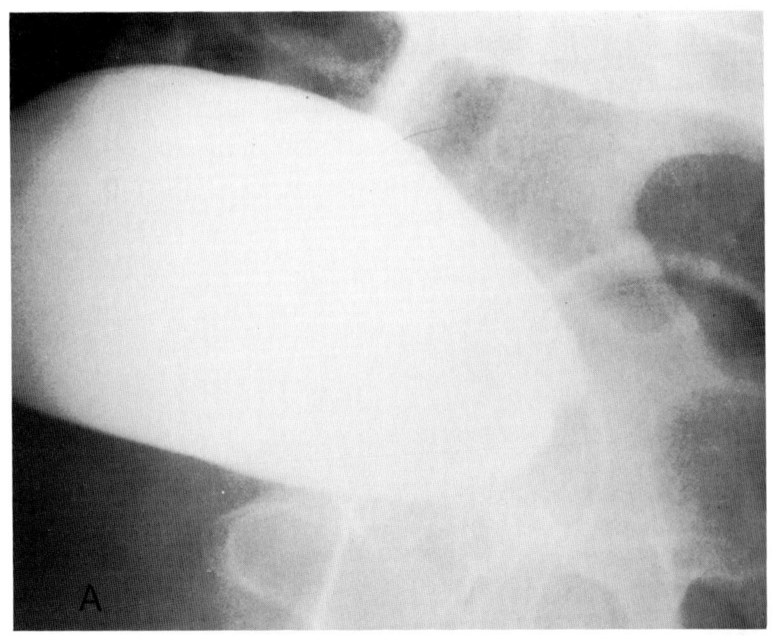

FIG. 8.3. Ledge posteriorly at the bladder neck due to the trauma of intermittent catheterization. (A) Radiological voiding cystourethrogram. The bladder neck fails to open. (B) Sonographic voiding cystourethrogram demonstrates that the bladder neck does open, but that there is a valvelike ledge posteriorly at the bladder neck, which had caused the obstruction seen in part A. Cases such as this would have formerly been misdiagnosed as detrusor bladder-neck dyssynergia, and the wrong therapy would have been administered.

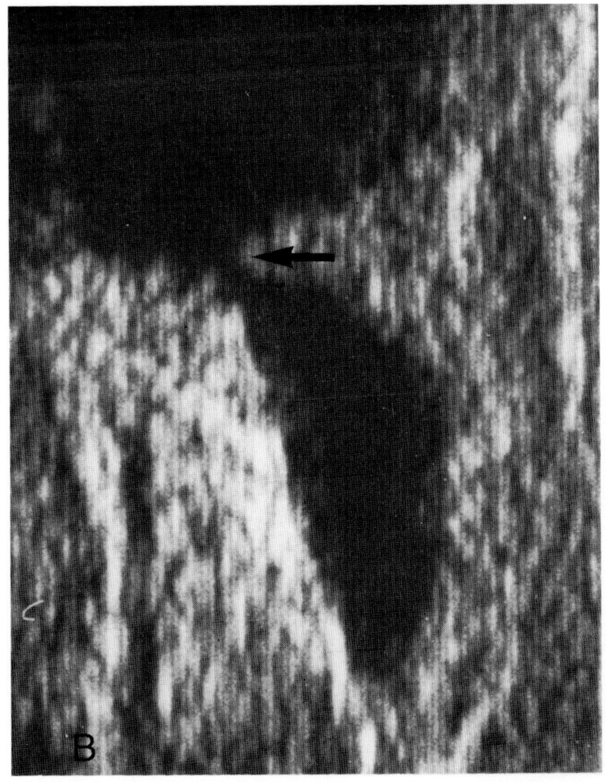

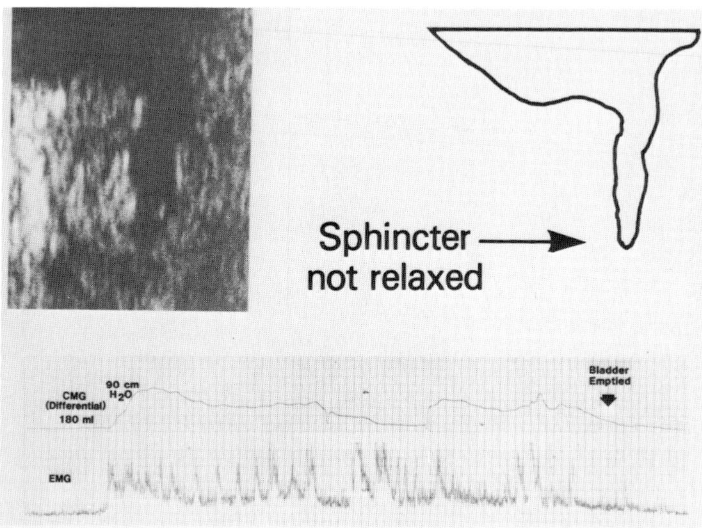

FIG. 8.4. Detrusor-sphincter dyssynergia. Simultaneous sonographic voiding cysto-urethrogram (top left) and differential cystometrogram (CMG) and electromyogram of the periurethral striated sphincter (bottom) performed on a patient with detrusor-sphincter dyssynergia. Note that the periurethral striated sphincter, which surrounds the lower two-thirds of the posterior urethra, fails to relax when the detrusor contracts.

Iatrogenic Hyperreflexia

Sonographic urodynamics has also made possible a new finding, that introducing a catheter into the bladder can make a reflex bladder hyperreflexic.[4] When catheters are introduced, they irritate these bladders, causing them to contract, even when very little fluid is present. Our patients who had hyperreflexic bladders when the catheter was introduced were later studied sonographically without catheters, and in about half the cases the apparent hyperreflexia disappeared (Fig. 8.6).

Bladder Saccules and Diverticula

Transrectal sonography clearly demonstrates bladder saccules and diverticula (Figs. 8.2, 8.7).

How to Investigate Patients with Neuromuscular Dysfunction of the Bladder

Our current approach is that, if the patient is able to walk, but neuromuscular dysfunction of the bladder is suspected, the patient should have a neurological examination, and a neurourological examination, and the voiding flow rate

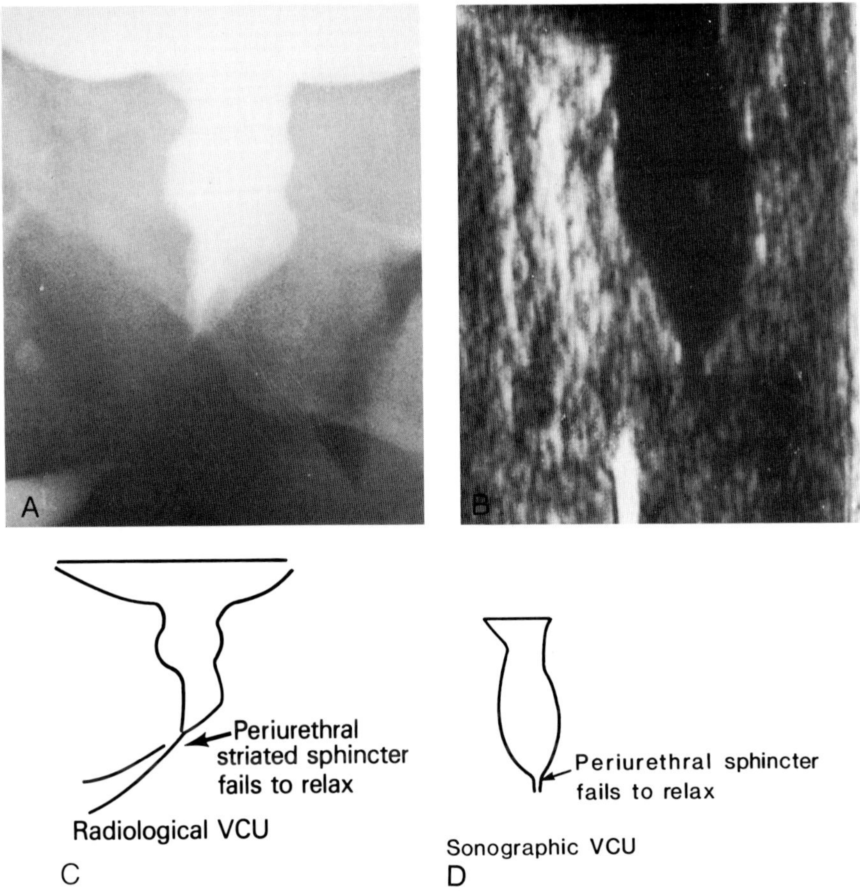

FIG. 8.5. Comparison of sonographic and radiographic voiding cystourethrogram in a patient with detrusor-sphincter dyssynergia. The sonographic study (B) demonstrates the detrusor-sphincter dyssynergia as well as the radiological study (A). (C) and (D) diagrammatic illustrations of parts (A) and (B).

should be measured. If these examinations are normal, the patient does not have neuromuscular dysfunction of the bladder. If the patient is paralyzed, or if the results from these tests are abnormal, the patient has neuromuscular dysfunction of the bladder, at which point we do an EMG of the periurethral striated sphincter and a simultaneous sonographic voiding cystourethrogram. If there is no dyssynergia, and if the bladder neck and urethra appear normal, there is no need for further investigation. If there is dyssynergia or if the bladder neck and urethra are abnormal, or if there is a large amount of urine remaining in the bladder after the patient has voided, a cystometrogram should be done. If that examination shows the bladder pressure is normal, there is

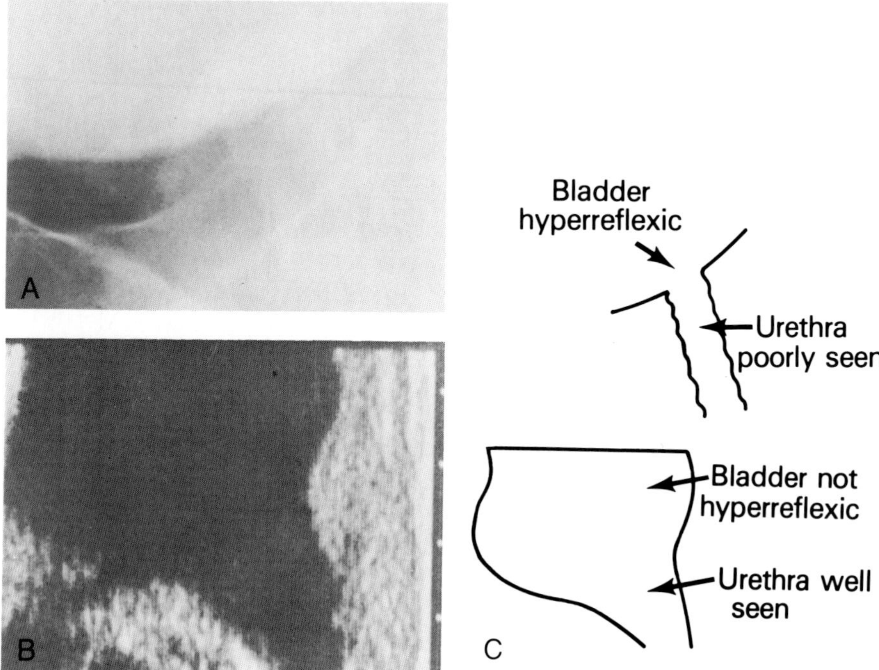

FIG. 8.6. Detrusor hyperreflexia. Radiological voiding cystourethrogram (A) does not show the bladder neck and posterior urethra well because the catheter has caused hyperreflexia. A sonographic voiding cystourethrogram performed in the same patient without a catheter (B) shows a wide bladder neck and posterior urethra. (C) Diagrammatic illustration of parts (A) and (B).

no need to investigate further, but if the bladder pressure is high, a radiological voiding cystourethrogram should be performed to check for reflux.

Management

Sonographic urodynamics can play at least three important roles in patient management. First, if the urologist thinks a sphincterotomy is necessary, sonographic urodynamics can direct the urologist about where and how to cut most appropriately. Second, if the patient is receiving drug therapy, sonographic urodynamics can help titrate the appropriate dose with great accuracy. Finally, the examination can help patients to retrain themselves to void after surgical or drug treatment.

The examination can aid the urologist in the following way: sonography can help locate precisely where the tip of the catheter is at any given moment while pressures are being recorded; if, for example, the catheter tip is in the urethra, its exact distance from the bladder neck can be measured. Thus, for

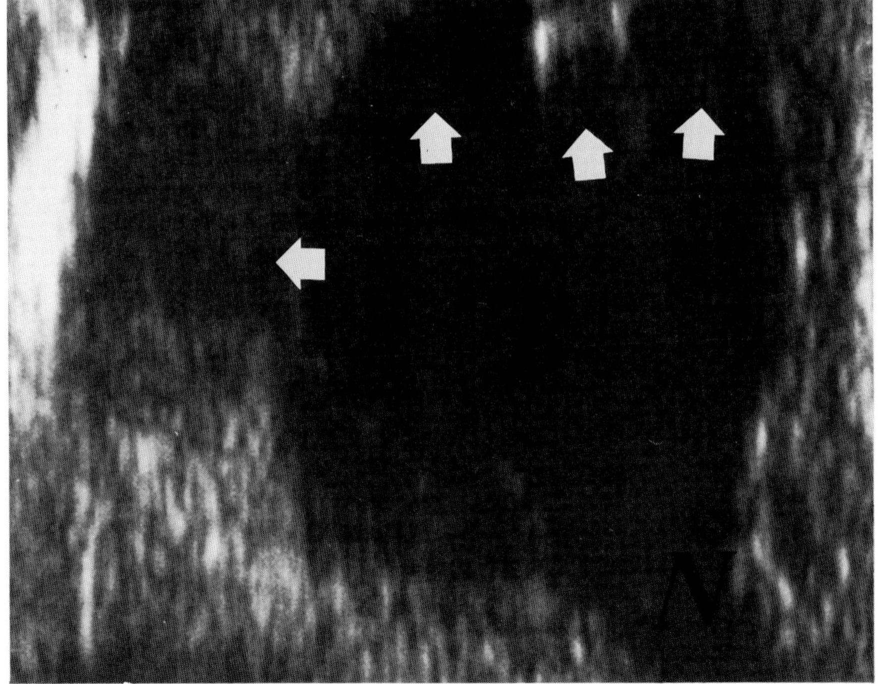

FIG. 8.7. Transrectal sonography showing several bladder diverticula (arrows). (B = bladder; N = bladder neck.)

the first time it is possible to determine exactly where abnormal pressures within the urethra are occurring, so that the results of this examination can help the urologist to determine whether to cut the bladder neck only, the periurethral striated sphincter only, or both. Previously, pressures were measured at multiple sites blindly or continuously while the catheter was being pulled out of the bladder and urethra, but either method is highly inaccurate as compared with this newer one.

If a patient with detrusor-bladder-neck dyssynergia has been given intravenous phentolamine, and the bladder neck relaxes, the patient can be treated further with oral prazocine. But it takes 2 to 3 days for that drug to take full effect; when that period has elapsed, sonographic urodynamics can be used to determine whether the bladder neck is as open as it had been under intravenous phentolamine. If it is not, the dosage can be increased; if it is, the dosage given was appropriate. In this way, sonographic urodynamics can help determine the results of drug therapy.

Sonographic urodynamics is extremely valuable for bladder retraining. Because of the urethral angle (Fig. 8.1) and the urethrosphincteric guarding reflex (Fig. 8.8),[2] the Credé maneuver tends to close the bladder neck in these patients, not open it. Suprapubic tapping, on the other hand, opens the bladder neck and posterior urethra. The tapping helps the patient initiate voiding, because

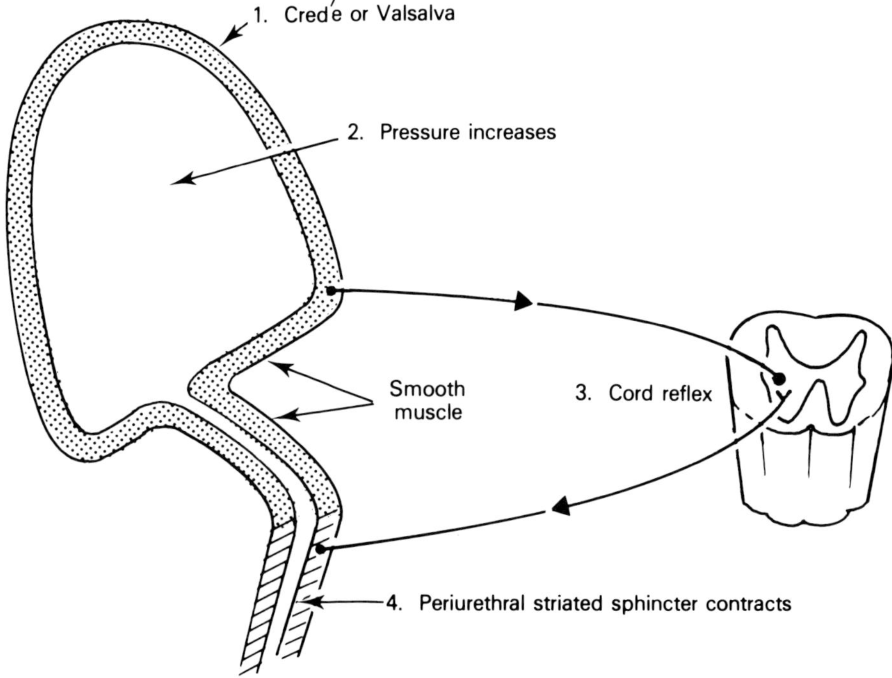

FIG. 8.8. The urethrosphincteric guarding reflex. When patients with an upper motor neuron lesion perform the Credé or Valsalva maneuver, the periuretheral striated sphincter contracts.

the periurethral striated sphincter contracts each time the patient taps; furthermore, striated muscle, unlike smooth muscle, becomes tired with repeated contractions, and will eventually relax after repeated contractions, in this case enabling the patient to void. As this procedure also does not elevate the bladder pressure as much as the Credé maneuver, it does not close the urethra. We therefore ask our patients to watch the video monitor during sonographic urodynamics, and they find that by tapping appropriately, they can learn to void. This tapping procedure is usually ineffective in two groups of patients: those with detrusor-bladder-neck dyssynergia where the muscle involved is smooth, not striated, and therefore will not relax with repeated contractions; and those patients with lower motor neurons lesions in whom the bladder, the bladder neck and urethra are flexic in any case. All the latter patients need to void, therefore, is a simple push on the bladder (the Credé maneuver).

CONCLUSIONS

Sonographic urodynamics, using the equipment and procedures as described, is as good as and sometimes better than the radiological voiding cystourethrogram. The advantages, however, are many. It complements urodynamic studies very well, and it allows the examiner to determine precisely where the pressures are being monitored. It does not radiate the patient or the examiners. It can determine the effects of drugs on the bladder neck and urethra during the procedure, and it allows the physician to follow patients receiving drug therapy to see if the drug treatment is effective. It can be done without catheterizing the patient, thus minimizing the risk of catheter-induced infection. Patients can be taught to retrain their bladders under sonographic control, and it permits the examination of soft tissue intraluminal projections and of the surrounding soft tissues as well.

For all these reasons, we are using this equipment and these procedures routinely at our institution, and have every confidence in their efficacy and safety.

ACKNOWLEDGMENT

We wish to thank Vickie Wolfe, R.N., for technical assistance.

REFERENCES

1. Friedland GW, Perkash I: Neuromuscular dysfunction of the bladder and urethra. Semin Roentgenol 18:255, 1983
2. Mahoney DT, LaFerte RO, Blais DJ: integral storage and voiding reflexes. Neurophysiologic concept of continence and micturition. Urology 9:95, 1977
3. McNeil JE: The prostate gland. Morphology and pathobiology. Monogr Urol 4:3, 1983
4. Shapeero LG, Friedland GW, Perkash I: Transrectal sonographic voiding cystourethrography. Studies in neuromuscular bladder dysfunction. AJR 141:83, 1983

9 Prostate Ultrasound

MATTHEW D. RIFKIN
ALFRED B. KURTZ

Prostatic malignancy is the second most common male cancer, with over 76,000 new cases and 25,000 deaths reported yearly.[1] Benign growth of the prostate is also very common, affecting over 80 percent of older men.[2] Although there are clinical symptoms that can be used to predict an enlarged prostate, including dysuria, frequency, and difficulty in attaining a normal urine flow, there are no specific signs of occult prostatic cancer. Clinically, the diagnosis of benign disease can often be suggested by rectal examination when the prostate feels rubbery and enlarged or by conventional imaging modalities where extrinsic compression upon the urinary bladder may be defined on an intravenous urogram or cystogram. Clinically, prostatic malignancy may be suspected only when a palpable hard area is noted on the rectal examination. Unsuspected metastatic prostatic disease may also be suggested by an elevation in the serum acid phosphatase levels. Radiographical evidence of adenopathy in the retroperitoneal and pelvic regions and sclerotic bone lesions are also suggestive but not diagnostic for prostatic carcinoma.

Although ultrasound can be utilized to demonstrate multiple processes involving the prostate, its major advantage is its ability to detect clinically unsuspected or subtle malignant changes of the gland. These small lesions are most commonly still contained within the prostatic capsule, and if they can be detected and removed prior to spread, prostatic carcinoma may be potentially curable.

ANATOMY

The prostate can be measured in three axes: the transverse (lateral), anteroposterior, and cephalocaudad. Normally the prostate measures approximately 4 cm in transverse diameter, 3.0 cm in anteroposterior dimension, and 3.8 cm in cephalocaudad projection,[3] and weighs approximately 20 g. It is situated in the pelvic cavity with the apex of the gland abutting the urogenital diaphragm. The posterior margin is adjacent to the anterior rectal wall, separated from it by Denonvilliers' fascia. The superoposterior portion is connected to the seminal vesicles, and the superoanterior margin is just inferior to the base of the urinary bladder.[5] The anterior prostatic margins abut on a collection of veins, fat, fascia, and vessels, termed the "anterior prostatic fat," and the lateral margins are bordered by the levator ani and obturator internus muscles (Fig. 9.1).[6]

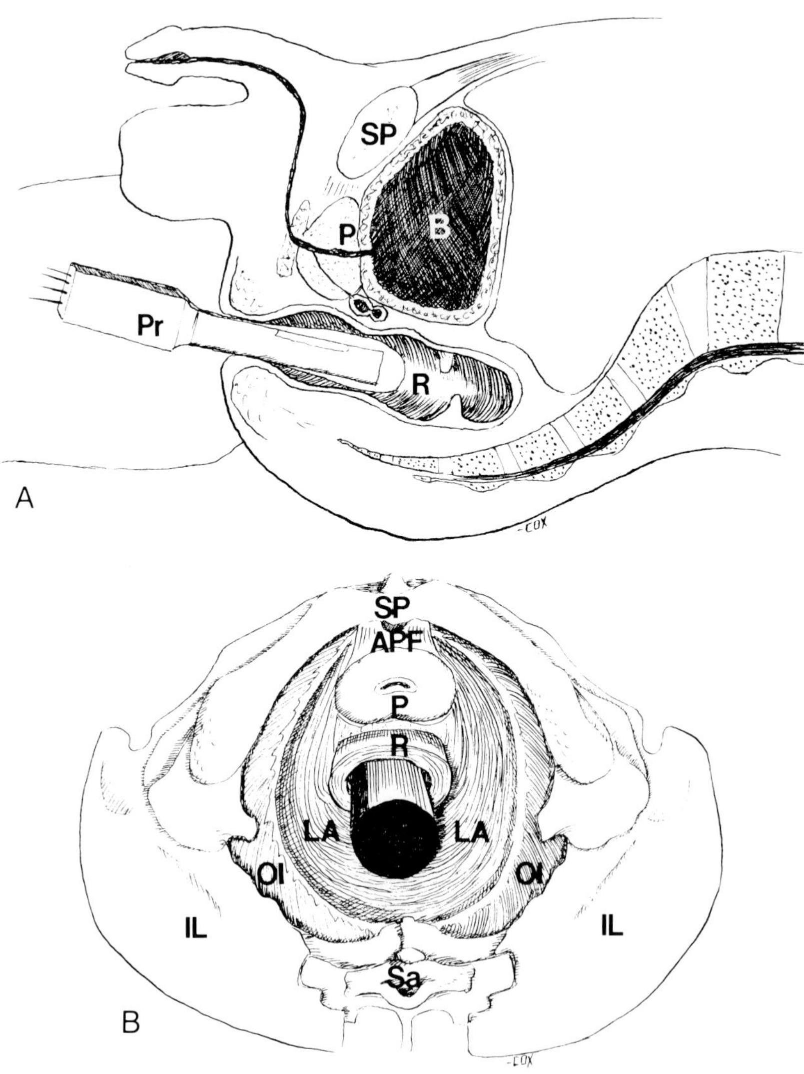

FIG. 9.1. Normal anatomy. (A) Line diagrams in sagittal and (B) transverse orientations with probes in the rectum (R) demonstrates normal anatomical orientation of the prostate (P). SP = symphysis pubis; B = bladder; P = prostate; R = rectum; Pr = probe; LA = levator ani muscle; OI = obturator internus muscle; IL = iliac bone; Sa = sacrum; APF = anterior prostatic fascia.

The prostate is enveloped by a thin, fibrous capsule, which is inseparable from the prostatic tissue.

The normal prostatic urethra courses in the middle of the gland running parallel to the rectum. The bilaterally symmetrical ejaculatory ducts extend from the seminal vesicles just lateral to the midline, and both drain into the prostatic urethra near the verumontanum at the prostatic utricle.

Histologically, the gland can be separated into the inner and outer prostate. The outer portion comprises all the glandular tissue. This glandular portion of the prostate is divided into 16 to 32 ducts composed of tubular alveolar tissue, with the majority of the lining cells of the simple or pseudostratified columnar epithelium type. The cells produce semen which is secreted into the prostatic urethra at the level of the prostatic utricle.[7] The inner prostate (endoprostate) extends from the bladder neck to the area of the verumontanum. It consists of periurethral mucosal and submucosal glands which empty into the prostatic urethra.

The seminal vesicles, which may be lobulated or smooth, are usually symmetrical and situated at the superoposterior aspect of the prostate. They extend from the midline and course laterally, either abutting on the entire cephalad portion of the prostate, termed the "base," or separated from the gland by fat and fascial material. The vas deferens, which transports sperm from the testes and epididymi, inserts into the medial aspect of the prostate at the same level as do the seminal vesicles.

ULTRASOUND TECHNIQUES

There are various ultrasound approaches used to evaluate the prostate. The simplest is the suprapubic examination which uses standard contact or real-time gray scale equipment with 3.5- or 5.0-MHz transducers. Prior to the examination, the urinary bladder is distended with fluid. The transducer is then placed on the anterior abdominal wall just superior to the symphysis pubis and angled inferiorly. The prostate, particularly when enlarged, can be defined as a relatively homogeneous structure (Fig. 9.2). To visualize the seminal vesicle, the transducer is angled slightly cephalad to the prostate.[10,11]

The transperineal approach uses the same equipment as the abdominal approach. The urinary bladder must be distended. The transducer is placed on the perineum (between the scrotum and the anus) and is angled directly cephalad. The prostate, particularly when enlarged or when involved with hyperechoic foci, can be identified just superior to the urogenital diaphragm (Fig. 9.3). Because of its limited value, this approach will not be discussed further.

Commercially available sonoendoscopic probes can also be used for evaluation of the prostate. These are specially designed instruments which can be utilized by insertion into the urethra (the transurethral approach) or in the rectum (the transrectal examination) (Fig. 9.4).

The transurethral examination is usually performed simultaneously with cystoscopic evaluation. Following insertion of a large (24-French or larger) cystoscope or resectoscope into the urinary bladder, a specially designed transducer

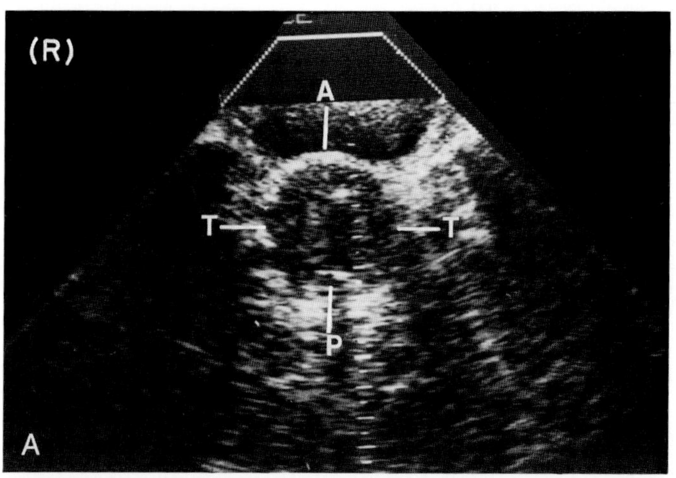

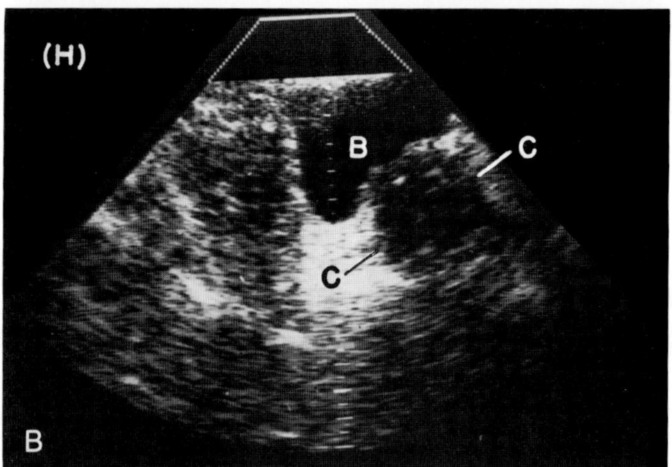

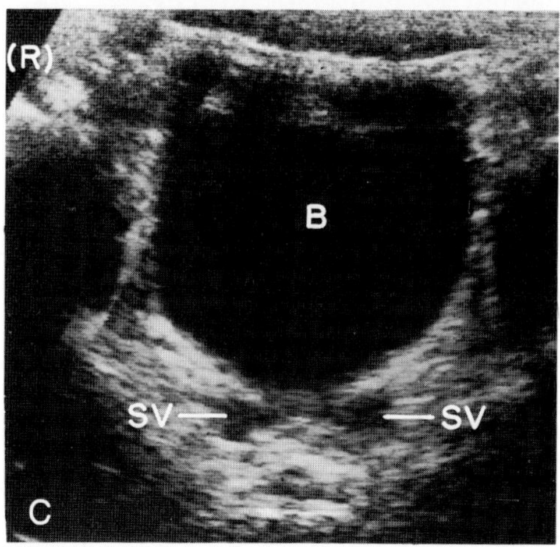

FIG. 9.2. Suprapubic prostate ultrasound. (A) Transverse and (B) longitudinal demonstrates the prostate to be defined through a fluid-filled urinary bladder (B). A hyperechoic focus is demonstrated. Without shadowing, calcification cannot be accurately assessed. Size measurements can be obtained by measuring the anteroposterior (AP) transverse (TT) and cephalocaudad (CC) dimensions. The seminal vesicles (SV) can best be demonstrated on (C) the transverse image just superior to the prostate. R = patient's right side; H = toward patient's head.

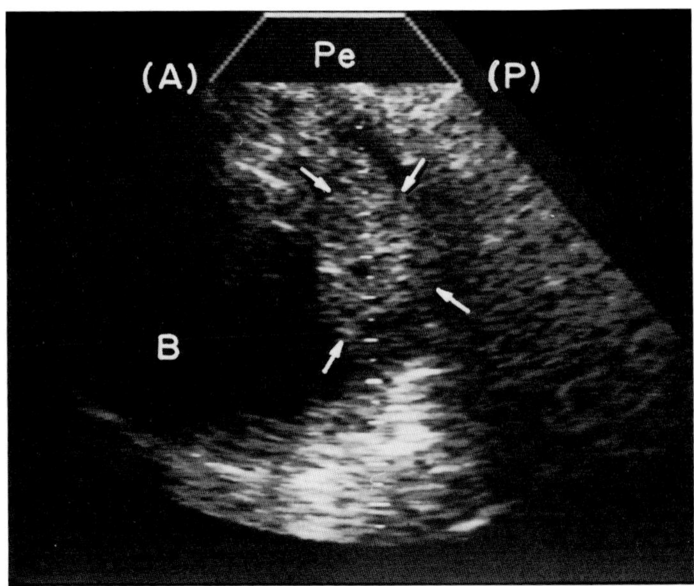

FIG. 9.3. Perineal prostate ultrasound. With the transducer placed on the perineum (Pe), the prostate (arrows) may be identified impinging upon the base of the fluid-filled urinary bladder (B). A = anterior aspect of patient; P = posterior aspect of patient.

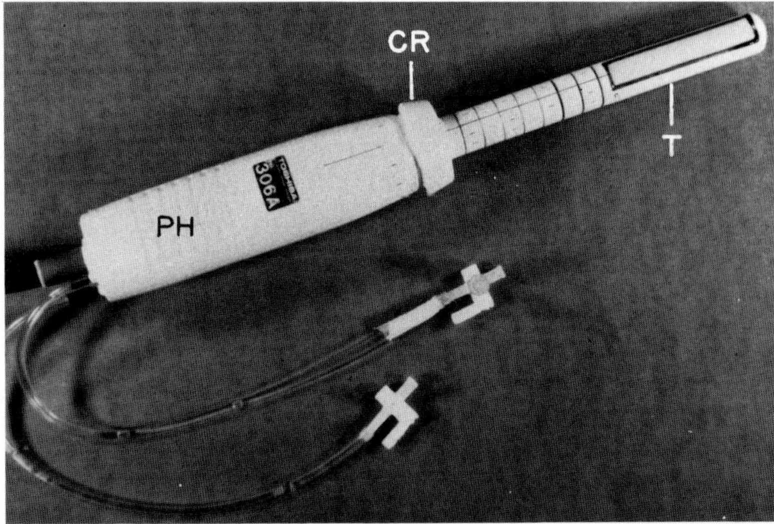

FIG. 9.4. Transrectal ultrasound probe. A longitudinal oriented linear-array endoscopic probe demonstrates the handle of the probe (PH) and the central ridge (CR) for securing the latex condom. The transducer crystals (T) are placed at the distal aspect of the insertable portion of the instrument.

is placed through the surgical instrument. The urinary bladder and the prostate can both be examined (Fig. 9.5). Once situated in the fluid-filled bladder, the transducer and cystoscope are removed slightly to examine the prostatic portion of the urethra and the prostate. Although commercially available units are restricted to the use of 5-MHz transducers, prototype equipment has a much wider variety of transducers. There are limitations to this procedure: First, imaging is only possible in transverse orientation ("radial" scanning plane). Second, because the examination is performed through the urethra, some peri-urethral prostatic abnormalities may not be imaged since the focal zone of these transducers is usually between 1 and 4 cm from the transducer surface. Third, this is an invasive procedure which requires either patient sedation or general anesthesia. This technique has limited value when compared with the transrectal scans for diagnosing prostatic lesions. As a result, it too will not be discussed further.

The transrectal sonoendoscopic approach requires no sedation. Commercially available units orient the image in either the radial (transverse) or longitudinal plane. No equipment is presently available which can image the prostate in both projections. The radial scans use 3.5- or 5.0-MHz transducers, although

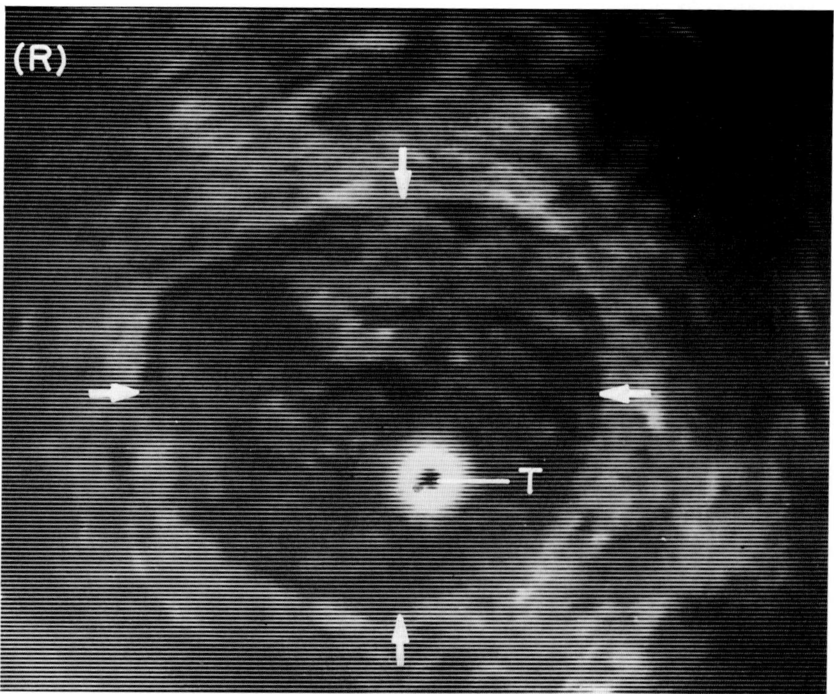

FIG. 9.5.   Transurethral prostate ultrasound. With the endoscopic probe with the transducer (T) placed within the urethra, the prostate (arrows) may be defined. The outer margins of the gland are clearly demonstrated. R = toward patient's right side.

higher-resolution prototype transducers are being developed. Images are generated at speeds of 1 to 10/sec, depending upon the equipment. The longitudially oriented images utilize a linear-array real-time system and are presently available with a choice of either 3.5- or 5.0-MHz transducer crystals.

The transrectal study can be performed in the lithotomy, lateral decubitus, or knee-chest positions. A digital rectal examination is performed prior to sonoendoscopic study to evaluate for prostatic impingement upon the rectum, possible rectal masses, or anal fissures, all of which may be relative contraindications to the procedure. Both types of transducers require the inserted portion of the probe be covered by a disposable rubber or latex condom which is secured at various places (depending upon the equipment) along the sonoendoscope probe. For proper acoustic contact, water is then inserted through specially designed orifices between the condom and the probe. The water is then removed, ensuring that no air remains to degrade the ultrasound image. Acoustic gel is then placed on the tip of the endoscope, and the probe is inserted into the rectum. Prior to insertion, the urinary bladder should be partly distended.

For the longitudinal examination, the endoscopic probe is placed deep enough into the rectum to identify the prostate. The probe is rotated clockwise and counterclockwise to evaluate the lateral lobes. If the entire gland cannot be demonstrated on a single image, the probe can be placed deeper to visualize the base of the gland.

When the transversely oriented radial units are used, the endoscopic probe should be placed deep enough into the rectum so that the fluid-filled urinary bladder can be identified. The probe is then withdrawn at 0.25- to 0.5-cm intervals until the seminal vesicles, the base of the prostate, the midportion of the gland, and finally the apex are identified and evaluated.

NORMAL ULTRASOUND IMAGING

The suprapubic abdominal approach images the prostate as a homogeneous structure with uniform low-level acoustic reflectivity. It is usually rounded or slightly ovoid in shape. The seminal vesicles are the same echogenicity or slightly less than the prostate. They may be demonstrated just superior to the prostate as symmetrically shaped structures extending laterally in a bow-tie or tubular configuration. The longitudinal image will demonstrate the seminal vesicle as a triangular protuberance extending from and often sonographically inseparable from the superior aspect of the prostate (Fig. 9.6A). Identification of the prostatic urethra is not possible by the suprapubic approach.[10]

The transrectal radial scan demonstrates the prostate as a symmetric, crescent-shaped, slightly ovoid gland with triangular-shaped posterolateral margins. The echogenicity is homogeneous and of moderate-to-low-level acoustic reflectivity.[12-15]

In certain instances, the endoprostate (inner prostate) can be identified as a slightly hypoechoic structure at the anterior periurethral region near the base of the gland (Fig. 9.6B).[16] The prostate broadens at the level of the midpor-

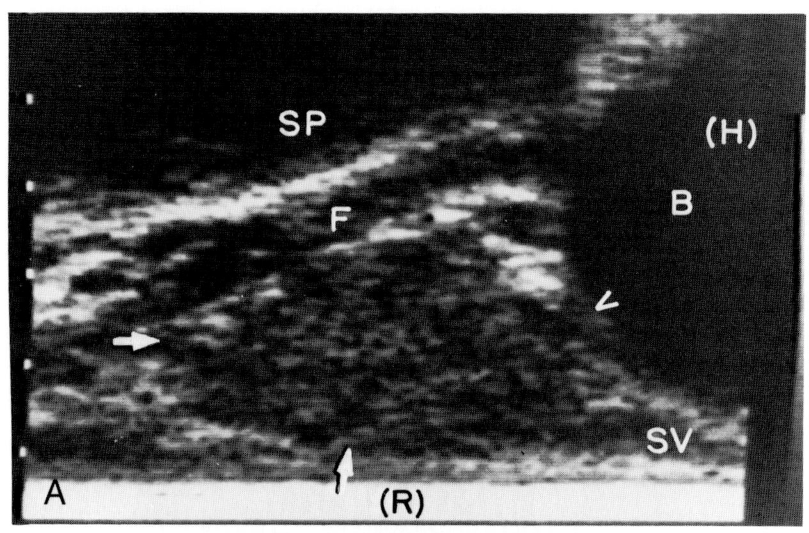

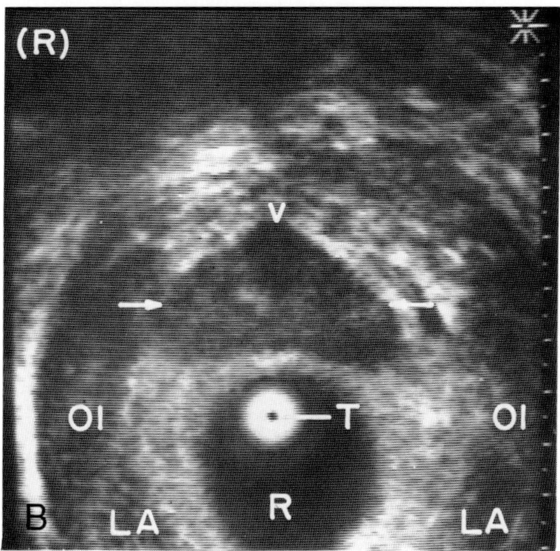

FIG. 9.6. Normal prostate. (A) Longitudinal-oriented transrectal prostate ultrasound with the transducer placed in the rectum (R), the prostate (arrows) is defined with low-level homogeneous echogenicity. The seminal vesicle (SV) is extending from the superior margin of the prostate, anterior to the rectum and posterior to the fluid-filled urinary bladder (B). The anterior prostatic fat (F) is situated between the prostate and the symphysis pubis (SP). The inner prostate (arrowhead) may be identified as a slightly hypoechoic structure at the area of the proximal urethra. H = toward patient's head. (B) Transrectal radial examination with the transducer (T) placed in the rectum (R), the acoustically homogeneous prostate (arrows) is defined. The hypoechoic inner prostate (arrowhead) is also demonstrated. The levator ani (LA) and obturator internus muscles (OI) are clearly demonstrated. (R) = toward patient's head.

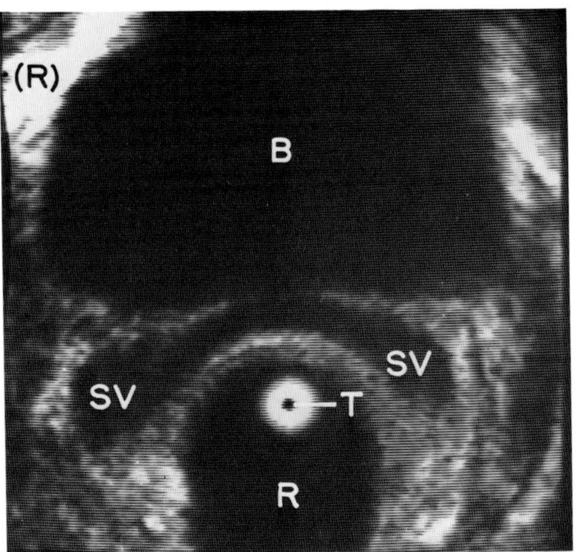

FIG. 9.7. Normal seminal vesicle—transrectal ultrasound radial approach. With the transducer (T) placed deeper in the rectum (R), the seminal vesicles (SV) are demonstrated posterior to the fluid-filled urinary bladder (B). R = toward patient's right side.

tion of the gland and narrows toward the apex, its caudal margin. The thin, fibrous capsule is not distinctly identified, but a combination of capsule and pericapsular tissue yields a bright hyperechoic margin. The prostatic margin at its base and apex are indistinctly seen. The normal prostatic urethra is usually not demonstrated. With the probe placed more deeply in the rectum, the normal

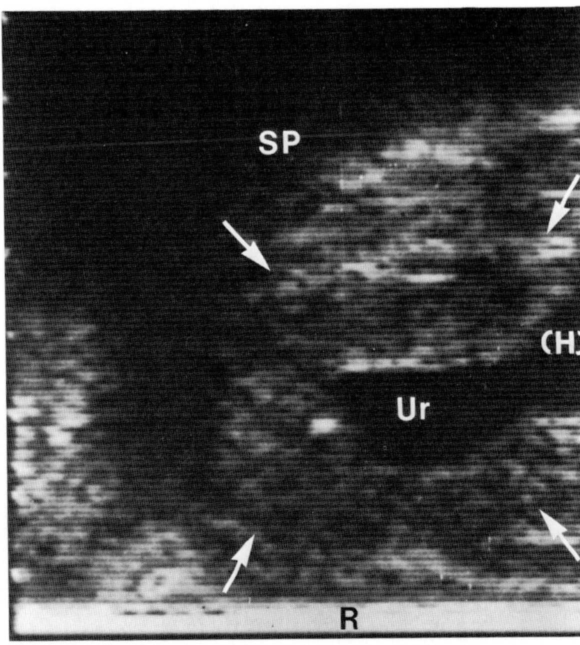

FIG. 9.8. Prostate ultrasound following transurethral resection of the prostate. A longitudinally oriented prostate ultrasound with the probe placed in the rectum (R) demonstrates the prostate (arrows) and the dilated proximal urethra (Ur) following partial resection of the gland. H = toward patient's head; SP = symphysis pubis.

seminal vesicles may appear bow-tie shaped, rounded, lobulated, or flattened (Fig. 9.7). They may extend directly lateral or surround the anterior rectal margin. The vas deferens may be seen as a rounded area toward its insertion at the medial aspect of the seminal vesicles. The surrounding pelvic musculature, the obturator internus and levator ani muscles, is usually well-defined posterolateral to the prostate.

Aside from different scanner orientation, the sonographic characteristics of the prostate are similar for the longitudinal linear array.[6,17,18] The normal prostate is rounded but has the same echogenicity. The peripheral zones are visualized, but the lateral capsule is not well seen. The margins of the apex and base are clearly demarcated. The seminal vesicles appear rounded and slightly more hypoechoic than the adjacent prostate. Unlike the radial scans, the prostatic urethra is well visualized. When empty, the prostatic urethra may be defined as parallel linear acoustic reflections representing the apposed walls of the tubular structure.[6] Similarly, portions of the ejaculatory ducts may be defined as acoustic reflectors parallel to the prostatic urethra. This appearance, similar to the empty urethra, is also due to reflections from the empty, apposed walls of the ducts. When distended with urine, while voiding or following a transurethral prostate resection, the bladder neck, proximal prostatic urethra, the area of the verumontanum, and the distal prostatic urethra immediately superior to the urogenital diaphragm are also identified (Fig. 9.8). In addition, the hypoechoic area of the endoprostate is also imaged with the linear-array scanner, at the superoanterior aspect of the gland. The adjacent pelvic musculature is not as clearly identified.

EVALUATION OF PROSTATE SIZE

An accurate preoperative estimation of the prostatic size and weight can help the urologist plan appropriate treatment. It has been suggested that glands larger than 60 g are more easily resected using a supra- or retropubic approach for the prostatectomy. Those with smaller glands, however, can be adequately treated by the transurethral approach.[19,20] Because of frequent asymmetrical enlargement, evaluation of prostatic size is highly inaccurate using conventional physical examination[21] and radiographic techniques.[22]

Ultrasound, on the other hand, has been shown to have a high degree of accuracy in predicting prostatic size and weight. The abdominal suprapubic approach is the easiest method to use. Transverse and longitudinal images are obtained (Fig. 9.2). When the gland is spherical in shape, a single radius can be measured with the formula for a sphere employed[23]

$$\text{Size} = 4/3\pi R^3$$

Since the specific gravity of prostatic tissue is 1.05 g/CC^3, the size of the gland is approximately equal to the weight. When the gland is asymmetrical in shape, the three different radii must be calculated separately[24]

$$\text{Weight} = 4/3\pi(R_1 R_2 R_3)$$

TABLE 9.1   Prostatic size—suprapubic sonogram

Degree of size	Diameter (cm)	Weight (g)
I	3.0–3.8	30
II	3.8–4.5	30–50
III	4.5–5.5	50–80
IV	>5.5	>85

Source: Aguirre CR, Tallada MB, Mayayo TD, Peroles LC, Romero JM: Evaluation comparison de volume protastique par l'echographie transabdominale, le profile uretral et la radiologie. J Urol 86:675, 1980.

Where R_1 = transverse radius, R_2 = longitudinal radius, and R_3 = lateral radius.

A further simplification of the technique has been recommended to assess prostatic size. The gland is examined in transverse orientation and an average of the two radii calculated. A chart has been prepared for rapid estimation of prostate weight (Table 9.1).[22]

The transrectal examinations require planimetric computation utilizing microprocessors.[25,26] This process is time consuming and more complicated than the simple abdominal approach.

BENIGN DISEASE

Benign prostatic hypertrophy can be subclassified into five distinct pathological entities, all with the same acoustic appearances.[27] All examples of prostatic hypertrophy originate from the inner, periurethral glandular tissue (central zone).[9] It should be stressed that it is the periurethral and mucosal tissue that hypertrophies sometimes asymmetrically, and that this may simulate specific lobar enlargement. The old description of actual enlargement of the middle lobe, anterior lobe, and so on is therefore inaccurate, as these specific lobes do not enlarge. The terminology is so ingrained, however, that it is still used today.

Any of the sonographic techniques described above can define the hypertrophied prostate, but with varying accuracy. The suprapubic sonogram can demonstrate the size and shape of the gland and image a diffusely altered and inhomogeneous acoustic texture (Fig. 9.9). Bright echogenic foci that shadow have been identified and are consistent with calculi. The suprapubic sonogram, however, often cannot consistently distinguish subtle benign nodules from the normal gland.[10]

Prostatic calculi are not diagnostic of specific disease processes. They may be seen as sequelae of prostatitis, healed necrosis, or as a nonspecific finding in benign hypertrophy. They may represent calcification of corpora amylacea, a proteinaceous material usually present within the normal prostate. Calculi are almost always related to benign diseases, although malignancy may occasionally but totally coincidentally develop in an area of previous calcification.[18]

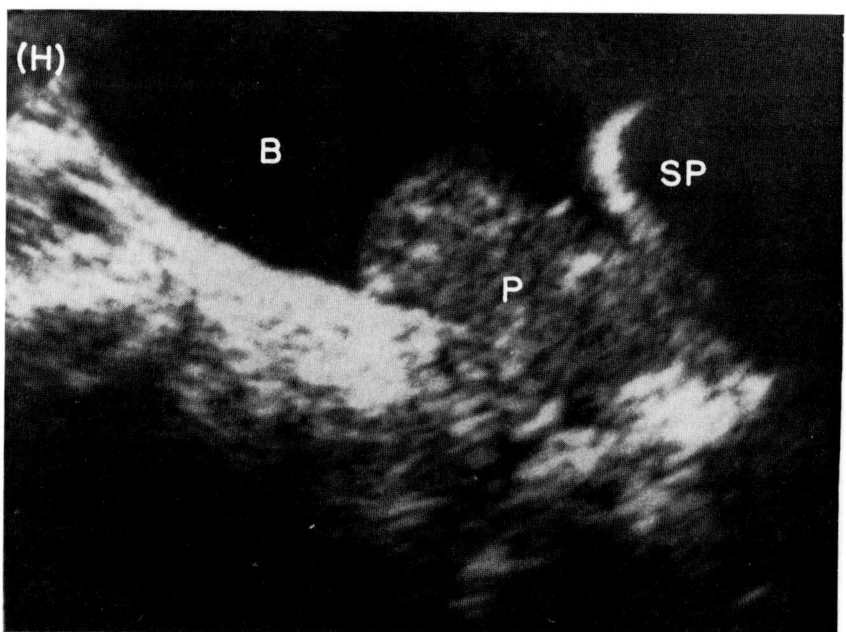

FIG. 9.9.   Benign prostatic hypertrophy, abdominal ultrasound. A large, echogenically homogeneous prostate (P) is noted impinging upon the urinary bladder (B) on this longitudinally oriented abdominal ultrasound. Bright acoustic reflectors and shadowing from the symphysis pubis (SP) are noted. H = toward patient's head.

A further distinction is that calculi most often develop, however, in the periurethral tissue, whereas malignancy occurs in the peripheral tissues. Unfortunately, there is overlap. Without shadowing on the sonogram, calculi cannot be definitively diagnosed, and thus the differentiation of the benign focus from cancer may not be possible.[18]

The transrectal ultrasound examination can often define benign prostatic hypertrophy. Both diffuse involvement and focal well-defined nodules (Fig. 9.10) have been demonstrated.[18,28] In addition, poorly demarcated benign nodules have also been encountered (Figs. 9.11 and 9.12). Any of these areas may be purely hypoechoic, of mixed acoustic reflectivity, or completely hyperechoic.[12,13,18,28,29] Although hypertrophy may appear sonographically to be situated anywhere within the gland, histologically it occurs in the periurethral area (Fig. 9.10). As these areas enlarge, they can distort the prostatic urethra and the peripheral portions of the prostate.

The foci or small areas within the hypertrophied nodules are important to analyze. The majority of these benign foci are hyperechoic. They are often thick scattered or diffusely bright (Table 9.2). Thin, subtly hyperechoic foci have also been described with benign disease, but are more frequently seen in cancer (Table 9.3).[18] Focal hypoechoic or isoechoic lesions may also be seen

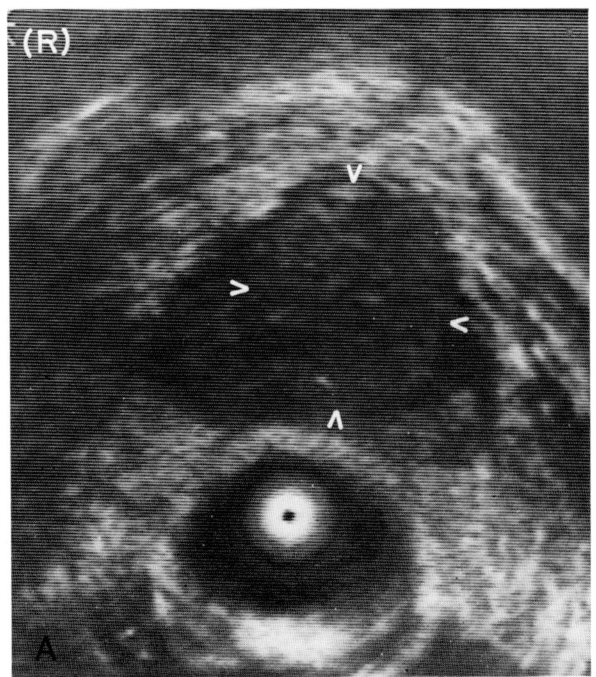

FIG. 9.10. Benign prostatic hypertrophy—transrectal ultrasound. (A) The transrectal transversely oriented ultrasound demonstrates a well-defined acoustically homogeneous nodule (arrowheads) situated in the region of the inner prostate. (B) The longitudinally oriented linear-array approach images a large well-defined nodule (arrowheads) in the region of the endoprostate. The benign lesions assume the major portion of the prostate. The seminal vesicle (SV) is also defined superior to the prostate. R = rectum; H = toward patient's head; R = patient's right side.

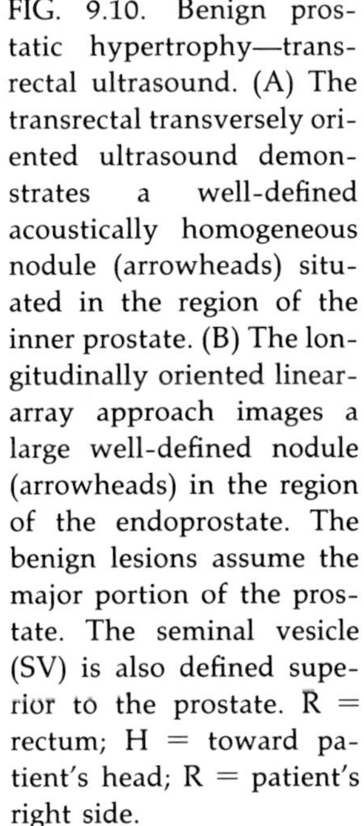

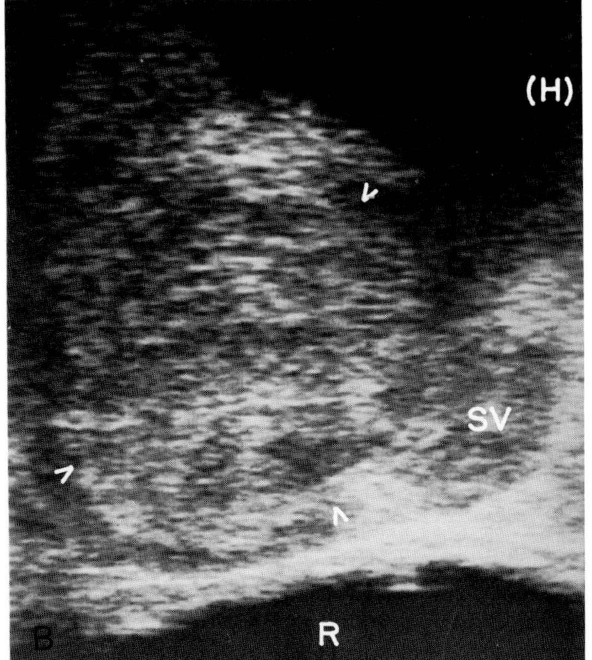

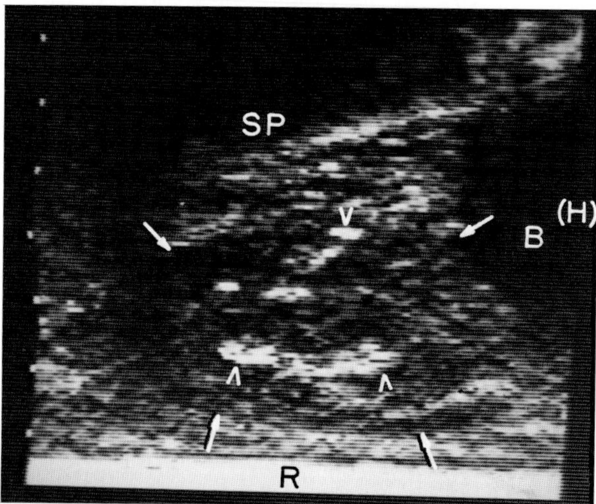

FIG. 9.11. Ill-defined hypertrophy. Longitudinally oriented transrectal ultrasound of the prostate (arrows) demonstrates grade III, thick and bright hyperechoic nonshadowing foci (arrowheads). These areas are not calcification and represent benign hypertrophy of the gland. R = rectum; SP = symphysis pubis; B = bladder; H = toward patient's head.

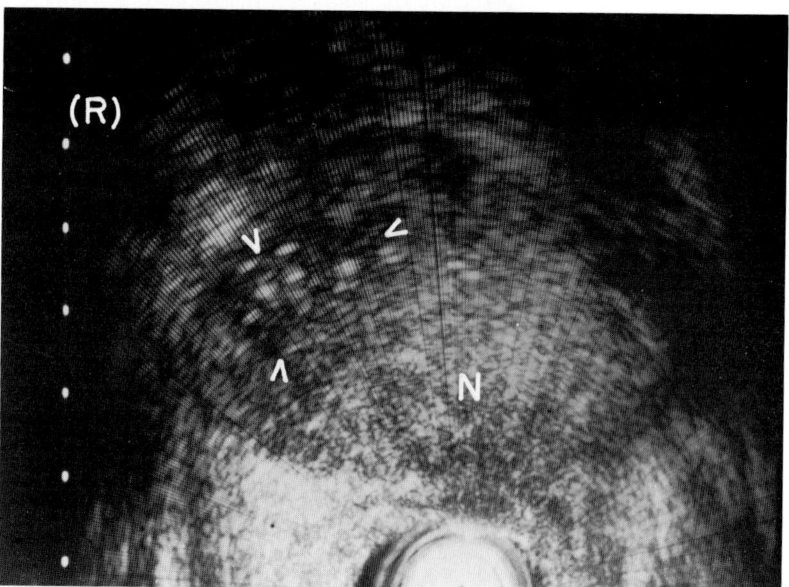

FIG. 9.12. Hypertrophy and prostatic carcinoma. A transversely oriented transrectal radial ultrasound of the prostate demonstrates a homogeneous but ill-defined benign nodule (N) of the prostate on the left side. There are scattered punctate hyperechoic grade I–II bright and thick foci (arrowheads) on the right side of the gland representing carcinoma. R = patient's right side.

**TABLE 9.2 Definition of echo thickness and brightness:
Transrectal prostate ultrasound**

Echo brightness
  I: Slightly more reflective than the acoustic texture of the normal
    prostate
  II: More reflective than I and less bright than III
  III: As hyperechoic as the reflection from the prostatic capsule
  IV: Brighter than the acoustic reflections from the prostate capsule
Echo thickness
  I: Punctate hyperechoic areas less than 2 mm in size; either separated
    or clustered
  II: Hyperechoic areas measuring 2 to 3 mm
  III: Hyperechoic foci as large as 3 to 4 mm
  IV: Hyperechoic foci greater than 4 mm in thickness

Source: Rifkin MD, Kurtz AB, Choi HY, Goldberg BB: Endoscopic ultrasonic evaluation of the prostate using a transrectal probe: Prospective evaluation and acoustic characterization. Radiology 149:265, 1983.

**TABLE 9.3 Acoustic characterization of the prostate:
Transrectal ultrasound**

	Benign disease foci (%)	Malignant foci (%)
Echo brightness		
I	7(15)	13(50)
II	8(17)	7(27)
III	14(29)	5(19)
IV	19(39)	1(4)
Echo thickness		
I	11(23)	16(62)
II	4(8)	6(23)
III	6(13)	4(15)
IV	27(56)	0(0)

Source: Rifkin MD, Kurtz AB, Choi HY, Goldberg BB: Endoscopic ultrasonic evaluation of the prostate using a transrectal probe: Prospective evaluation and acoustic characterization. Radiology 149:265, 1983.

in benign disease. When present, these lesions are often more clearly and sharply demarcated than the benign hyperechoic lesions.

PROSTATIC MALIGNANCY

Prostate cancer develops in the peripheral glandular tissue.[30] Although it had been previously stated that the posterior lobe was the major site to undergo malignant change, this was a clinical impression caused solely by the region of the prostate that could be palpated. It has now been shown that all the peripheral tissue (i.e., the posterior, lateral, and portions of the anterior lobes of the prostate) have equal propensity to develop cancer.[8]

The major benefit of prostatic ultrasound is the ability to demonstrate clinically unsuspected cancer. Although many of these subtle focal abnormalities may be malignant, there is, however, overlap with benign pathology. To differentiate the clinically nonpalpable lesions, an accurate biopsy technique is essential. Accurate ultrasound-guided biopsy techniques have been developed, are easily mastered, and will be described in the next section. While preliminary research with magnetic resonance imaging has suggested the possibility of detecting clinically unsuspected focal malignancy of the prostate, a biopsy to prove such pathology is often not possible.

PROSTATE BIOPSY

Transrectal ultrasound guidance can be used for a transperineal prostatic biopsy. Although the radial scan does utilize specially designed guides that can place the needle within suspected areas of abnormality, the needle is not defined until it has entered the suspicious area, and the tip may not always be identified.[31,32] Thus, deviation of the needle course cannot be ascertained, and alteration of the needle tract cannot be easily or quickly performed.

The longitudinally oriented linear-array examination permits immediate correction of an aberrantly placed needle. With the patient in the lithotomy position, the area of abnormality is ascertained with transrectal ultrasound. Under aseptic conditions, the biopsy needle, either small-gauge for cytological evaluation[33] or large bore[34,35] (i.e., a Travenol tru-cut needle) for tissue diagnosis can be utilized. The needle should be positioned in the midline of the perineum. As it is inserted, it is kept parallel to the course of the transrectal prostate probe until the needle tip is identified by sonography at the urogenital diaphragm. The needle is then advanced under continuous ultrasound guidance into the apical region of the prostate and placed into the suspected area of disease (Fig. 9.13). The course of the needle can be altered at any stage of the insertion as needed to perform the biopsy.[36,39]

Transrectal biopsy guides have also been developed for transrectal prostate biopsy. These require flexible needles; the largest presently available is 20 gauge. The needle is placed within the specially designed device over the linear-array sonoendoscopic probe. The needle curves as it is placed through the

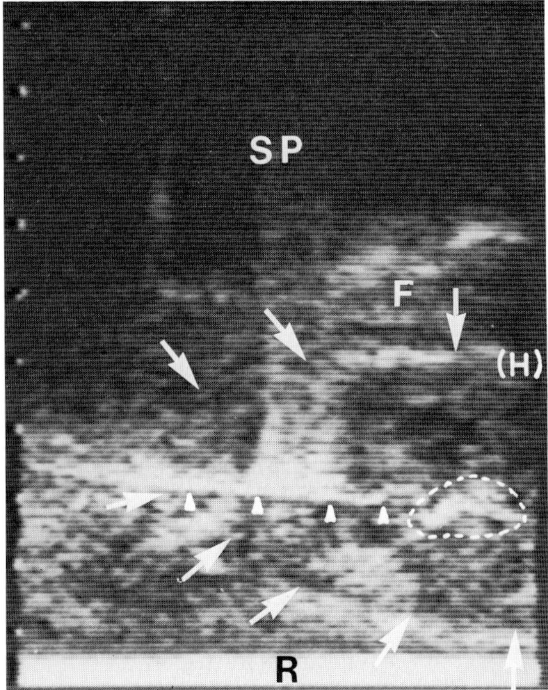

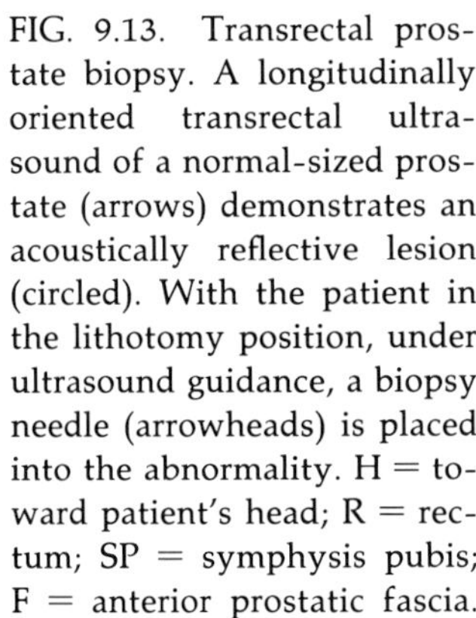
FIG. 9.13. Transrectal prostate biopsy. A longitudinally oriented transrectal ultrasound of a normal-sized prostate (arrows) demonstrates an acoustically reflective lesion (circled). With the patient in the lithotomy position, under ultrasound guidance, a biopsy needle (arrowheads) is placed into the abnormality. H = toward patient's head; R = rectum; SP = symphysis pubis; F = anterior prostatic fascia.

rectal mucosa, the rectal wall, and into the areas of prostatic abnormality. Tissue is then obtained for cytological and/or tissue diagnosis.

DIFFERENTIATION OF MALIGNANCY FROM BENIGN DISEASE

Large, diffuse prostatic cancers can be diagnosed with multiple imaging modalities, including computed tomography and magnetic resonance imaging. Both the radial and longitudinal linear-array examinations can define these areas of abnormality. The radial scan can define extension to the lateral wall to a better degree than the linear-array examination (Fig. 9.14).

The major benefit of transrectal prostate ultrasound is its ability to identify the clinically unsuspected or nonpalpable lesion or the subtly suspicious area that was palpated on digital rectal examination.[18] By defining these focal areas, biopsy with ultrasound guidance is then possible.

While malignancy may present as an irregular area of abnormal echogenicity compared to normal prostate, many untreated cancers will be seen as slightly more hyperechoic foci than the normal prostatic tissue. The foci are usually ill-defined with thin, punctate scattered areas (Fig. 9.15).[18] Only rarely is very thick and bright hyperechoic carcinoma defined (Table 9.3). Some cancers may change acoustic characteristics following treatment.

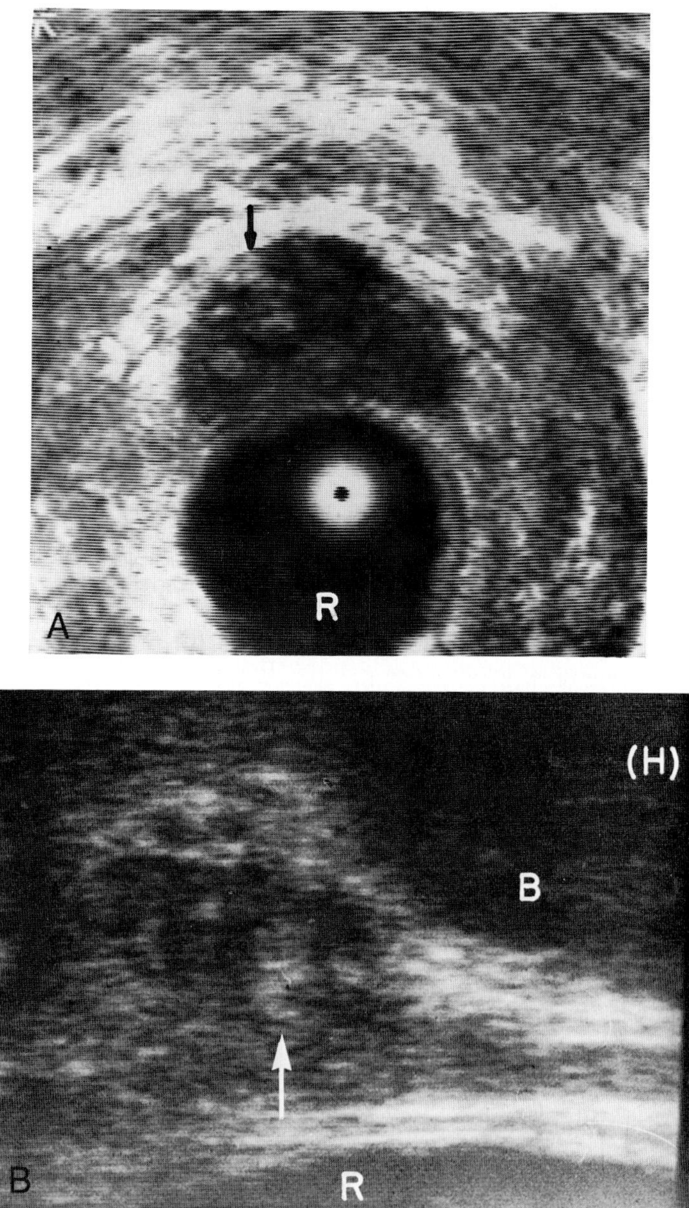

FIG. 9.14.   Prostate cancer. (A) A transrectal radial scan demonstrates an acoustically mixed lesion with a hyperechoic area (arrow) extending to, but not beyond, the right lateral margin of the prostate. (B) The longitudinally oriented image also demonstrates the scattered acoustic reflectors (arrow) due to malignancy but to the capsule is less clearly defined. R = rectum; B = bladder; H = toward patient's head.

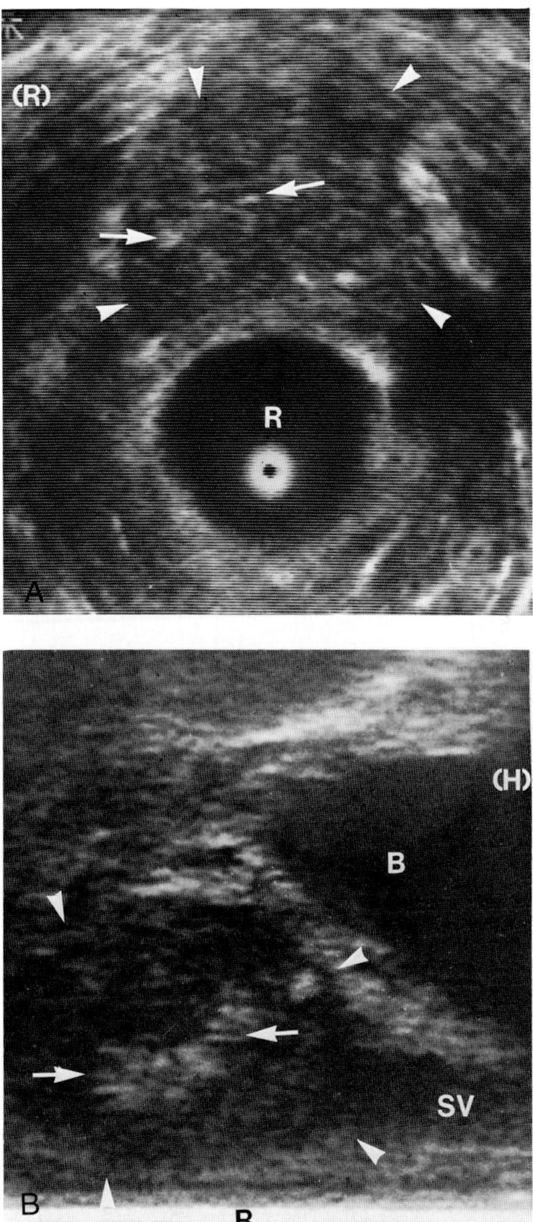

Carcinoma does not calcify. However, malignancy may develop, as previously described, in an area of previous dystrophic calcification. We have observed that calcifications are better defined on the linear-array examination than the radial approach (Fig. 9.16). This is most likely due to the physical features of reflections of the acoustic beam from the fluid-filled condom surrounding the tip of the probe. If a bright hyperechoic focus causes shadowing, the diagnosis of a prostatic stone is obvious. However, without shadowing, differentiation between other pathological processes, particularly carcinoma, cannot always be done by ultrasound.

It must be emphasized that there is some overlap between the benign lesion and malignancy. With the use of transrectal ultrasound-guided biopsies, however, focal areas of abnormality can be accurately diagnosed.[12-15,17,18,28,29]

Differentiating between prostatic carcinoma and benign prostatic hypertrophy may be suggested as follows:

1. Diffuse involvement suggests benign disease.
2. A well-defined nodule suggests benign disease.
3. Bright and thick hyperechoic foci suggest benign disease.
4. Shadowing from a hyperechoic focus is diagnostic of calcification, consistent with benign disease.
5. Cysts suggest benign disease (Fig. 9.17).

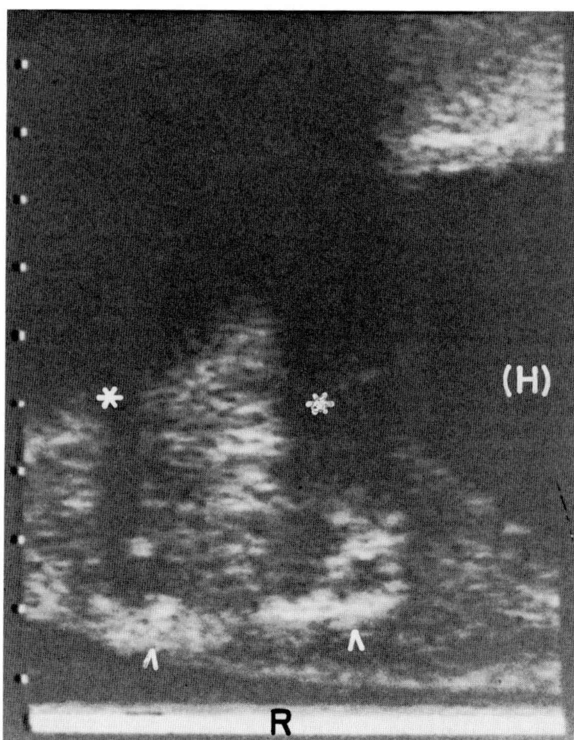

FIG. 9.16. Prostatic calculi. Longitudinally oriented linear array transrectal ultrasound of the prostate demonstrates bright echoes (arrowheads) with acoustic shadowing (*) from calculi. With the transducer in the rectum (R), acoustic shadowing or acoustic enhancement is noted extending toward the anterior abdominal wall. H = toward patient's head.

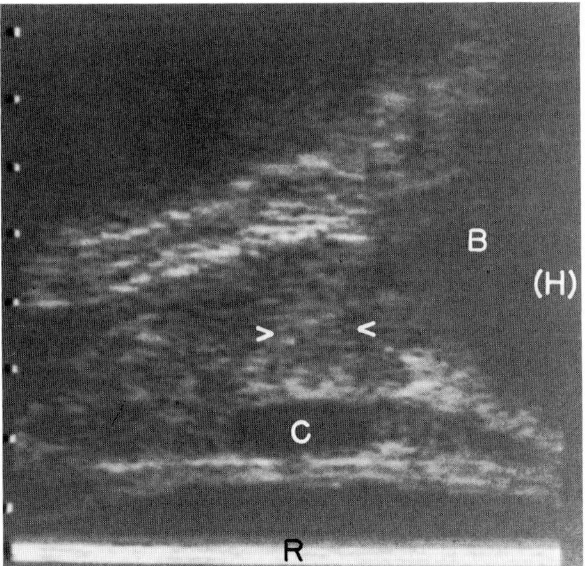

FIG. 9.17. Prostatic cyst. Longitudinally oriented transrectal examination demonstrates the probe and covering condom, which is distended with water, within the rectum (R). The prostate is not enlarged but a well-defined anechoic cyst (C) with sharp margination and posterior acoustic enhancement (arrowheads) is noted. A digital rectal examination was highly suspicious for malignancy which was not present. B = urinary bladder; H = toward patient's head.

6. An ill-defined area of subtle hyperechoic texture suggests malignancy, although benign disease may occasionally cause similar findings.

7. Irregular capsular margins suggest malignancy.

8. An ill-defined focus suggests malignancy.

The differences of the transrectal radial and transrectal linear-array approaches can be summarized as follows:

1. The radial scan can define the lateral margins of the gland better than the longitudinal examination.

2. The radial scan can define asymmetry and asymmetrical involvement of the prostate better than the longitudinal scan.

3. Periprostatic malignancy with invasion of the lateral capsule or pelvic musculature can be seen by the radial scan more accurately.

4. The linear-array longitudinal orientation can define the base and apex of the gland better than the radial scan.

5. The linear-array examination better defines prostatic calcifications.

6. Biopsies are more accurately performed with the longitudinal linear-array examination.

7. Both units can identify the anterior and posterior margins of the prostate.

8. Depending upon the resolution of the transducer, both techniques can define malignancy equally well.

In summary, ultrasound can accurately measure the size of the prostate, and transrectal ultrasound can clearly define areas of unsuspected or clinically suspected disease of the prostate better than any clinically available imaging instrumentation at this time. With transrectal longitudinal-oriented ultrasound, accurate biopsies of clinically nonpalpable lesions can be performed to secure needed tissue for definitive diagnosis.

REFERENCES

1. Silverberg E: Cancer statistics 1984. CA 34:7, 1984
2. Walsh PC: Benign prostatic hyperplasia. p. 949. In Campbell's Urology. 4th Ed. W.B. Saunders, Philadelphia, 1979
3. Snyder WS: Report of the Task Group on Reference Man. Pergamon Press, Oxford, 1974
4. Leissner KH, Tisell LE: The weight of the human prostate. Scand J Urol Nephrol 13:137, 1979
5. Gray H: Gray's Anatomy. 28th Ed. Goss CM (ed): Lea & Febiger, Philadelphia, 1966
6. Rifkin MD, Kurtz AB: Ultrasound of the Prostate. p. 95. Sanders RC (ed): In Ultrasound Annual 1983. Raven Press, New York, 1983
7. Weyrauch HM: Surgery of the Prostate. W.B. Saunders, Philadelphia, 1959
8. McNeal JE: Regional morphology and pathology of the prostate. Am J Clin Pathol 49:347, 1968
9. McNeal JE: The prostate and prostatic urethra: A morphologic synthesis. J Urol 107:1008, 1972
10. Greenberg M, Neiman HL, Brandt TD, Falkowski W, Carter M: Ultrasound of the prostate. Radiology 141:757, 1981
11. Greenberg M, Neiman HL, Vogelzang R, Falkowski W: Ultrasonographic features of prostatic carcinoma. J Clin Ultrasound 10:307, 1982
12. Peeling WB, Griffiths GJ, Evans KT, Roberts EE: Diagnosis and staging of prostatic cancer by transrectal ultrasonographic system. Ultrasound Med Biol 5:129, 1979
13. Gammelgaard J, Holm HH: Transurethral and transrectal ultrasonic scanning in urology. J Urol 124:683, 1980
14. Harada K, Tanahashi Y, Igari D, Numata I, Orikasa S: Clinical evaluation of inside echo patterns in gray scale prostatic echography. J Urol 124:216, 1980
15. Brooman PJC, Griffiths GJ, Roberts E, Peeling WB, Evans K: Per rectal ultrasound in the investigation of prostatic disease. Clin Radiol 32:669, 1981
16. Rifkin MD: The lower genitourinary tract and testes. p. 425. Goldberg BB (ed): In Abdominal Gray Scale Ultrasonography. 2nd Ed. John Wiley, New York, 1984
17. Sekine H, Oka K, Takehara Y: Transrectal longitudinal ultrasonotomography of the prostate by electronic linear scanning. J Urol 127:62, 1982
18. Rifkin MD, Kurtz AB, Choi HY, Goldberg BB: Endoscopic ultrasonic evaluation of the prostate using a transrectal probe: Prospective evaluation and acoustic characterization. Radiology 149:265, 1983
19. Hohenfellner R: Suprapubic prostatectomy. In Marberger H, Haschenk H, Schirmer HKA, Colston JAC, Witkin E, Liss AR, (eds): Prostatic Disease. A. R. Liss, New York, 1976
20. Melchior J, Valk WL, Foret JD, Mebust WK: Transurethral prostatectomy: Computerized analysis of 2,223 consecutive cases. J Urol 112:634, 1974
21. Bissada NK, Finkbeiner AE, Redman JF: Accuracy of preoperative estimation of resection weight in transurethral prostatectomy. J Urol 116:201, 1976
22. Aguirre CR, Tallada MB, Mayayo TD, Perales LC, Romero JM: Evaluation comparative du volume prostatique par l'echographie transabdominale, le profil uretral et la radiologie. J Urol. 86:675, 1980

23. Henneberry M, Carter MF, Neiman HL: Estimation of prostatic size by suprapubic ultrasonography. J Urol 121:615, 1979

24. Abu-Yousef MM, Narayana AS: Transabdominal ultrasound in the evaluation of prostate size. J Clin Ultrasound 10:275, 1982

25. Hastak SM, Gammelgaard J, Holm HH: Transrectal ultrasonic volume determination of the prostate—A preoperative and postoperative study. J Urol 127:1115, 1982

26. Bartsch G, Egender G, Hubscher H, Rohr H: Sonometrics of the prostate. J Urol 127:1119, 1982

27. Franks LM: Benign prostatic hyperplasia: Gross and microscopic anatomy. In p. 63. Grayhack JT, Wilson JD, Scherbenske MJ, (eds): Benign Prostatic Hyperplasia. NIH Workshop, DHEW Publication (NIH) 76–1113, 1975

28. Watanabe H, Saitoh M, Mishina T, Igari D, Tanahashi Y, Harada K, Hisamichi S: Mass screening program for prostatic diseases with transrectal ultrasonotomography. J Urol 117:746, 1977

29. Harada K, Igari D, Tanahashi Y: Gray scale transrectal ultrasonography of the prostate. J Clin Ultrasound 7:45, 1979

30. McNeal JE: Origin and development and carcinoma in the prostate. Cancer 23:24, 1969

31. Holm HH, Gammelgaard J: Ultrasonically guided precise needle placement in the prostate and the seminal vesicles. J Urol 125:385, 1981

32. Hastak SM, Gammelgaard J, Holm HH: Ultrasonically guided transperineal biopsy in the diagnosis of prostatic carcinoma. J Urol 128:69, 1982

33. Fornage BD, Touche DH, Deglaire M, Faroux MJC, Simatos A: Real-time ultrasound-guided prostatic biopsy using a new transrectal linear-array probe. Radiology 146:547, 1983

34. Rifkin MD, Kurtz AB, Goldberg BB: Sonographically guided transperineal prostatic biopsy: Preliminary experience with a longitudinal linear-array transducer. Am J Roentgenol 140:745, 1983

35. Rifkin MD, Kurtz AB, Goldberg BB: Prostate biopsy utilizing transrectal ultrasound guidance: Diagnosis of nonpalpable cancers. J Ultrasound Med 2:165, 1983

10 Scrotal Ultrasound

HEDVIG HRICAK
WILLIAM K. HODDICK

A variety of imaging modalities have been utilized to complement the clinical presentation and physical findings in the differential diagnosis of scrotal pathology. Clinical evaluation of intrascrotal pathology depends primarily on careful bimanual palpation. Clinical signs and symptoms are nonspecific, variable, and commonly misleading.[1] Radiological modalities including thermography, radionuclide scanning,[2] diagnostic ultrasound, and more recently magnetic resonance imaging[3] have all been described as valuable adjuncts in differentiating scrotal pathology.

Diagnostic ultrasound is exceptionally well suited for studying the scrotum.[4-20] Sonography is simple to perform, causes no patient discomfort, is noninvasive, relatively inexpensive, and widely available. When the clinical diagnosis is in question, sonography is a reliable adjunct in differentiating intra- and extratesticular causes of scrotal enlargement, evaluating various etiologies of painful scrotum (e.g., spermatic cord torsion versus epididymitis versus tumor), and determining testicular integrity in cases of trauma. Additionally, ultrasound is helpful in determining testicular size, searching for the undescended testicle, demonstrating occult testicular neoplasms, and following patients after unilateral orchiectomy for recurrent testicular neoplasms.

TECHNIQUE

A wide variety of ultrasound units have been utilized for scrotal scanning. Although dedicated high-resolution "small parts" scanners have been strongly advocated, it is not imperative to have access to a small parts scanner in order to evaluate the scrotum.[5-11] Static scanners or either linear-array or sector real-time scanners can reliably detect the majority of scrotal abnormalities. In general, high-frequency transducers are used, either 5.0, 7.5, or 10.0 MHz.[16,22] Because of the superficial position of the testes, beam attenuation is minimal, and short-focus high-frequency transducers are routinely employed for scanning. This minimizes near-field resolution problems. In exceptional cases, a

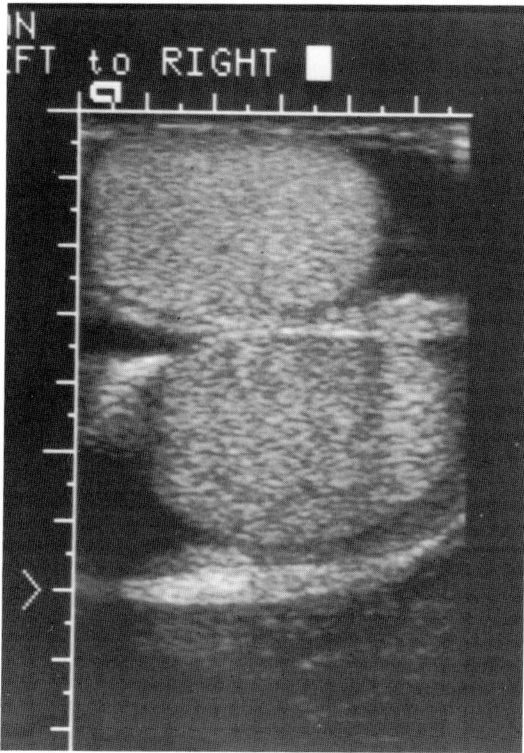

FIG. 10.1. Coronal scan facilitates visualization of the testicle, particularly when near-field resolution presents a problem. Note the small bilateral hydroceles.

small-diameter probe can be utilized. Additionally, scanning using the contralateral testis as an acoustic window (coronal orientation) may prove useful (Fig. 10.1).

A number of sonographic techniques have been used, including water-immersion scanning, water-path scanning, and contact scanning.[4,10,22]

Water-immersion techniques require a special form of equipment in which the transducer is actually within the water path.[8] Water-path scanning involves interposition of a fluid path between the transducer and the scrotum.[4] Many real-time sector scanners have a short fluid path incorporated into the transducer head. This technique enjoys considerable popularity as it offers the technical advantage of "retracting" the testicle directly within the focal zone of the ultrasonic beam. The disadvantages are that the depth of the water must be calculated so as not to result in reverberative artifacts and so that the focal zone will cover the testicular region. Additionally, this technique is more cumbersome than contact scanning, and it is difficult to simultaneously palpate and position the testis during scanning.

When performing contact scanning, the ultrasonographer can elevate the scrotum by a towel draped over the thighs and/or by inserting a rolled towel between the thighs if additional elevation is needed. The penis is placed onto the anterior abdominal wall and covered by a drape. This results in minimal exposure of the patient while retaining maximal access to the area of interest.

Prior to scanning, a concise history is obtained while the scrotum is gently palpated and the epididymis is positioned posteriorly. Correct anatomical positioning facilitates accurate localization of intratesticular lesions and various peritesticular fluid collections and allows thorough examination of testis and epididymis.

It is preferable to begin scanning the presumed normal testis first in order that the gain and gray scale may be assigned properly. As the testes are paired organs, the normal side may then be used as a comparison for any contralateral abnormality. It is important to obtain closely spaced (0.5 cm) sequential images in both the transverse and longitudinal planes.

NORMAL ANATOMY

The testis is a compound gland enclosed within the dense fibrous connective tissue capsule of the tunica albuginea. Along the posterior aspect of the testis, the tunica albuginea invaginates into the testis as the mediastinum testis.[1] On the transverse images of the testes the mediastinum is seen as an echogenic line either at the 3- or 9-o'clock position. On the longitudinal images, the mediastinum appears as an echogenic line, usually extending from the cephalic aspect of the testicle. The length of the mediastinum is variable. Extending radially from the mediastinum to the periphery of the tunica albuginea are the fibrous septula testes which divide the organ into 250 pyramidal components, the lobulae testes.

On sonography, the testis appears with uniformly distributed medium-level echoes. It measures 3 to 5 cm in length, 3 to 2 cm in anteroposterior diameter, and 2 to 3 cm in width. The lobular testes cannot be individually resolved with ultrasound.

Each testis has an outpouching of peritoneum, the tunica vaginalis propria testis, which envelops it. It forms a serous cavity around the testis, and normally a few millimeters of clear amber fluid are present between the two layers.[1] Often, the opposed layers of the tunica vaginalis can be seen as a brightly echogenic line surrounding the testis.

The epididymis lies along the posterior aspect of the testis. The testis and epididymis are easily rotated, and the epididymis must be manually positioned posteriorly in order for the scrotal contents to be viewed in an anatomically correct position. The epididymis is customarily subdivided into three regions: the head (caput, globus major), body (corpus), and tail (caudo, globus minor). Sonographically, the head of the epididymis is seen posterior and superior to the testicle. The spatial distribution of the epididymal echoes is more course than that of the testis, and the amplitude of the echoes is similar to or higher than that of the testis. The body of the epididymis is seen dorsal to the testicle, has a coarse distribution of echoes, and the echogenicity of the corpus epididymis is at the posterior and interior aspect of the testis. The echo characteristics of the tail of the epididymis are similar to that of the body. Often, the ductus deferans is visualized on the transverse scan along the medial aspect of each testis as a circular hypoechoic area.

TESTICULAR PATHOLOGY

Acquired Atrophy

Acquired testicular atrophy occurs secondary to a wide variety of pathological conditions including infertility, senility, prolonged hyperpyrexia, debility, avitaminosis, cirrhosis of the liver, hypothyroidism, schizophrenia, exogenous hormones, endocrine diseases, and crytorchidism.[23] Additionally, acute atrophy, a painful condition, has been reported as a complication after renal transplantation.

Sonographically, the testicle appears normal except for its diminutive size. It measures less than 3 cm in length and 2 cm in anteroposterior diameter. The epididymis is not involved. As the epididymis maintains its normal size, it may falsely appear enlarged relative to the small testicle. A false diagnosis of epididymitis will be avoided by consistently measuring testicular size.

Undescended Testis (Cryptorchism)

The testes develop from an elongated embryonic gonad that lies ventral to the mesonephric ridge. Internal descent brings the testes to the site of the future internal inguinal ring. The external descent begins with the migration through the inguinal canal into the scrotum. Arrest of descent of the testicles may occur anywhere along their pathway.[1]

In the absence of a clinically palpable testicle within the scrotum, sonography should be used as a screening modality.[8] In 70 percent of cases, the undescended testicles will be located in the inguinal canal, where they can be effectively demonstrated ultrasonographically. The sonographic diagnosis is based on the demonstration of a mass with uniformly distributed, medium-level echoes. The mass is elliptical in configuration and present along the expected path of the testicular descent (Fig. 10.2). In the inguinal region, normal structures are usually bilaterally symmetric, and a discrete tissue mass, even as small as 1 cm, can be detected. Outside the inguinal canal, sonography is not often successful in detecting cryptic testicles. In cases where ultrasound cannot resolve the problem, computed tomography (CT)[24] and testicular angiography have demonstrated some efficacy.[25,26]

Testicular Neoplasms

Testicular tumors are the most common neoplasm in men between 25 and 35.[1] An additional peak incidence is noted near 2 years of age. In the vast majority of cases (97.6 percent), testicular tumors are malignant germinal cell

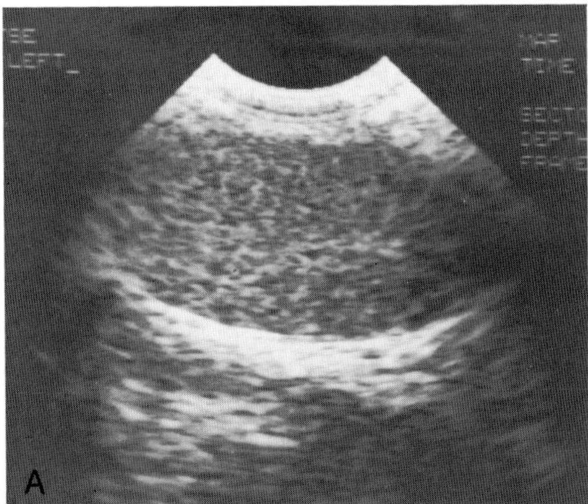

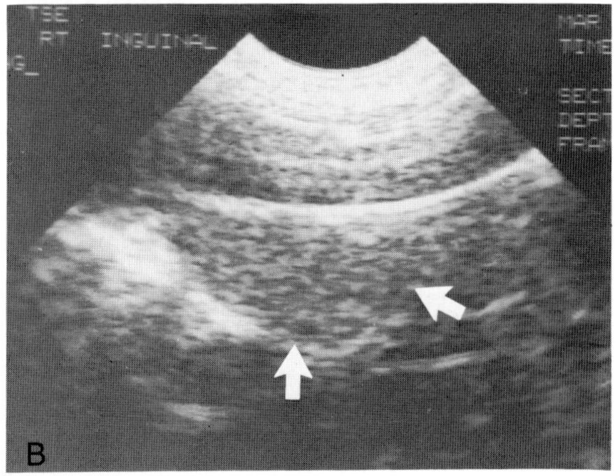

FIG. 10.2.   Right-sided unde-scended testis. (A) Normal left testicle within the scrotum. No right testicle was identified within the scrotum. (B) Examination of the right inguinal canal revealed the hypoplastic right testicle within the canal (arrows).

tumors with one of four histological patterns: (1) seminoma, 37.8 percent; (2) embryonal carcinoma, 31.6 percent; (3) teratomas, 26.5 percent; or (4) choriocarcinoma, 1.8 percent.[21,27]

The symptoms of testicular neoplasm are variable and unfortunately misleading. They include swelling, induration, focal lump, and secondary hemorrhage. Ten percent of patients with testicular neoplasm will have symptoms of extratesticular extension at the time of presentation.[1] Testicular tumors are usually confined to the glandular elements of the testis. The exception is embryonal carcinoma which oftens distorts the contour of the testicles because of its tendency to invade the capsule and epididymis.[24]

The homogeneous, medium-level echogenicity of the normal testis represents an excellent background for the detection of testicular pathology. In the vast majority of cases, neoplasms will disrupt the normal homogeneous architecture throughout the testicles. A localized tumor is seen as a circumscribed hypo-, hyper-, or mixed echogenic nidus in an otherwise uniform testicular echo structure[5,6,11,17,18] (Figs. 10.3–10.5). The hypoechoic appearance of the neoplasm

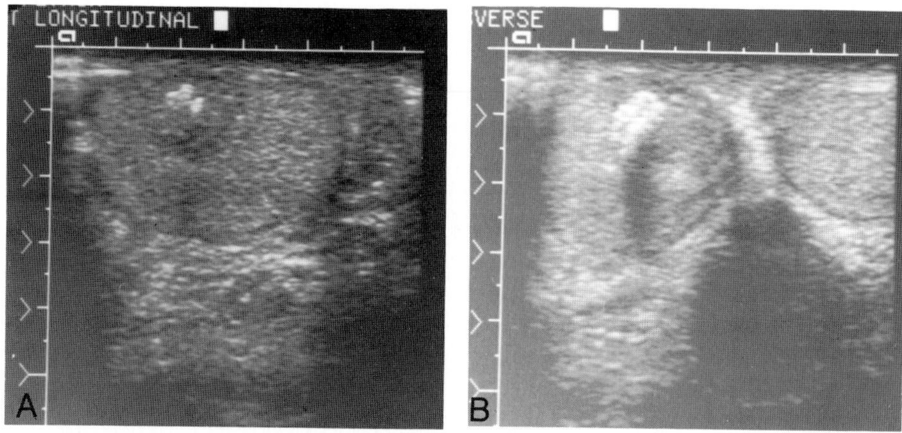

FIG. 10.3.   Embryonal testicular tumor. Mixed echogenicity region disrupting the otherwise homogeneous testicular architecture represents the neoplasm. Longitudinal (A) and transverse (B).

is seen more commonly. Enlargement of the testicle with uniform decrease in the echogenicity is seen with lymphoma. If the tumor is confined by the tunica albuginea, the testis typically retains its own shape. If the tunica or epididymis is invaded, the contour of the testis will be distorted. Unfortunately, there is no specificity to the sonographic findings, and based exclusively on sonographic findings, neoplasm cannot be accurately differentiated from orchitis, hemorrhage, infarction, abscess, or chronic torsion. However, the false-

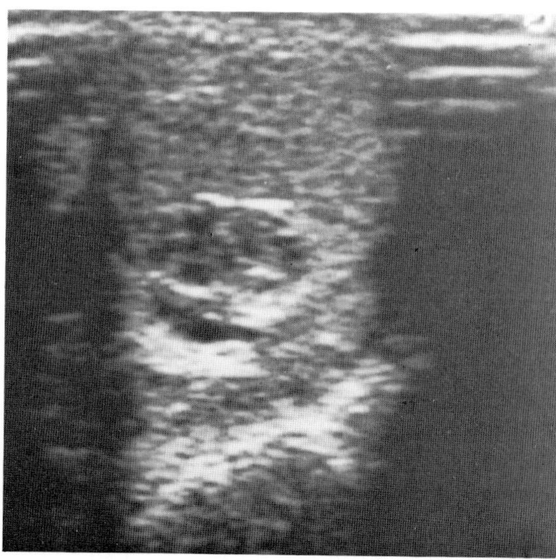

FIG. 10.4.   Epidermoid cyst. The homogeneous testicular architecture is disrupted by the inhomogeneous tumor.

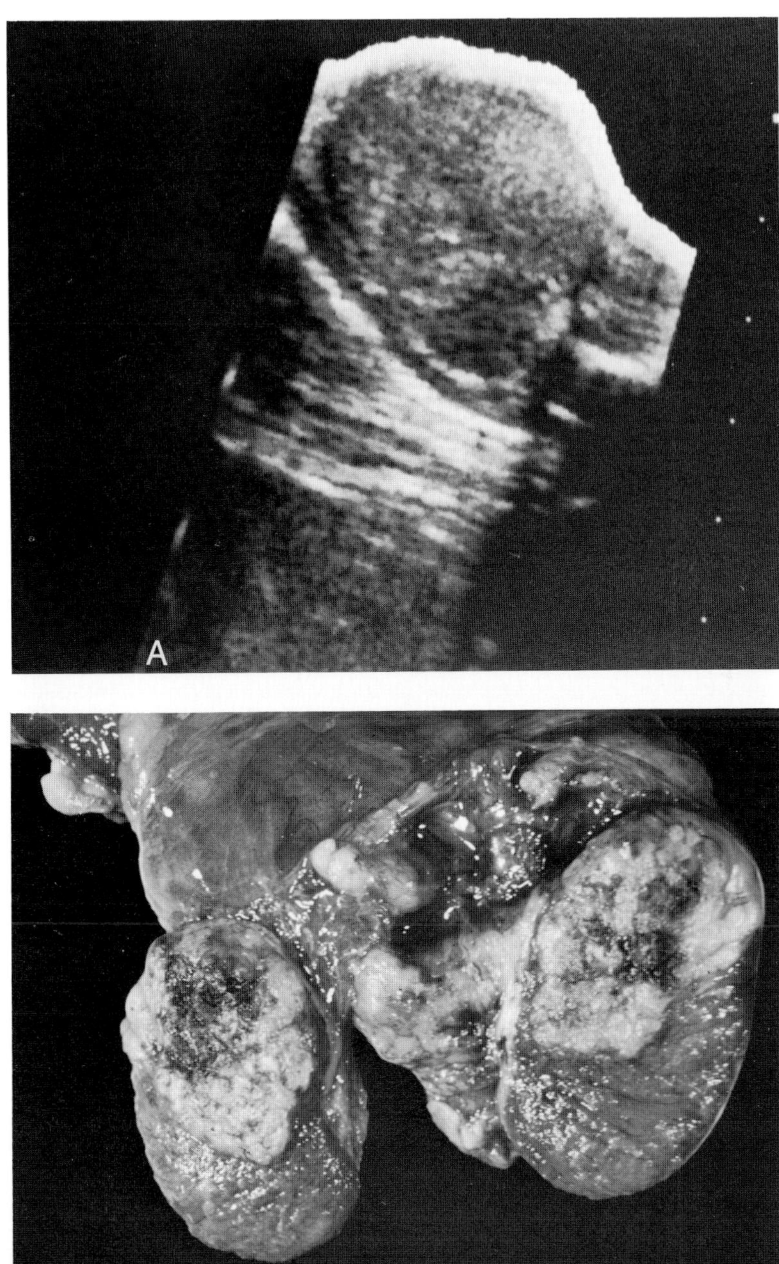

FIG. 10.5.   (A) Longitudinal sonogram and (B) cut gross pathological specimen demonstrating a seminoma.

negative rate for tumor detection is low, and the accuracy in detecting testicular neoplasms has been reported as high as 80 to 90 percent.[17,18] When germ cell tumor metastases are encountered in the presence of testicles that appear normal on palpation, ultrasonography is invaluable in detecting an occult testicular malignant neoplasm.[8,19,28] Correct sonographic identification of the abnormal testis not only discloses the pathology but facilitates surgical removal and precludes unnecessary excision of the contralateral normal testes.

Acute Nontraumatic Scrotal Abnormalities

In the nontraumatized patient, a swollen, acutely painful hemiscrotum represents a medical emergency, since prompt surgical intervention is often indicated.[29,30] The pain is often so severe that only a superficial physical examination of the involved side is obtainable. Sonography can be helpful in differentiating the two most common causes of acute pain, acute torsion of the spermatic cord and acute epididymitis.

Spermatic Cord Torsion

Torsion of the spermatic cord results from the faulty development such that the epididymis lacks its strong attachment to the scrotum. This allows the testis to rotate freely within the scrotum. The testis must be freely movable in order for the spermatic cord to become twisted.

Clinically, torsion of the spermatic cord presents with the sudden onset of

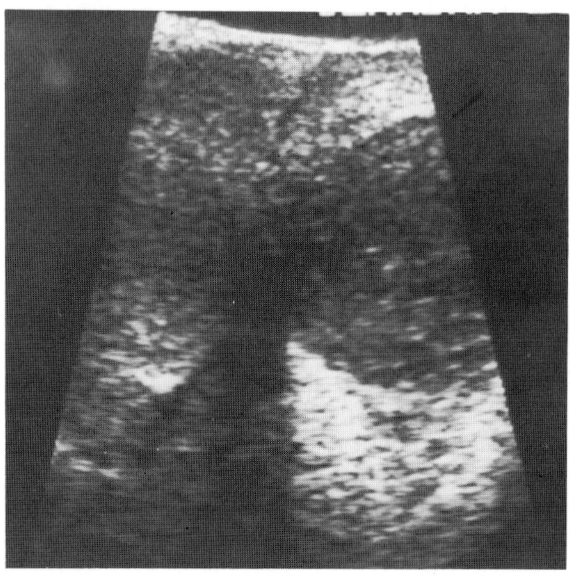

FIG. 10.6. Nine-year-old boy with acute spermatic cord torsion. The left testicle is enlarged and hypoechoic on this transverse image. Right testis is normal.

severe scrotal pain, typically in young or adolescent patients. The pain often occurs when the patient is at rest or asleep. In the newborn, spermatic cord torsion is characterized by swelling and redness of the scrotum, often with an apparent lack of symptoms. Differentiation of torsion from epididymitis may be difficult and has been reported as being impossible in 50 percent of cases.[1]

A spectrum of ultrasonographic changes becomes manifest in the scrotum following acute spermatic cord torsion.[1,9,14,29,31-34] The appearance of the testicle depends on the duration of the torsion. Definite sonographic abnormalities have been documented within 1 hour following experimental torsion in experimental animals. The spectrum of findings includes testicular enlargement, diminished echogenicity of the testicular parenchyma, enlargement of the epididymal body, scrotal wall thickening, and occasionally hydrocele formation (Fig. 10.6). The sonographic changes have been shown to precede the associated histological changes,[34] indicating that sonographic manifestations are evident before testicular necrosis occurs when the testis can still be salvaged.

Doppler ultrasound has also been used to determine the presence of intratesticular and spermatic cord arterial pulsations. With torsion of the cord, the arterial pulse is lost, indicating a lack of perfusion of the testicle. Doppler analysis of the testicle and spermatic cord in conjunction with gray scale evaluation of the scrotum facilitates the correct diagnosis.[12,16] Radionuclide scintigraphy can be a useful adjunctive study in the evaluation of these patients (Fig. 10.7).

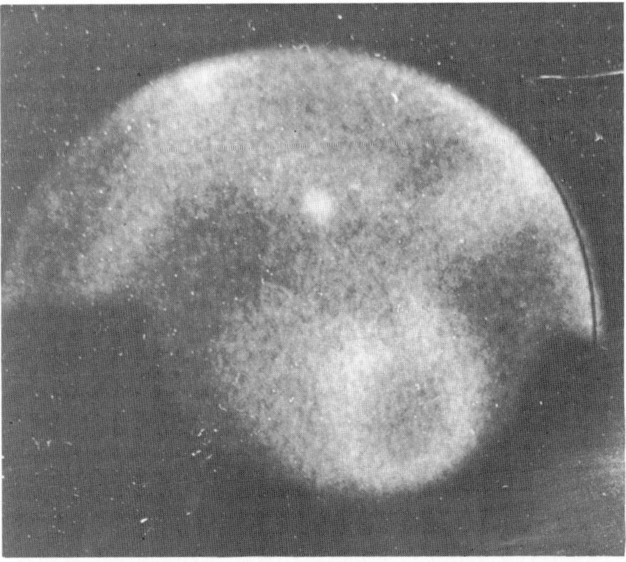

FIG. 10.7.   Radionuclide study demonstrating the hypoperfused testicle surrounded by a hyperemic halo.

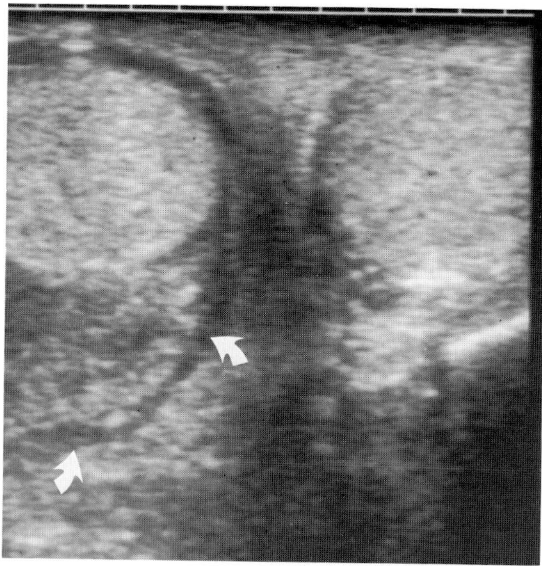

FIG. 10.8. Longitudinal ultrasonogram in patient with acute right-sided epididymitis. The epididymis is enlarged, inhomogeneous (arrows), and hypoechoic as compared with the ipsilateral testis.

Epididymitis

Acute epididymitis is the most common inflammatory lesion of the scrotum. Epididymitis is often associated with prostatisis and generally responds to appropriate antibiotic therapy. The history can be misleading, and physical exami-

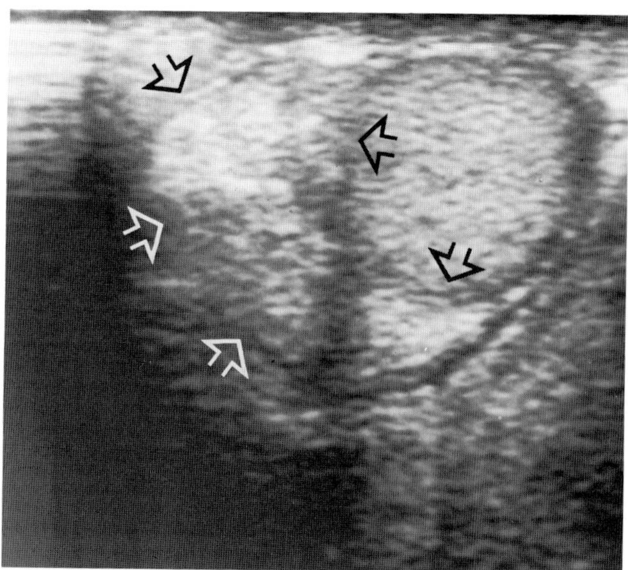

FIG. 10.9. Longitudinal ultrasonogram in patient with epididymitis. The epididymis (arrow) is enlarged and inhomogeneous.

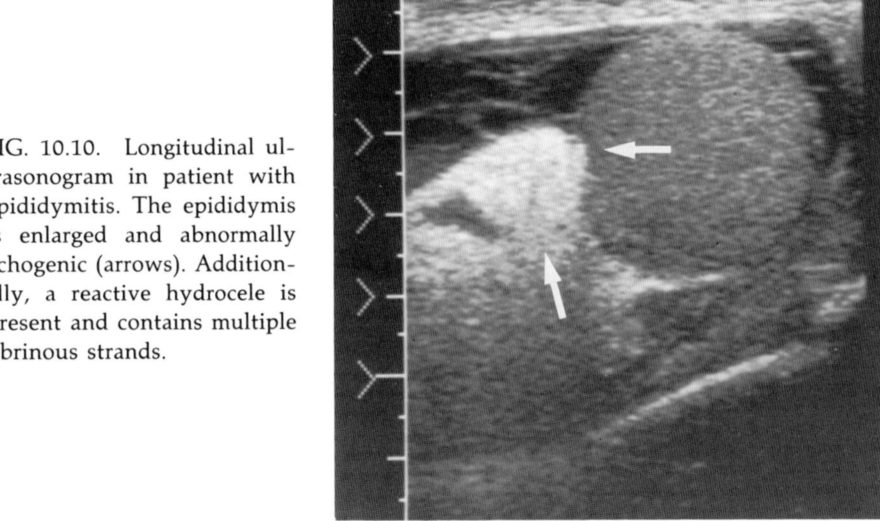

FIG. 10.10. Longitudinal ultrasonogram in patient with epididymitis. The epididymis is enlarged and abnormally echogenic (arrows). Additionally, a reactive hydrocele is present and contains multiple fibrinous strands.

nation is often limited because the scrotum may be extremely tender to palpation. On clinical grounds, the differentiation of epididymitis from acute spermatic cord torsion is extremely difficult in up to 50 percent of cases. Additionally, in 10 percent of cases, testicular tumors may mimic the clinical presentation of acute epididymitis. Ultrasonography can be extremely helpful in re-

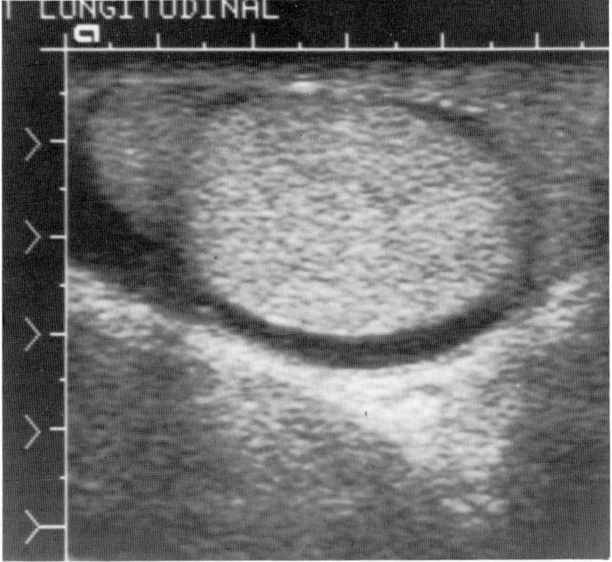

FIG. 10.11. Longitudinal ultrasound examination of left scrotum in patient with epididymitis. The head of the epididymis is enlarged and slightly hypoechoic. A hydrocele is present.

solving these clinical dilemmas. Acute epididymitis manifests as an enlarged epididymis with altered echo texture. Although the process may be localized to the head of the epididymis, both the head and body are commonly involved. Homogeneous or inhomogeneous diminuition in the echogenicity of the epididymis is often demonstrated. In chronic epididymitis, the echogenicity of the epididymis may be increased. In up to 20 percent of patients with acute epididymitis, there is associated orchitis. When orchitis is present, the testis is enlarged and echogenicity diminished. Focal hypoechoic areas of either the testis or epididymis suggests suppuration and early abscess formation (Figs. 10.8–10.13).

Orchitis

Isolated orchitis (unless caused by viral infections) is rare because it is almost always associated with epididymitis (Figs. 10.14, 10.15). A heterogeneous texture of the testicular echo pattern with a normal-appearing epididymis always raises the possibility of testicular tumor regardless of history. Approximately one-half of the patients with testicular tumors have pain as a presenting symptom.[1] In an individual case, it may not be possible by sonography to distinguish a testicular abscess from neoplasm. Resolution after antibiotic therapy is important to document sonographically in cases of suppurative orchitis in order to exclude an associated underlying tumor from diagnostic consideration.

Benign Scrotal Masses

Hydrocele

A hydrocele is an abnormal accumulation of serous fluid between the visceral and parietal layers of the tunica vaginalis. A hydrocele may be congenital, in which case there is a direct communication with the abdominal cavity as a result of failure of closure of the funicular process. Secondary hydroceles may be idiopathic, or often they are associated with epididymitis, orchitis, as well as chronic or missed spermatic cord torsion. Additionally, scrotal trauma is often associated with hydrocele formation.[27,35] In less than 10 percent of cases is hydrocele associated with neoplasm.

An acute hydrocele has a thin wall and always transilluminates. Chronic hydroceles usually have a thick wall and therefore will not transilluminate. Sonography can play a significant role in these cases.

Hydroceles present sonographically as an echo-free zone with strong sound transmission (Fig. 10.16). The sac of the hydrocele is typically single chambered, but a multichambered structure with septation may be present. The wall of the hydrocele is variously thickened. High-amplitude echoes representing calci-

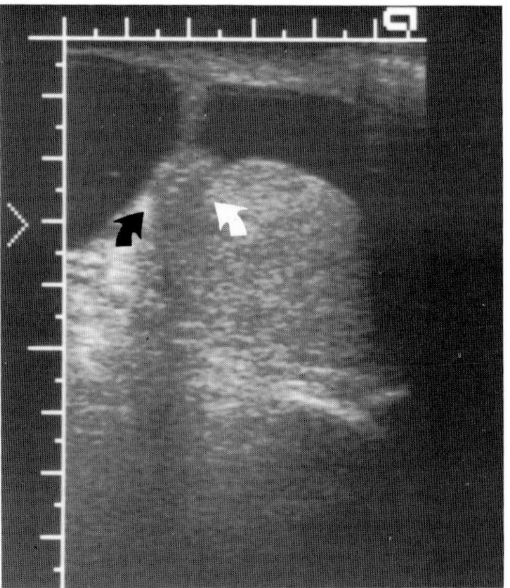

FIG. 10.12. Longitudinal scan in patient with epididymitis. The epididymis (arrows) is enlarged and the echogenicity slightly diminished. Bilateral hydroceles are also present.

fications may be present. In some cases, low-level echoes may be present within the hydrocele cavity. The echoes represent fibrous strands that originate either from a detached villous projection or organizing proteinaceous material in cases of infection or hemorrhage. Septations within the hydrocele may be idiopathic but more commonly are associated with hemorrhage or infection.[1,21] The under-

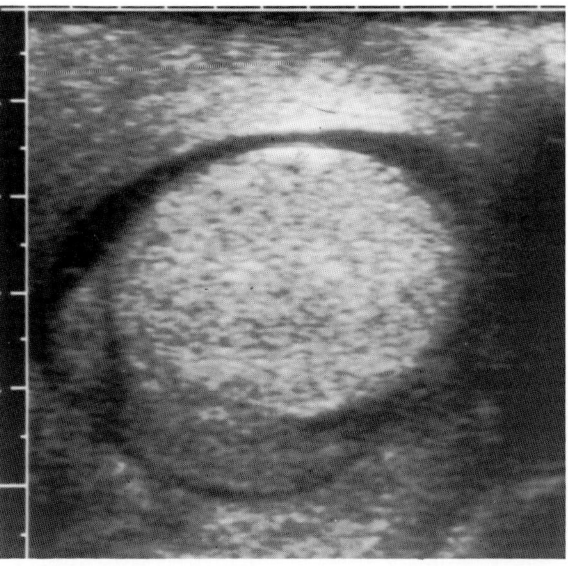

FIG. 10.13. Longitudinal scan in patient with epididymitis. The epididymis is enlarged and the echogenicity slightly diminished. A hydrocele is also present, and the scrotal skin is thickened.

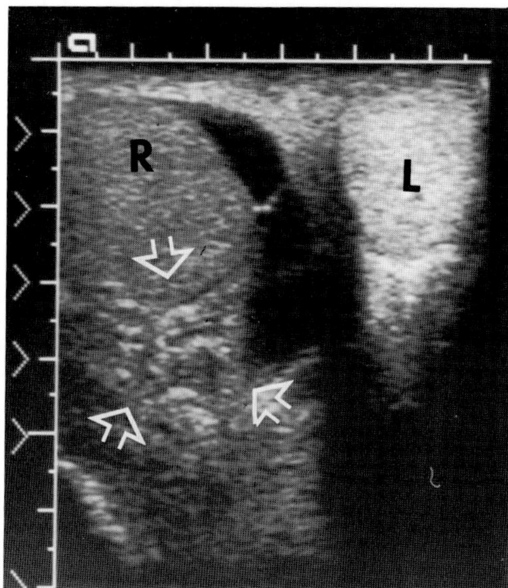

FIG. 10.14. Transverse ultrasonogram in patient with acute right side epididymal orchitis. The right testicle (R) is enlarged and hypoechoic. The body of the epididymis (arrows) is enlarged with inhomogeneous echogenicity. A hydrocele is also present with some fibrinous strands.

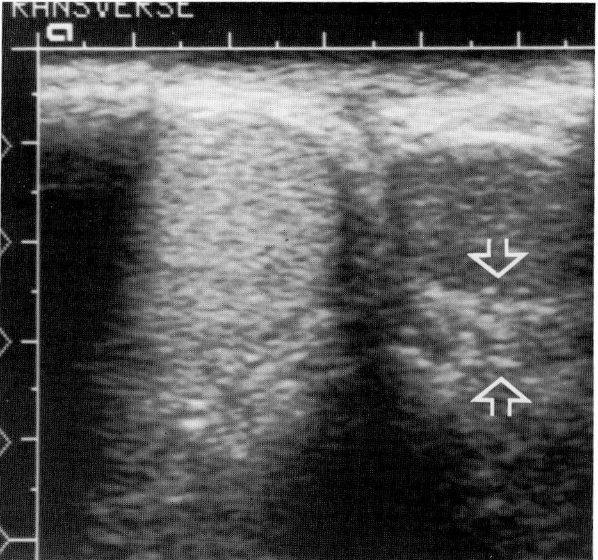

FIG. 10.15. Transverse ultrasonogram in patient with resolving epididymal orchitis. The left testicle is diminished in size and echogenicity relative to the normal right testicle. The left epididymis is prominent (arrows).

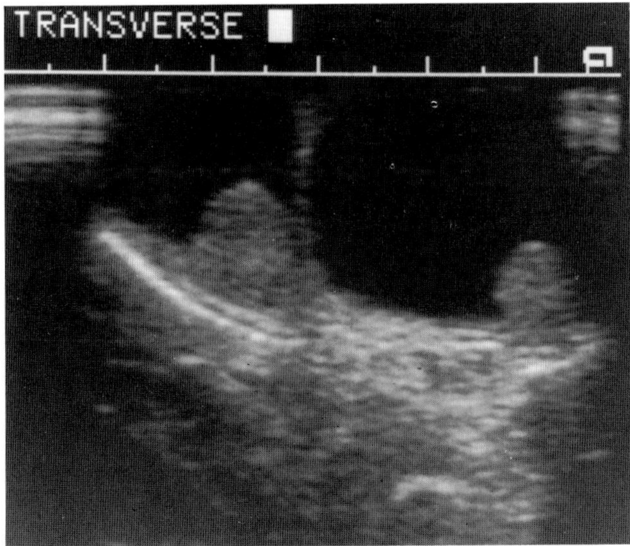

FIG. 10.16. Transverse scan in newborn with large bilateral hydroceles.

lying testis is well visualized and is smoothly surrounded by fluid, except on its posterior surface, where the testis is attached to the epididymis.

Spermatocele

Spermatocele is a retention cyst of small tubules within the epididymis most commonly present in the head of the epididymis. A spermatocele may be unilateral or bilateral, unilocular or multilocular.[22] Sonographically, a spermatocele is seen as an echo-free fluid collection in the region of the epididymis (Fig. 10.17). Based on its anatomical landmarks, a spermatocele may be differentiated from a hydrocele. As the spermatocele is located within the epididymis, the testicle is displaced anteriorly, whereas a hydrocele is usually seen anteriorly surrounding the testicle.[6] Occasionally, a spermatocele may be very large and difficult to distinguish from a hydrocele by sonography. Spermatoceles may demonstrate low-level echoes representing sediment composed of cellular debris, fat, or spermatozoa.[22]

Varicocele

Varicocele is a condition in which the veins of the pampiniform plexus are enlarged and elongated, and their tortuosity is increased.[21,27,36] Although it has been reported that the left side of the scrotum is involved in the vast majority of cases, our experience has demonstrated the incidence of ultrasonographically demonstrable right-sided varicoceles to be substantially higher than that anticipated from clinical series as well as physical examination.[38,39] Varicocele may be primary idiopathic or secondary. Secondary varicoceles may result from pressure on the spermatic vein or its tributaries by an enlarged liver or

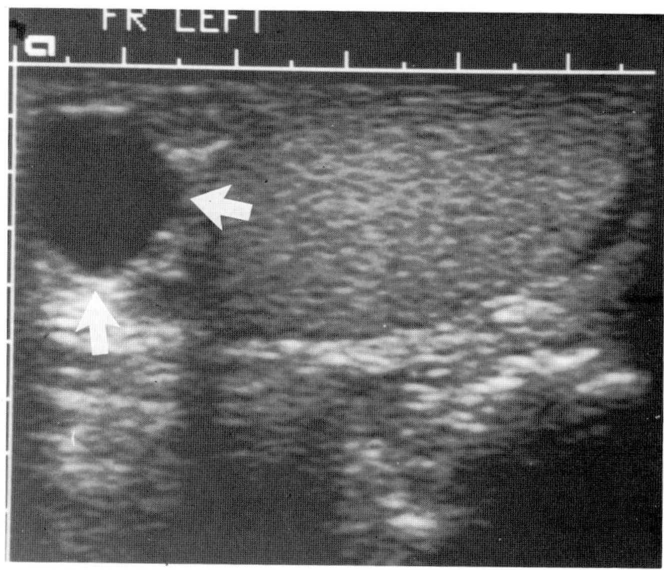

FIG. 10.17.   Longitudinal ultrasonogram of the left scrotum. A spermatocele is present in the head of the epididymis (arrows).

spleen, by pronounced hydronephrosis, muscle strain, or abdominal tumors. Primary varicoceles are predominantly seen in young boys. On sonography, a varicocele is imaged as tubular, serpiginous anechoic fluid collections in the region of the epididymis (Fig. 10.18). Patients with varicoceles and internal spermatic vein reflux have a significant reduction in sperm density which has been implicated as a cause of infertility. Doppler ultrasound examination for venous reflux may be performed.[40]

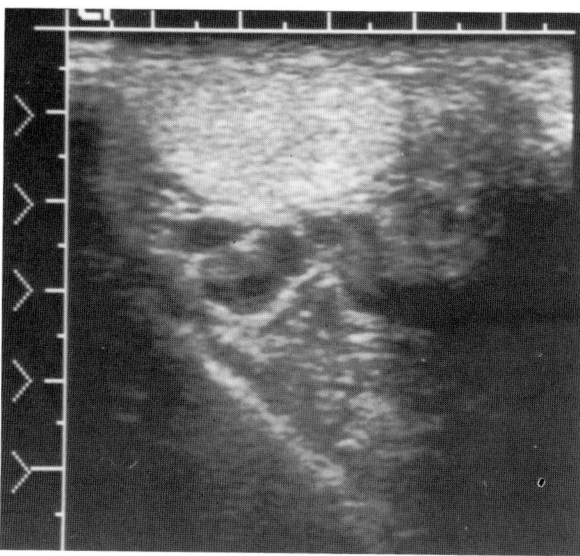

FIG. 10.18. Longitudinal ultrasonogram demonstrating a large right-sided varicocele.

Scrotal Hernia

Scrotal hernia in most instances is a clinical diagnosis. However, physical examination may be quite limited if the accompanying pain is sudden and severe. In these instances, sonography may prove helpful. Sonographically the scrotal hernia appears as a complex intrascrotal mass separate from the testicle.[41] The finding of a normal testis and epididymis is important. However, visualization of the normal testicle can sometimes be difficult because of air and fat within the hernia, leading to high reflectivity as well as attenuation and scattering of the sound. In addition to demonstrating a complex mass within the scrotum, scanning the inguinal region facilitates the diagnosis. Particularly with real-time sonography, it is possible to identify intestine or omentum within the inguinal canal and display the extension of the bowel or omentum into the scrotum.

Epididymal Abscess

Epididymal abscess presents ultrasonographically as a complex intrascrotal mass, most commonly located within the tail of the epididymis (Fig. 10.19). Evaluation of the underlying testis is of paramount importance since the status of underlying testicle influences surgical approach.

Epididymal Tumors

Most neoplasms of the epididymis are benign adenomatoid tumors.[22] Very rarely are such tumors demonstrated to be malignant. They typically appear

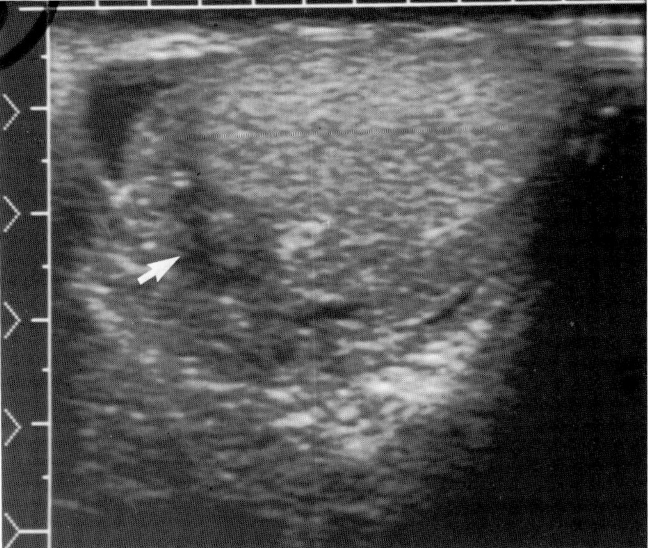

FIG. 10.19.   Longitudinal ultrasonogram in patient with enlarged epididymis secondary to epididymitis. The focal regions of hypoechogenicity represent liquification in regions of abscess formation (arrow).

on ultrasound examination as sharply demarcated masses separate from the testis. They have homogeneously distributed medium- to high-level echoes. The echogenicity is often increased as compared with the testicle. The spatial distribution of the echoes within the tumors is less coarse than that of the epididymis.

Trauma to the Scrotum

Blunt trauma to the scrotum generally results from athletic injuries or industrial or vehicular accidents. Less commonly it results from violence or self mutilation by psychiatric patients.[1] Patients with scrotal lacerations or penetrating scrotal injuries undergo emergency surgery and are generally not candidates for sonography. In cases of blunt trauma, the main role of sonography is to exclude an intrinsic testicular abnormality such as rupture.[32,42-44]

Scrotal Hematoma

Hematoma of the scrotum is an effusion of blood within the scrotal wall. The blood may collect beneath the tunica dartos, between the tunica vaginalis and fibrous coat, or in the scrotal septum. The sonographic appearance of the hematoma depends on its age and location. In the acute stage, the hematomas located within the tissue of scrotal wall will demonstrate only thickening of the wall (Fig. 10.20). Hypoechoic areas within the wall due to liquification of the hematoma can be seen after 48 to 72 hours.

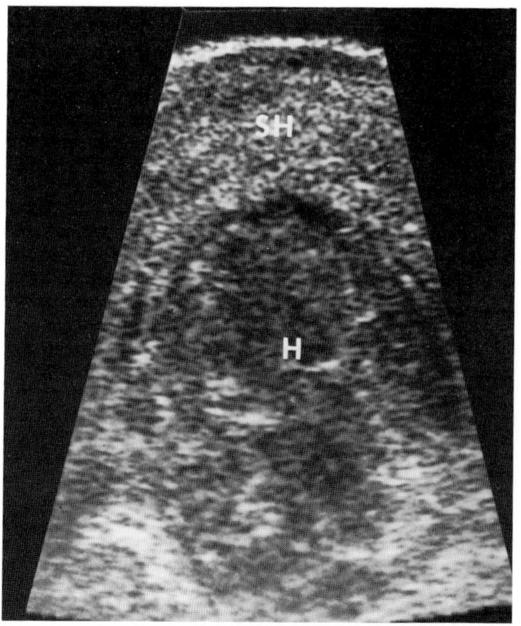

FIG. 10.20. Transverse ultrasonogram in a patient with a large scrotal hematoma (SH) and a complex hematocele (H).

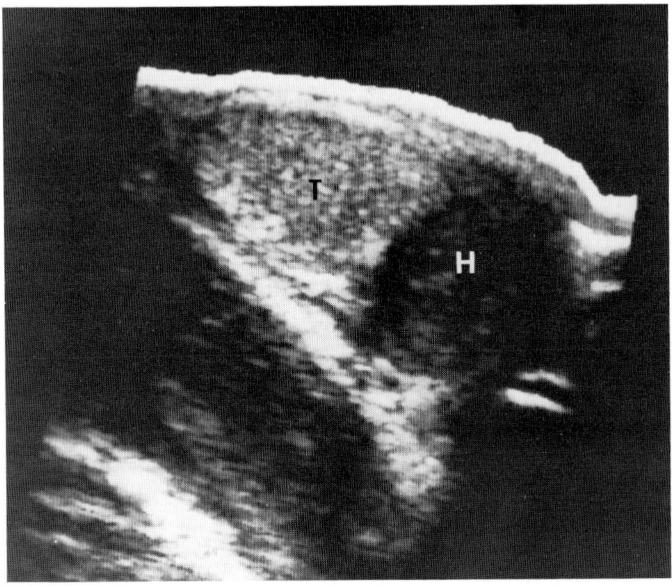

FIG. 10.21. Longitudinal ultrasonogram with hematocele (H) along the lower pole of the intact testicle (T).

Hematocele

Hemorrhage in the sac of the tunica vaginalis is known as a hematocele. It may develop spontaneously, in which case it is slow and insidious in its development. A rapidly developing hematocele is invariably the result of trauma. The diagnosis is suggested by a history of injury and by finding a hydrocele that does not transilluminate. It presents sonographically as a complex fluid collection containing numerous echoes (Figs. 10.20, 10.21). In a longstanding hematocele, the tunica vaginalis becomes abnormally thickened with dense fibrous tissue and sonographically appears as a thick-walled fluid collection that is indistinguishable from chronic hydrocele or abscess. Occasionally, the tunica vaginalis becomes partially calcified.

Urinary Extravasation

When the bulbous urethra is perforated, the rupture may involve the deep fascia of the penis so that extravasating urine can extend in to the superficial perineal compartment of the scrotum. Sonographically, it is seen as an anechoic fluid collection within the scrotal cavity that is indistinguishable from hematocele or hydrocele in some cases. However, as the extravasated urine dissects along the soft tissue planes, it may create a characteristic onion-peel appearance (Fig. 10.22).

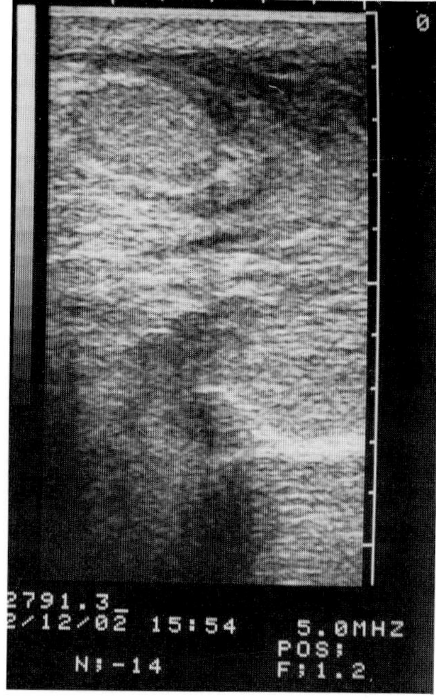

FIG. 10.22. Longitudinal view of urinoma. The urine has extravasated along the soft tissue planes inducing the characteristic onion-peel appearance.

Intratesticular Hematoma

Hemorrhage within the testicle can occur with the tunica albuginea remaining intact. The injury appears ultrasonographically as a heterogeneous focus of diminished echogenicity, within the intact but often swollen testicle (Fig. 10.23).

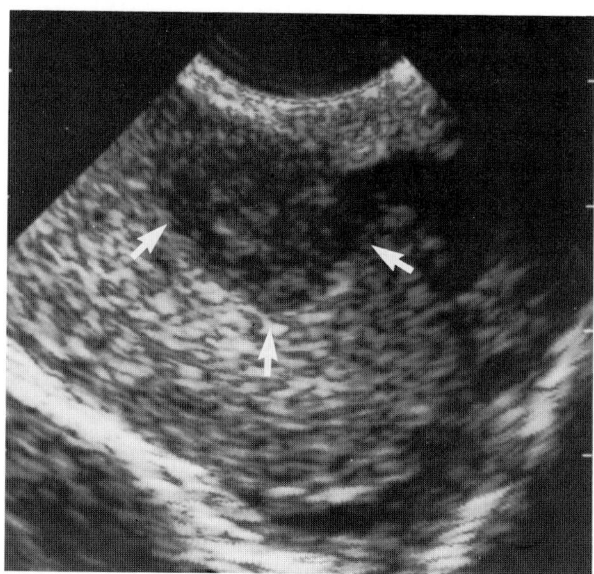

FIG. 10.23. Longitudinal scan demonstrating intratesticular hematoma (arrows). The tunica albuginea at surgery was intact.

Such a hematoma sonographically is indistinguishable from tumor. Scrotal hematomas and hematoceles are often present.

Testicular Rupture

Testicular rupture occurs when the inelastic tunica albuginea is torn, resulting in extrusion of testicular contents into the scrotal sac. The process is frequently accompanied by hematocele formation. The goal of surgical intervention is to repair and salvage the involved testicle. Discrete fracture planes often are not identified by sonography in cases of testicular rupture. Therefore, any alteration of the normal testicular echogenicity in traumatized patients suggests testicular rupture and requires surgery.

REFERENCES

1. Bunce PL: Scrotal abnormalities. p. 232. In Glenn JF (ed): Urologic Surgery. Harper and Row, New York, 1975

2. Holder LE, Melloul M, Chen D: Current status of radionuclide imaging. Semin Nucl Med 11, 1981

3. Hricak H: Pelvis. In Margulis AR, Kaufman L, Crooks LE (eds): Clinical Magnetic Resonance Imaging. San Francisco, University of California, 1983

4. Pederson JR, Holm HH, Hald T: Torsion of the testis diagnosed by ultrasound. Jr Urol 113:66, 1975

5. Sarti DA, Sample WF: Renal, adrenal, retroperitoneal and scrotal ultrasonography. p. 386. In Sarti DA, Sample WF (eds): Diagnostic Ultrasound, Text and Cases. John Wiley, New York, 1980

6. Phillips GN, Schneider M, Goodman JD et al: Ultrasonic evaluation of the scrotum. Urol Radiol 1:157, 1980

7. Leopold GR, Woo UL, Scheible FW et al.: High resolution ultrasonography of scrotal pathology. Radiology 131:719, 1978

8. Hricak H: Sonography of the scrotum. p. 371. In Margulis AR, Gooding CA (eds): Diagnostic Radiology. University of California, San Francisco, 1982

9. Freidrich M, Claussen CD, Felix R: Immersion ultrasound of testicular pathology. Radiology 141:235, 1981

10. Orr OP, Skolnick MC: Sonographic examination of the abnormal scrotum. Clin Radiol 31:109, 1980

11. Arger PH, Mulhern CB, Coleman BG et al.: Prospective analysis of the value of scrotal ultrasound. Radiology 41:763, 1981

12. Gohcoman E, Sample WF, Skinner DG, Ehrlich RM: Diagnostic ultrasound in the evaluation of scrotal masses. J Urol 18:601, 1977

13. Miskin M, Bain J: B-mode ultrasonic examination of the testes. J Clin Ultrasound 2:307, 1974

14. Bird KI Jr: Emergency testicular scanning. Diagnostic ultrasound in emergency medicine. p. 264. In Clinics in Ultrasound. Churchill Livingstone, New York, 1981

15. Deukota J: Testicular sonogram. J Natl Med Assoc 72:806, 1980

16. Goodman JD, Haller JO: The scrotum. Diagnostic ultrasound in pediatrics. p. 264. In Clinics In Ultrasound. Churchill Livingstone, New York, 1981

17. Gronval S, Brunner M, Jacobsen GK et al.: Ultrasound in the detection of testicular tumors. Int J Androl, suppl., 4:185, 1981

18. Graunthoff H, Weisbach L: Zur sonographischen diagnostik bei hodenerkrandungen. Nuc Compact 11:93, 1980

19. Peterson LJ, Catalona WJ, Kochler RE: Ultrasonic localization of a non-palpable testis tumor. J Urol 122:843, 1979

20. Miskin M, Buckspan M, Bain J: Ultrasonographic examinations of scrotal masses. J Urol 117:135, 1977

21. Jeffrey RB, Laing FC, Hricak H, McAninch JW: Sonography of testicular trauma. AJR 141:993, 1983

22. Hricak H, Filly RA: Sonography of the scrotum. Invest Radiol 18:112, 1983

23. Mostof FK: Testes, scrotum and penis. p. 1013. In Anderson WAD, Kissure JM (eds): Pathology. C.V. Mosby, St. Louis, 1977

24. Stanley RJ, Lee JKT, McClennan BL: Searching for the cryptic testis: The role of computed tomography. p. 80. In The Society of Uroradiology 3rd Annual Postgraduate Course, (Syllabus) Uroradiology, January, 1981

25. Glickman MG, Weiss RW, Itzchak Y: Testicular venography for undescended testis. AJR 129:67, 1977

26. Khademi MS JJ, Falls A: Selective spermatic arteriography for localization of an impalpable undescended testis. Radiology 136:627, 1980

27. Bloom W, Fawcett DW: Male reproductive system. p. 805. In Textbook of Histology. W.B. Saunders, Philadelphia, 1975

28. Glazer HS, Lee JKT, Melson LG, McClennan BL: Sonographic detection of occult testicular neoplasms. AJR 138:673, 1982

29. Cass AS, Cass BP, Veeraraghaven K: Immediate exploration of the unilateral acute scrotum in young male subjects. J Urol 124:829, 1978

30. Williamson RCN: Death of the scrotum: Testicular Torsion. N Engl J Med 296:338, 1977

31. Donahue RE, Utley WLF: Torsion of the spermatic cord. Urology 11:33, 1978

32. Friedman SG, Rose JC, Winston MA: Testicular trauma. J Urol 125:748, 1978

33. Carroll BA, Gross DM: High frequency scrotal sonography. AJR 140:511, 1983

34. Hricak H, Lue T, Filly RA, et al.: Experimental study of the sonographic diagnosis of testicular torsion. J Ultrasound Med 2:349, 1983

35. Jeffrey RB, Laing FC, Hricak H, McAninch JW: Sonography of testicular trauma. AJR 141:993, 1983

36. Rifkin MD, Foy PM, Kurtz AB, Pasto ME, Goldberg BB: The role of diagnostic ultrasonography in varicocele evaluation. J Ultrasound Med 2:271, 1983

37. Wolverson MK, Houttuin E, Heiberg E, Sundaram M, Gregory J: High resolution real time sonography of scrotal varicocele. AJR 141:775, 1983

38. McClure RD, Hoddick WK, Abber JC, Hricak H: Scrotal ultrasound. Its usefulness before and after varicolelectomy. Urology, in press

39. Oster J: Varicocele in children as adolescents: An investigation of the incidence among Danish school children. Scand J Urol Nephrol 5:27, 1971

40. Hirsch AV, Kellett JM, Robertson G, Pryor JP: Doppler flow studies, venography, and thermography in the evaluation of varicoceles of fertile and subfertile men. Br J Urol 52:560, 1980

41. Sabramangam BR, Bathazar EJ, Raghaverdra BM et al.: Sonographic diagnosis of scrotal hernia. AJR 139:535, 1982

42. Albert MI: Testicular ultrasound for trauma. J Urol 72:806, 1980

43. Anderson KA, Jeffrey RB, Laing FC et al.: Ultrasonography for the diagnosis and staging of blunt scrotal trauma. J Urol 130(5):933, 1983

44. Jeffrey RB, Laing FC, Hricak H, McAninch JW: Sonography of testicular trauma. AJR 141:993, 1983

11 Doppler in Urology

HEDVIG HRICAK
KENNETH J. W. TAYLOR
KENNETH MARICH
TOM F. LUE
PETER BURNS

Since the first description of the Doppler effect by Christian Johann Doppler in the 1840s, this principle has gained widespread use for applications in radar, astronomy, and medicine. Doppler demonstrated that when sound of a particular frequency strikes a moving object, it is reflected back at a different frequency, and this frequency shift is related to the velocity of the moving object. The first medical application of Doppler ultrasound was reported by Satomura[1] in 1959 in which the Doppler effect was used to measure arterial blood flow. Since then, numerous medical applications for Doppler ultrasound have emerged and have become established modes of diagnostic investigation. The use of Doppler ultrasound is well established for diagnosis in cardiology, peripheral vascular and cerebrovascular disease, and obstetrics. More recent developments in quantitative Doppler spectrum analysis have increased the clinical utility and diagnostic accuracy of Doppler techniques. Technological innovation is now helping to extend the utility of Doppler to new clinical areas including deep abdominal flow evaluation, organ transplantation, tumor assessment, and urological applications, to name a few. This chapter presents the most recent clinical investigations for the use of Doppler ultrasound to evaluate renal disease, spermatic cord torsion, and vasculogenic impotence.

TECHNICAL ASPECTS

Doppler Principle

Doppler ultrasound has gained clinical acceptance due to a better understanding of sound wave theory, more effective techniques for signal processing, and easier-to-use Doppler systems. The Doppler effect exists for ultrasonic waves.

This effect is a change in frequency—the Doppler shift (Δf)—defined as the difference between the reflected frequency (f_R) and the transmitted frequency (f_0).

$$\Delta f = f_R - f_0$$

Simple, nondirectional Doppler systems only detect the presence or absence of flow and are frequently used for pressure measurements. Bidirectional Doppler systems separate Doppler shift information into two channels and distinguish structures as either moving toward or away from the transducer. If the object is moving toward the sound source, f_R will be greater than f_0. If it is moving away from the source, f_R will be less than f_0. The Doppler shift is directly related to the velocity of the moving object, as shown in the following equation:

$$\Delta f = f_R - f_0 = \frac{2f_0 V}{C}$$

where V is the velocity of the moving object and C is the speed of sound in the medium.

In clinical application, the Doppler probe is coupled to the skin with gel, and the sound beam is transmitted toward the vessel or area of interest. Moving structures, such as red blood cells, serve as scatterers, and the reflected echoes are detected by the transmitting transducer. Therefore, the Doppler frequency shift is not only a function of the velocity of the moving structures but is also influenced by the angle of the incident sound beam as given by

$$\Delta f = \frac{2f_0 V}{C} \cos \theta$$

where θ is the angle between the incident sound beam and the direction of blood flow (see Fig. 11.1).

Since velocity has both a speed and direction component, the magnitude of the Doppler frequency shift will vary with the cosine of the angle (θ) between the probe and artery. As the angle becomes smaller, the frequency shift increases; and as the angle approaches 90° a minimal wave form is obtained (Fig. 11.2).

Theoretically, when the objects move at right angles to the sound beam, the Doppler shift is zero. In practice, angles of 30 to 70° are used for most clinical applications.

Since depth of penetration of sound through tissue is inversely related to the fundamental Doppler frequency (f_0), high-frequency sound is attenuated at a faster rate than low-frequency sound. In general, attenuation as a function of frequency and tissue depth is given by the following relationship, 1 db/cm/MHz. Thus, to optimize the Doppler analysis, it is important to choose an appropriate fundamental frequency (f_0) for each clinical application, dependent on the depth of the vessel of interest.

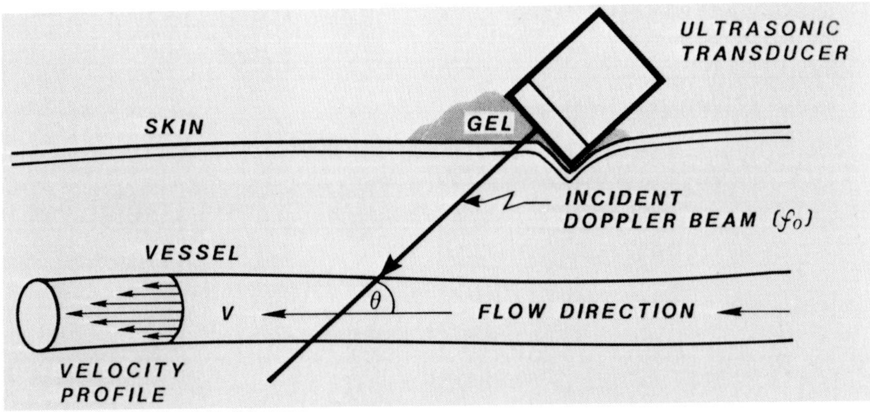

FIG. 11.1   The ultrasonic transducer is coupled to the skin with gel and is oriented to optimize the Doppler shift from the vessel of interest.

Continuous-Wave Doppler

Continuous-wave (CW) Doppler probes utilize two piezoelectric crystals. One continuously transmits sound, whereas the second crystal continuously receives the reflected sound waves. Thus, CW Doppler systems detect all moving objects in the beam path (Fig. 11.3), and their major limitation is lack of range resolution.

The Doppler frequency spectrum obtained with CW systems represents signals derived from all sources of movement in the beam path (arteries and

θ	$\cos$	
30°	0.87	
60°	0.5	
80°	0.17	

FIG. 11.2   The Doppler shift frequency and wave form are directly related to the cosine of the angle of incidence of the Doppler beam with respect to the flowing blood (θ).

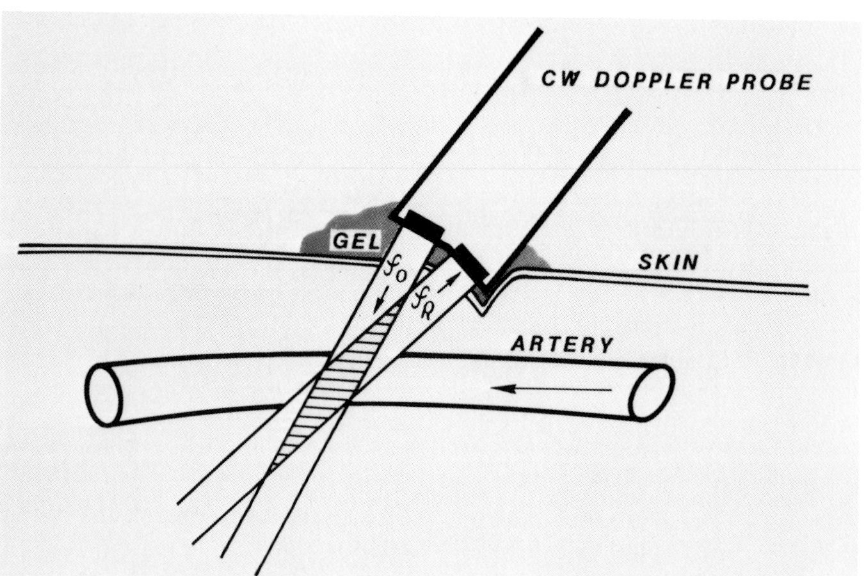

FIG. 11.3 Continuous-wave Doppler probes have two piezoelectric crystals; one continuously transmits sound (f_O) whereas the other continuously receives the reflected echoes (f_R). Echoes are detected from the entire sample volume region (lined area).

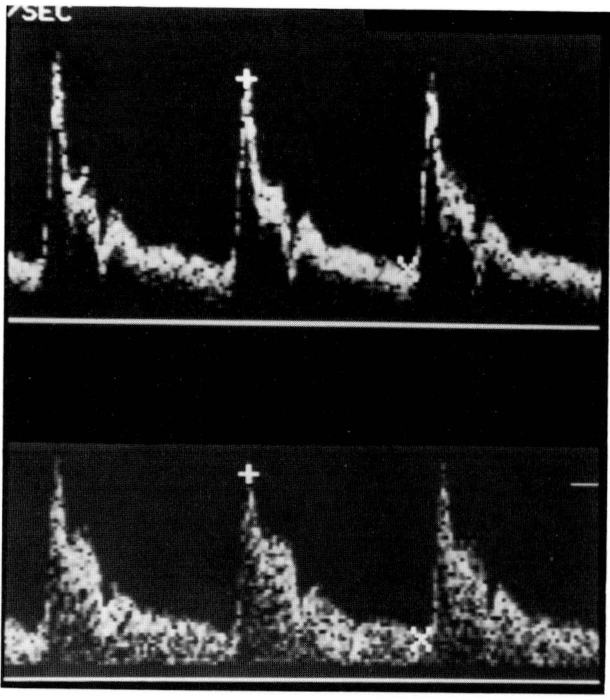

FIG. 11.4 Gray scale spectra derived from a pulsed Doppler (upper trace) and continuous-wave Doppler (lower trace). Note the spectral broadening in the continuous-wave trace due to sampling velocities across the entire vessel.

veins). It is difficult to select Doppler shift data from a specific vessel or region of interest in that vessel. For this reason, CW Doppler spectra are relatively broad (Fig. 11.4).

Pulsed Doppler

Pulsed Doppler systems consist of only one piezoelectric crystal that is used alternatively to transmit and receive ultrasound signals. The sound pulse or burst is very short (microseconds), and the pulses are spaced at fixed time intervals to allow detection of the reflected sound wave before the next transmitted pulse. Given that the speed of sound in tissue is 1,540 m/sec, the crystal is activated to "listen" for the reflected sound at a specific time after pulse transmission. This technique is called "range gating," and by adjusting the time interval between pulse transmission and gate activation, flow signals from a given range or depth can be evaluated (Fig. 11.5).

Pulsed Doppler systems, therefore, provide the capability of precisely locating a desired vessel and allow discrete sampling of flow within that vessel. The velocities detected represent all of the velocities within a small area called the "sample volume." The size and shape of the sample volume depend on the pulse length and the beam width of sound in the region of interest. The depth at which the velocities are analyzed is controlled by the amount of delay in the range gate. More advanced Doppler systems provide operator control of the sample volume length for specific quantitative applications. Due to discrete sampling, the pulsed Doppler technique greatly reduces noise artifacts and provides analysis of center-stream blood flow. In normal flow profiles, most of the red blood cells have similar velocities, resulting in a narrow band of frequencies. Abnormal flow conditions can result in a wide band of frequencies due to turbulence and are detectable with pulsed Doppler systems.

When pulsed Doppler is combined with static scan imaging (duplex scanner), the position of the sample volume is visualized for accurate placement in vessels or organs (Fig. 11.6).

Doppler Spectrum Analysis

Spectrum analysis is a process of analyzing the component frequency elements of sound over a period of time or pulse cycle. The audible Doppler shifts vary in pitch over the cardiac cycle and occur in the frequency range of 20 Hz to about 16 kHz. The Doppler shift contains all of the frequencies (except those removed by high- and low-pass filters) that have resulted from movement of scatterers (RBCs) present in the sample volume. For some applications, experienced users can audibly distinguish arterial from venous flow and also differentiate normal flow from disturbed flow associated with disease. For more quantitative analysis, visual display of the Doppler wave forms can be analyzed. The most common displays include strip chart recordings and real-time spectra presented on a television monitor.

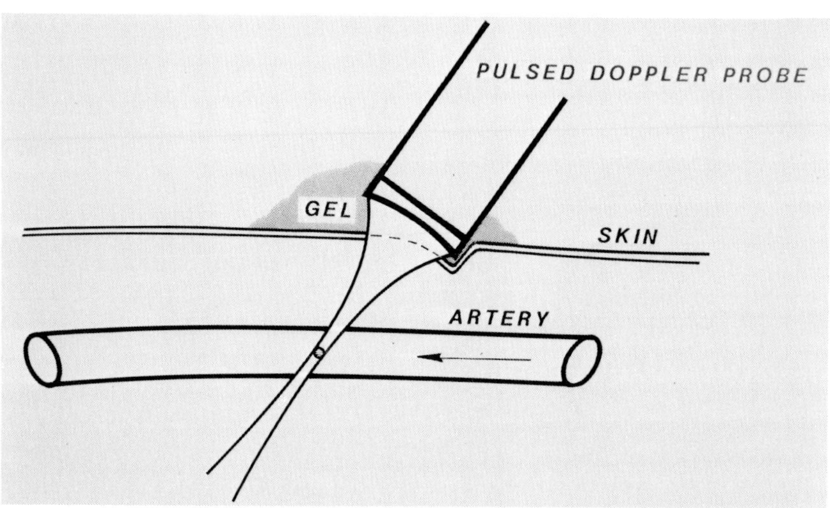

FIG. 11.5   Pulsed Doppler probes use one focused piezoelectric crystal and allow discrete sampling of blood flow from a specific location within the selected vessel of interest.

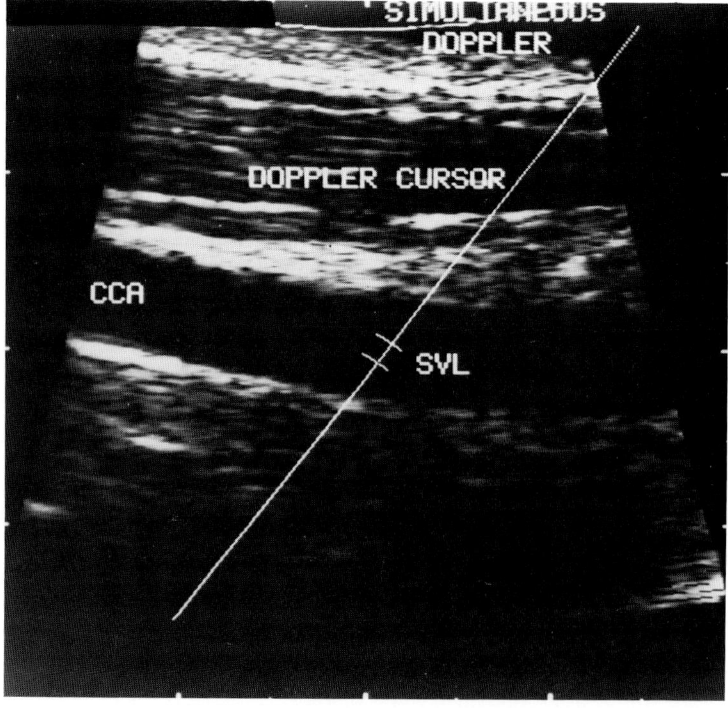

FIG. 11.6   Sagittal image of the common carotid artery (CCA) shows the position of the incident Doppler beam and the location of the range-gated sample volume (SVL). The duplex scanner offers the advantage of accurate placement of the Doppler sample volume.

246

Zero-crossing detectors[2] provide an analog tracing that can be recorded using a simple strip chart recorder. The analog tracing displays bidirectional information in a compressed, single-line wave form and does not display the entire Doppler spectrum; therefore, important diagnostic spectral data are lost. The analog wave form can be used as a qualitative indicator of the Doppler signal frequency response. However, it should be noted that the output of the zero-crossing detector is proportional to the root mean squared Doppler frequency and does not truly represent either the peak or mean frequency[3] and is inadequate for quantitative analysis. In addition, due to the complex blood velocity patterns found in most vessels, the resulting Doppler signal is complex and requires a more rigorous analysis, such as frequency spectrum analysis.

Real-time spectrum analysis is the method of choice for processing all of the frequency components in the wave form. Spectrum analysis is a process that separates the sound signal into its individual frequency components and shows the relative contribution (amplitude) of each of these components in relationship to the total signal over a period of time. This analytical process

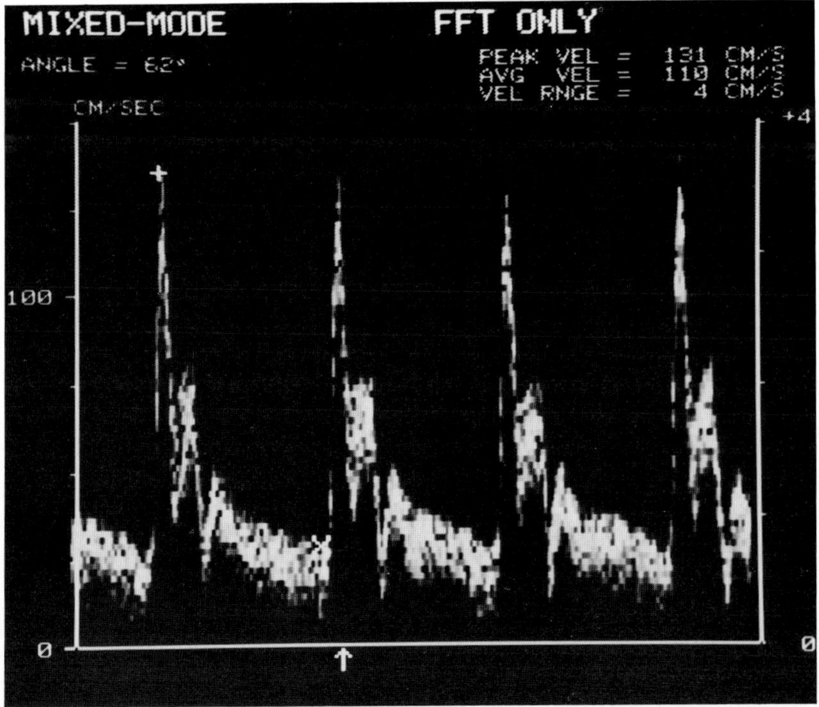

FIG. 11.7   Real-time, gray scale spectrum analysis display shows velocity wave forms over a 4-second period. Movement of cursor (arrow) allows automatic calculation of peak velocity (131 cm/sec), average velocity (110 cm/sec), and velocity range or bandwidth (4 cm/sec) at peak systole. Advanced analyzers allow quantification at any point in the cardiac cycle.

can be performed by a number of methods including multiple filters,[4,5] time compression analysis,[6] or fast Fourier transform (FFT) analysis.[7,8] The advent of digital electronics has greatly improved spectrum analysis through the use of FFT techniques used for rapid quantification of spectral characteristics associated with disease. As illustrated in Fig. 11.7, the FFT display shows frequency on the vertical axis (Y axis), time on the horizontal axis (X axis), and the amplitude of the reflected signals as different degrees of gray scale density (Z axis). Through analysis of all the Doppler information, signal artifacts (i.e., background noise, vessel wall movement, probe movement) can be eliminated, and specific spectral components can be quantitatively evaluated.

The ability to quantify accurately Doppler spectral characteristics associated with disease has been the basis for objective correlative studies leading to new clinical procedures in peripheral vascular, cardiac, deep abdominal, and fetal applications. Quantitative evaluation of gray scale wave forms and measurement of spectral parameters such as peak velocity, average velocity, band width (spectral broadening), velocity ratios, and pulsatility indices can be used as objective criteria to determine the presence of disease and to grade its severity. Advanced signal-processing techniques are opening new diagnostic potential for clinical investigation to determine the significance of volume blood flow

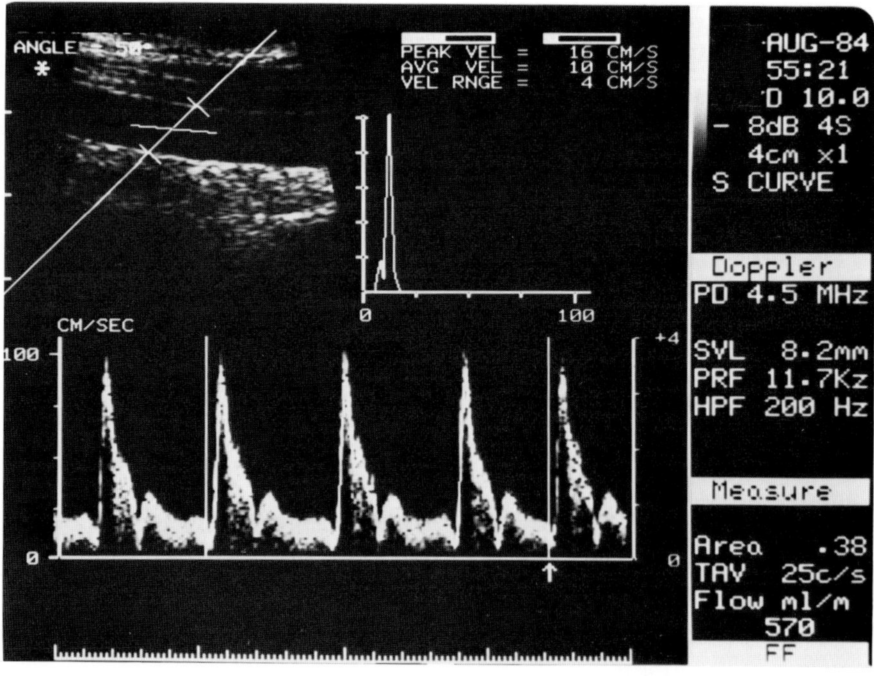

FIG. 11.8 Volume blood flow of 570 ml/min (right lower text field) is calculated based on a time average velocity (TAV = 25 cm/sec) over the three cardiac cycles and the vessel area (0.38 cm²). Automatic determination of volume blood flow promises new diagnostic potential.

(Fig. 11.8) and the analysis of spectral components of blood flow patterns using methods such as transfer function analysis and principal component analysis.

RENAL DOPPLER APPLICATIONS

The deep position of the kidneys and the presence of numerous surrounding vessels make the use of pulsed Doppler essential to isolate the blood flow signals arising only from the renal vessels. Thus, a duplex system which allows both imaging and Doppler is optimal for this application. An ATL Mk 600 and a prototype Technicare ultrasound system were used for the renal studies presented. The sector scanners allows optimal access for imaging, although the angle between the renal vessels and the interrogating Doppler ultrasound beam frequently approaches 90°, which is unfavorable for the acquisition of good Doppler signals. Nichols et al.[9] have reported the successful detection of renal artery stenosis using the duplex technique. They identified 59 of 61 normal vessels and 10 of 12 stenosed vessels, including 1 of 3 occluded vessels, resulting in a specificity of 97 percent, and a sensitivity of 83 percent, and 33 percent for significant stenoses and occlusion, respectively.

Visualization of the left renal vessels of the normotopic kidney is often limited due to air in the intervening gut. Even access to the right renal vessels can be difficult; in practice, it is often impossible to succeed in excluding a left renal artery stenosis. Because of these difficulties of access to the proximal renal arteries, parenchymal vascular Doppler signals in the normotopic kidney were studied; then the study was extended to transplanted kidneys, in which access is invariably excellent.

Duplex Doppler can be used in several different ways with varying degrees of sophistication in the investigation of renal vascular integrity. For the most simple application, the presence or absence of flow can be used to diagnose renal artery or vein occlusion. Spies et al.[10] have recently reported on the difficulties involved in the diagnosis of complete occlusion of the renal artery by static scanning alone. In segmental occlusion, the presence of segmental changes on the static scan indicates such a vascular accident. Duplex Doppler allows reliable diagnosis of renal artery or vein occlusion. Even where access to the renal vessels is limited, the absence of parenchymal signals allows the reliable diagnosis of vascular occlusion.

More sophisticated applications of duplex Doppler include FFT spectrum analysis of the signal to yield a time-velocity spectrum. The studies presented have defined the typical time-velocity spectra in all subdivisions of the renal vasculature from the main renal artery down to the arcuate branches. Tracing the renal vessels distally, the signal becomes less pulsatile and more damped (see below). FFT spectral analysis allows the reliable diagnosis of renal artery stenosis, providing there is access to the entire renal artery. Again, the anastomosed renal artery in renal transplants is easier to visualize than are the normotopic vessels. Renal artery stenosis is characterized by high-velocity turbulent jet with evidence for poststenotic turbulence. The recognition of such abnormal

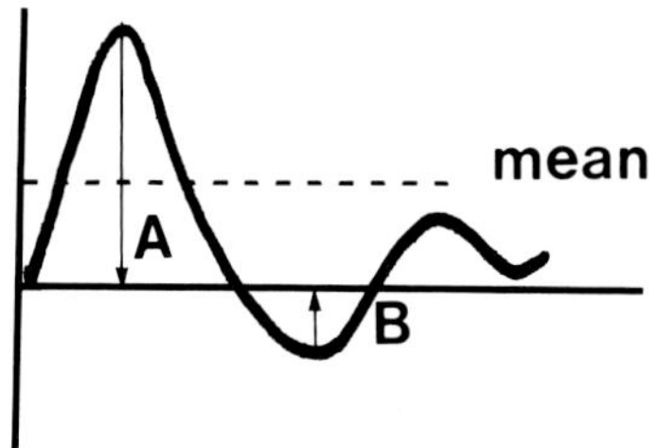

FIG. 11.9 Pulsatility index (PI) equals A minus B divided by the mean.

signals and their return to normal allow documentation of successful angioplasty.

Renal vascular signals can be quantitatively analyzed using the pulsatility index (PI). This is the peak-to-peak excursion of the maximum Doppler shift frequency divided by the mean (Fig. 11.9). It is a quantitative measure of pulsatility of the flow velocity; a lower distal vascular impedance gives rise to a more damped flow signal with a lower PI. Preliminary studies have indicated increasing PI as being characteristic of acute renal rejection.

Finally, the signals can be quantified further into an estimate of absolute blood flow. First, the angle between the vessel axis and the beam must be measured to calculate the velocity of red cells within the renal vessels. To calculate absolute blood flow, it is necessary to measure, in addition, the renal artery diameter. In such small vessels, there is inevitably a considerable error involved in this measurement so that, in practice, renal blood flow measurement is unlikely to be accurate. In view of the magnitude of these errors, it was decided not to try to measure this quantity clinically, although this has been achieved by others.[11]

Normal Kidney

Vascular Doppler signals arising from the renal vessels and renal parenchyma have been examined in over 30 normal individuals. The signals were elicited from the main renal artery and vein, the branches in the renal sinus, the interlobar arteries, and the arcuate arteries located at the corticomedullary junction. Slight movement of the Doppler sample volume in all these positions provides signals derived from the renal veins as well as arteries. The Doppler spectra are shown in Fig. 11.10. There is a major difference between the vascular signals seen in the aorta and those found in the renal artery originating from the aorta. Numerous different signals in the many branches arising from the aorta can be seen, indicating that the Doppler spectrum is more dependent upon the characteristics of the receiving circulation than the input signal from the aorta.[12] In the aorta, there is plug flow—that is, all red cells move at the same velocity at any instant in time (Fig. 11.10C). Thus, there is a flat velocity profile passing down the aorta, and the time-velocity spectrum shows a clear "window" under the spectrum. There is a small reverse-flow component, due

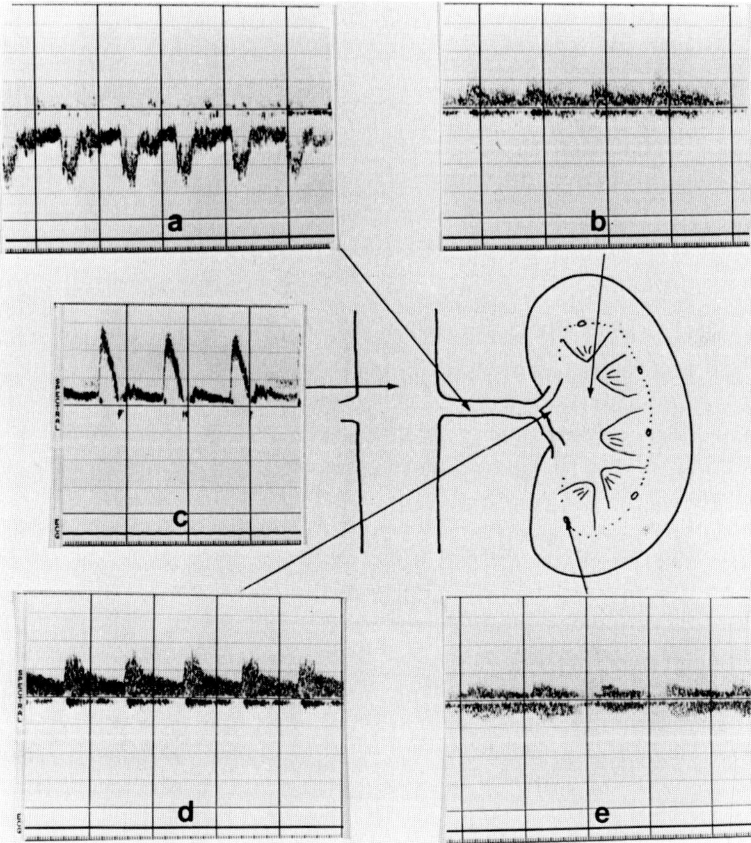

FIG. 11.10 Normal renal time-velocity spectra. (a) Main renal artery. (b) Interlobar artery. (c) Midaortic artery. (d) Renal sinus vessels. (e) Arcuate vessels. (Reproduced courtesy of Taylor KJW, Burns PN: Abdominal and pelvic duplex scanning. Ultrasound Med Biol, in press.)

to the high impedance of the lower limbs, which maintains diastolic flow to the kidneys. The Doppler spectrum in the renal artery shows much more forward flow during diastole (Fig. 11.10A), and this dampening of the signal becomes more marked as the smaller branches of the renal vascular tree are examined (Fig. 11.10B and D), down to the arcuate arteries (Fig. 11.10E). In the latter, the flow is almost continuous with little systolic modulation. In contrast, the renal vein signals are in the opposite direction and are continuous in the smaller vessels but show the same variation with respiration and cardiac cycles that are seen in the inferior vena cava more proximally. The presence of these parenchymal signals makes possible the successful detection of renal vascular occlusion, providing the equipment used is sufficiently sensitive to detect the normal signals.

Transplanted Kidney

In the transplanted kidney, the kidney is virtually always transplanted into the iliac fossa and the anastomosed renal artery can be easily seen and traced to its anastomosis using the duplex combination of imaging and pulsed Doppler (Fig. 11.11). The external iliac artery can easily be seen, usually lying on the medial aspect of the transplanted kidney. The typical plug flow, with a well-marked reverse component, is important to recognize since this may be the only signal demonstrated near the kidney in renal vascular occlusion (Fig. 11.12A). It must be recognized as being nonrenal in origin. It is also important to limit the width of the Doppler sample volume gate to around 2 mm so that there is accurate anatomical localization of the site of the signals. The pulsations of the anastomosed renal artery can be detected on dynamic scanning, and signals can be sampled at multiple points along the path of the vessel (Fig. 11.12C). Note that in this particular patient there was some turbulence in the anastomosed renal artery during diastole. This appears to be quite common, and it is presumably due to some roughening of the artery associated with the anastomosis. It is therefore important to obtain a baseline soon after surgery so that any subsequent change in the degree of turbulence associated with developing stenosis is appreciated. The renal veins and external iliac veins tend to be more easily visualized than the arteries and can similarly be sampled. The renal vessels can be sampled at multiple points within the renal sinus

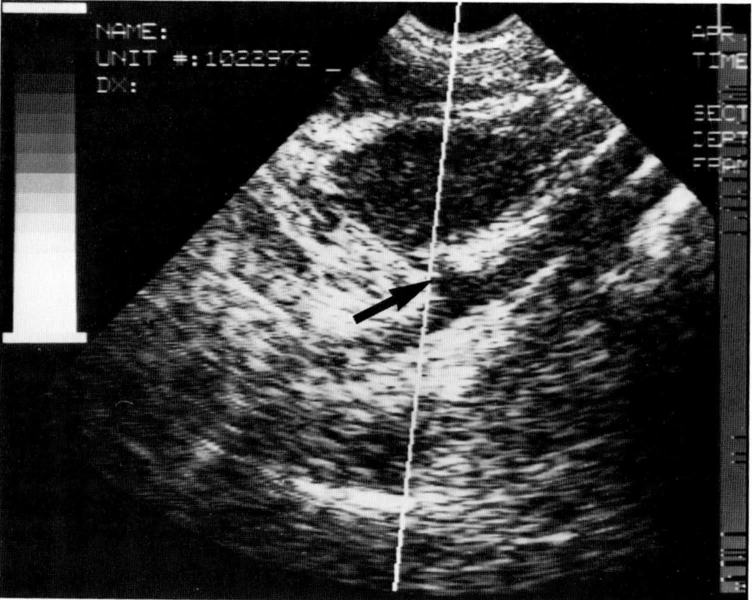

FIG. 11.11 Duplex scan of renal artery (arrow) which has been anastomosed to the external iliac artery.

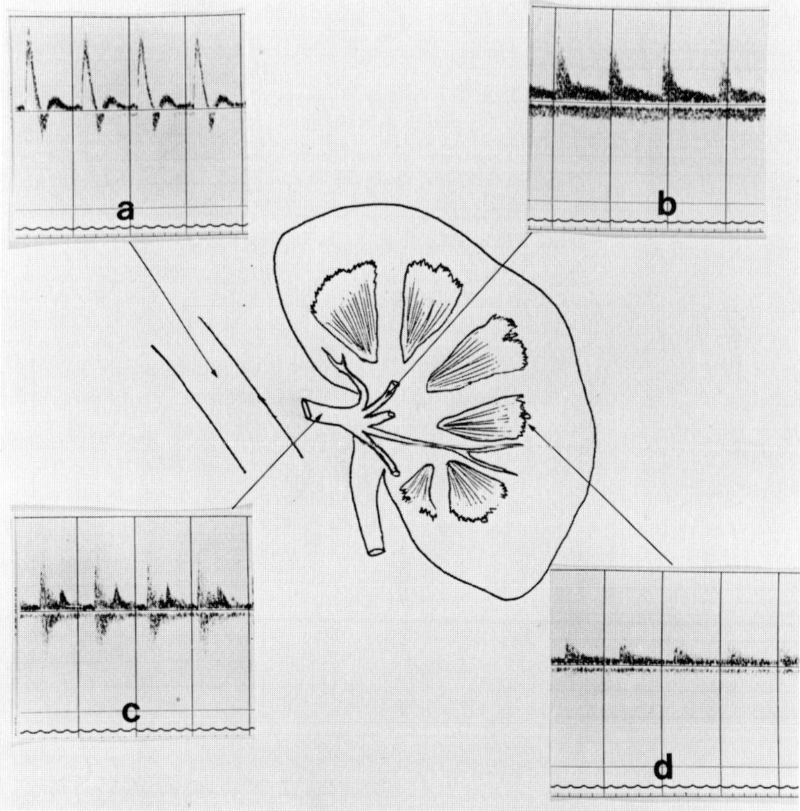

FIG. 11.12 Time-velocity spectra in normal renal transplant. (a) External iliac artery. (b) Renal sinus vessels. (c) Anastomosed renal artery which shows some turbulence during diastole. (d) Arcuate artery. (Reproduced courtesy of Taylor KJW, Burns PN: Abdominal and pelvic duplex scanning. Ultrasound Med Biol, in press.)

(Fig. 11.12B), in the midzone of the kidney, and also at the level of the arcuate vessels (Fig. 11.12D) lying at the corticomedullary junction. In 80 examinations performed on 30 patients, all patients with patent vessels demonstrated these normal vascular signals at all levels. As in the normotopic kidney, it should be noted that the Doppler signals become more damped as the more distal vessels become smaller in diameter.

Renal Artery Stenosis

A 44-year-old male presented 4 months after a successful renal transplant with renewed hypertension. The transplanted renal artery was well visualized and was searched throughout its entire length for an abnormal signal. The proximal artery demonstrated normal velocity (Fig. 11.13). A very localized,

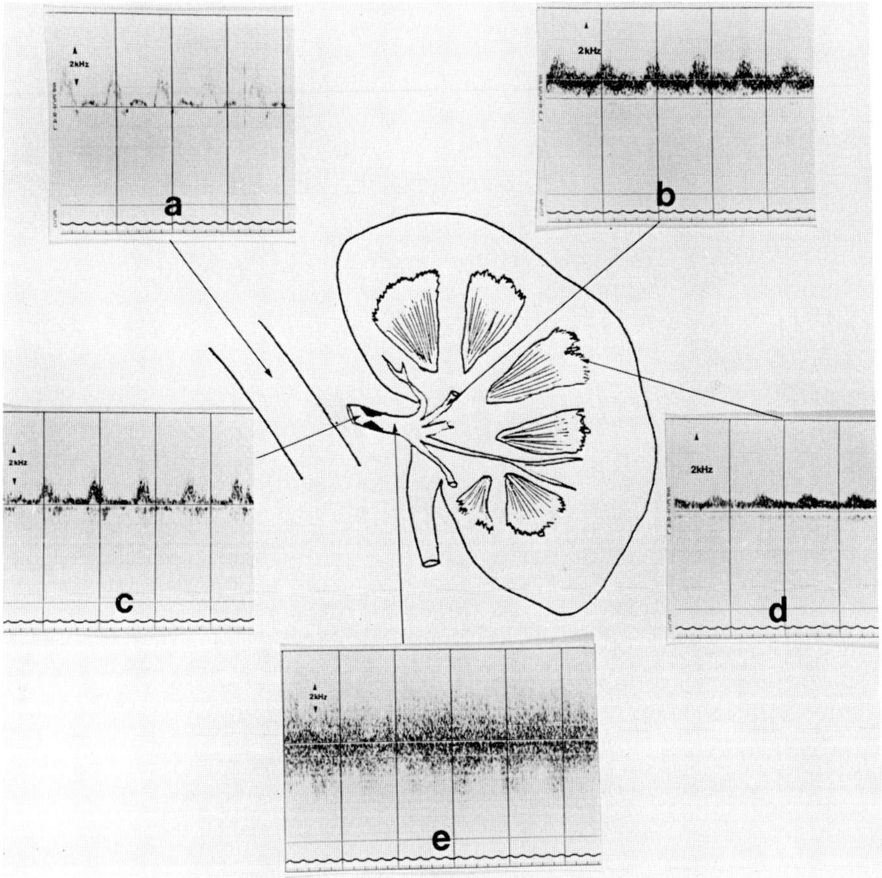

FIG. 11.13   Time-velocity spectra in renal artery stenosis. (a) External iliac artery. (b) Renal sinus vessel. (c) Proximal anastomosed renal artery. (d) Arcuate artery. (e) Turbulent poststenotic renal artery. (Reproduced courtesy of Taylor KJW, Burns, PN: Abdominal and pelvic duplex scanning. Ultrasound Med Biol, in press.)

high-pitched jet was heard but could not be localized for a sufficient time to permit recording. Gross turbulence was seen immediately distal to this jet (Fig. 11.13E). The presence of vortices and eddy currents gave rise to both forward and reverse flow. There was still turbulence in the renal sinus (Fig. 11.13B), but more distally the arterial spectra were normal (Fig. 11.13D). Digital intra-arterial angiography demonstrated significant renal artery stenosis, and an angioplasty was performed. Following successful angioplasty, completely normal signals were found throughout the renal artery branches (Fig. 11.14). This noninvasive diagnosis was most valuable as far as patient management was concerned. In fact, this patient was referred back some time later with a possibility of recurrent renal artery stenosis presenting with renewed hypertension.

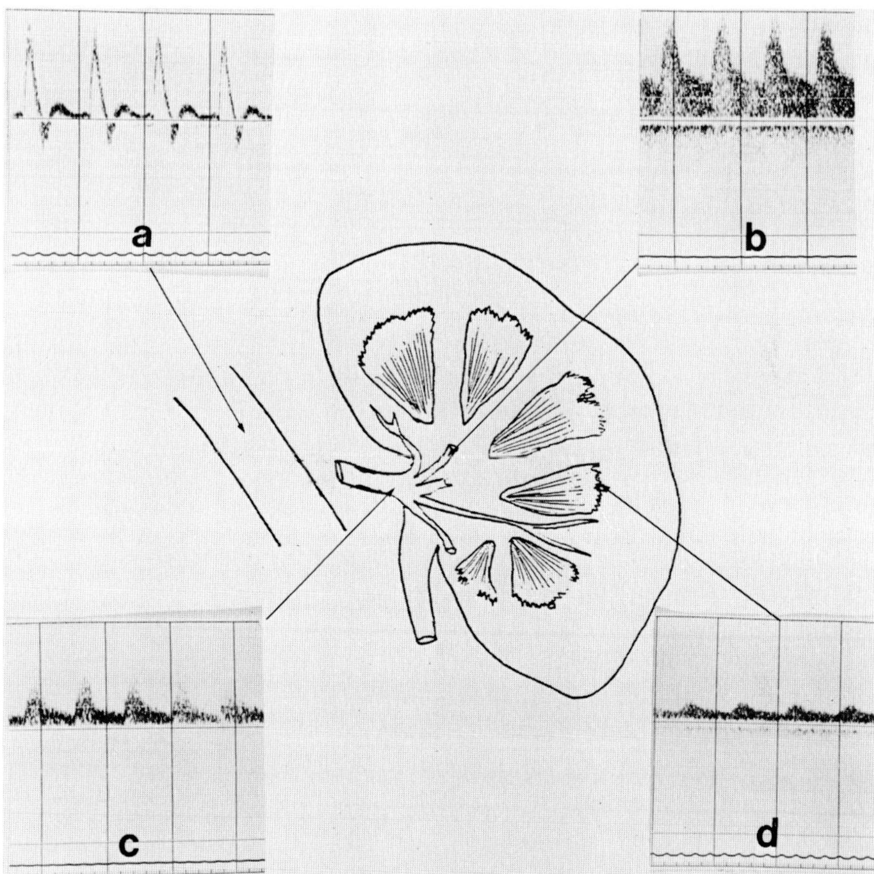

FIG. 11.14   Time-velocity spectra in renal transplant after angioplasty. (a) External iliac artery. (b) Renal sinus. (c) Main renal artery. (d) Arcuate vessels. (Reproduced courtesy of Taylor KJW, Burns, PN: Abdominal and pelvic duplex scanning. Ultrasound Med Biol, in press.)

On this occasion, there was no evidence of high-velocity jets or of turbulence, and the patient was taken off cyclosporine with resolution of his hypertension.

With other patients we have been less successful. One patient was erroneously considered to have renal artery stenosis based on highly turbulent signals which were due to noise. With increasing experience in obtaining these signals, fewer false-positive diagnoses will be made. In another patient with a high-velocity, turbulent jet, digital intravenous arteriography demonstrated a nonsignificant stenosis in an accessory renal artery. Our transplant team successfully uses ultrasound to screen for renal artery stenosis. When the Doppler examination is technically adequate, this diagnosis can be excluded. Doppler analysis may result in some false-positive diagnoses due to nonsignificant stenoses, but it does provide a useful triage mechanism in patients with renewed hypertension of unknown origin. Since renal artery stenosis may occur in up to 25 percent of patients with renal transplants[13-15] at varying times after transplantation, such a screening method is useful.

Renal Vascular Occlusion

A 48-year-old woman with a 30-year history of hypertension and diabetes presented with end-stage renal disease and dialysis for 2 years. She received a cadaveric renal transplant on July 24. Baseline Doppler on the following day demonstrated good vascular signals throughout the transplant, which initially functioned well. On the seventh day, the patient's creatinine and BUN were rising, and a renal scan demonstrated no perfusion of the lower pole. The renal scan was considered to be consistent with rejection. She developed small bowel obstruction and was explored 2 days later. On August 7, no Doppler signals were obtained at any point throughout the kidney, and the only vascular signal obtained on the medial edge of the kidney was typical of the external iliac artery (Fig. 11.15). At surgery, renal artery thrombosis was found, and a

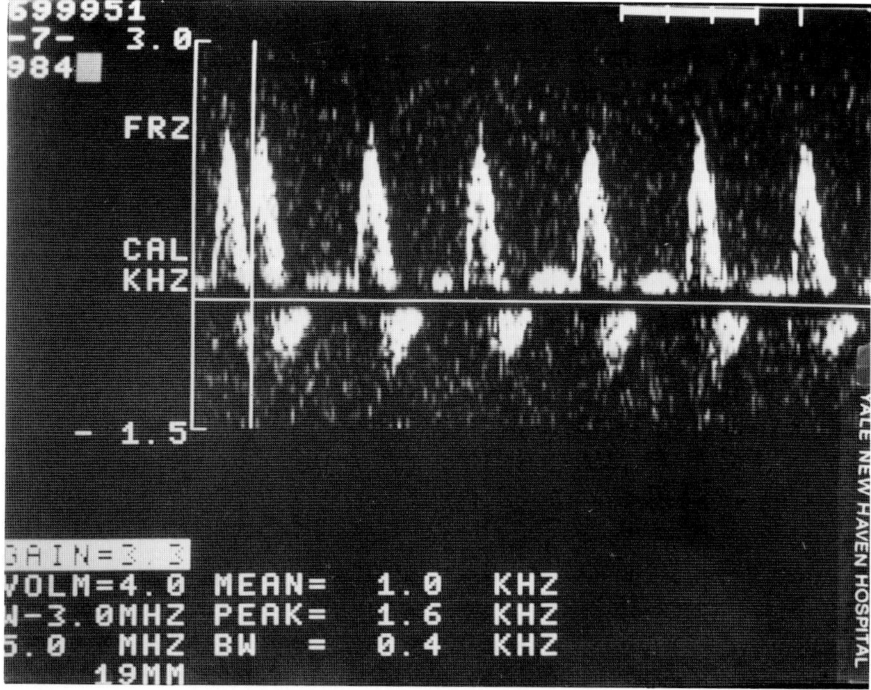

FIG. 11.15 Doppler signal obtained from medial edge of transplanted kidney. Note plug flow and reverse component are characteristic of external iliac artery (compare with Fig. 11.12A).

nephrectomy was performed. A pale hemorrhagic kidney was found with an intact anastomosis but renal artery thrombosis.

Renal Transplant Rejection

Two previous authors have reported abnormal Doppler vascular signals in patients with renal transplant rejection. Both Berland et al.[16] and Arima et al.[17] reported more pulsatile signals in rejecting kidneys. In 5 of 30 patients with transplants, we have noted dramatic changes in the renal vascular signals associated with rejection.

A 38-year-old female with probable Alport's syndrome underwent a renal transplant on June 20. This was followed by a period of oliguria considered to be due to acute tubular necrosis (ATN). A perfusion scan done immediately after surgery demonstrated good flow but subnormal function compatible with ATN and, in fact, the patient produced only 8 ml of urine in 24 hours. Duplex Doppler analysis on the following day demonstrated a high impedance in the arcuate arteries (Fig. 11.16A), suggestive of acute rejection. The following day, it was decided on clinical grounds that her ATN was not responding, and the patient was dialyzed. Six days after surgery, the nuclear scan appeared abnormal with decreased perfusion indicating renal rejection. Doppler studies were repeated on the following day and showed severe spectral changes. There was little systolic flow and no evidence of diastolic flow (Fig. 11.16B). Renal biopsy demonstrated vascular infiltration with lymphocytes consistent with vascular rejection. She was treated with appropriate therapy and improved, producing 1,200 ml of urine and decreasing creatinine and BUN. Posttreatment Doppler studies demonstrated excellent and normal flow in the arcuate vessels (Fig. 11.16C).

This patient is one of the more dramatic examples showing the utility of Doppler to assess vascular integrity of renal transplants. In 5 of 30 patients to date, ultrasound has demonstrated early rejection in patients assumed to have ATN on clinical grounds. These changes have generally preceded deterioration of the perfusion scan, and, in these patients with early rejection, the nuclear scan is usually interpreted as being consistent with ATN. It is notable that the changes seen on Doppler examination have been in patients with vascular rejection as opposed to those with interstitial rejection. Although more experience is required, abnormal Doppler signals in renal transplants are already becoming an accepted indication for renal biopsy and instituting antirejection therapy.

Patients with renal transplants frequently suffer numerous complications. Such complications include the abnormal accumulation of biological fluid including urine, lymph, or blood. These can all be successfully imaged by ultrasound. Patients with renal transplants also develop hydronephrosis which can be reliably detected by ultrasound, although an early baseline is required to note the degree of normal pelvicalyceal dilatation which occurs in the many patients with renal transplants. Thus, ultrasound has been used successfully

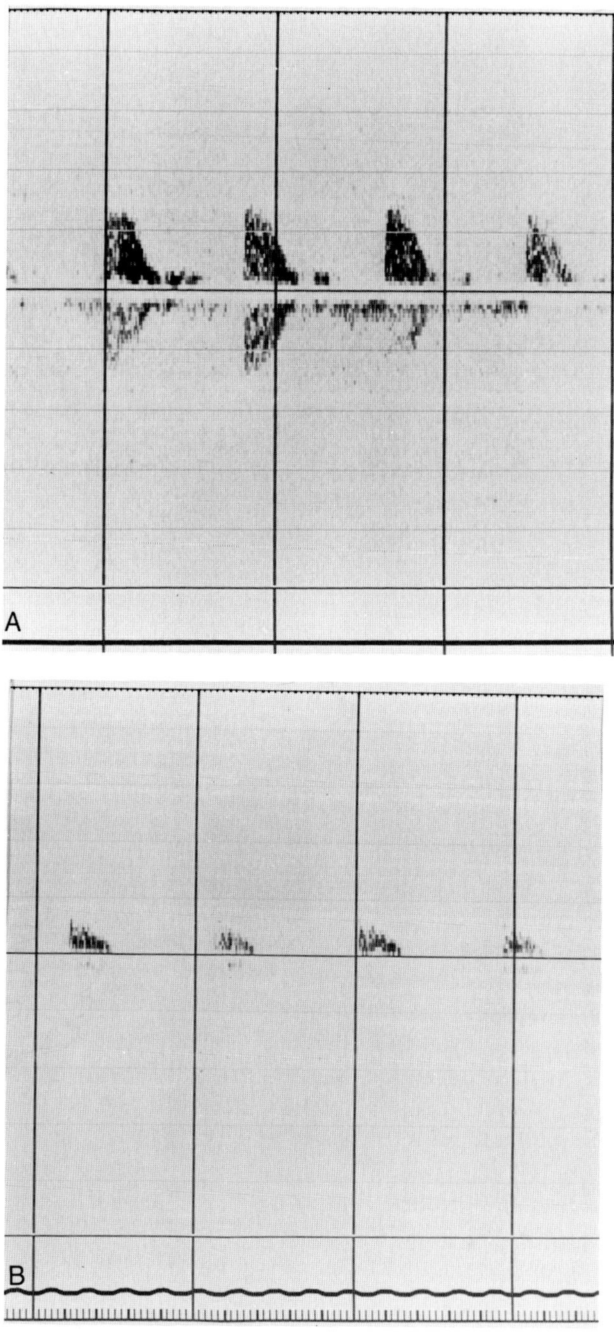

FIG. 11.16   (A) Highly pulsatile time-velocity spectrum with little diastolic flow indicates high impedance in an arcuate artery. (B) Low-amplitude signal with absent diastolic flow indicates high vascular impedance in severe transplant rejection (Figure continues).

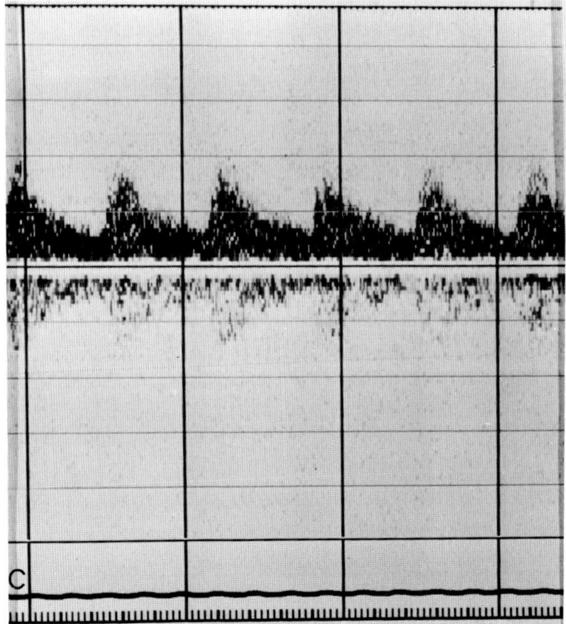

FIG. 11.16   (Continued). (C) Normal spectra after successful treatment of rejection.

to image the anatomy of the transplant and the surrounding anatomy. Vascular complications, however, are also common and include renal artery stenosis, occlusion, rejection, and acute tubular necrosis. Nuclear scanning is only of modest help, particularly in differentiating rejection from ATN in the early postoperative period. In practice, clinical evaluation with judicious serial biopsy remains an important means to manage these patients. With the ability to detect renal vascular occlusion, stenosis, and acute vascular rejection, duplex Doppler spectrum analysis now allows the evaluation of renal vascular integrity in addition to mere anatomical imaging. Much more experience is required to delineate the final use of duplex Doppler in evaluation of transplants, but already important applications are being defined.

SPERMATIC CORD: DOPPLER APPLICATIONS

The clinical diagnosis of spermatic cord torsion relies upon a history of sudden onset of severe unilateral scrotal pain and swelling, usually while the patient is at rest or asleep. In the absence of a typical history, differentiation of torsion from acute epididymitis is difficult and, in practice, the two are indistinguishable in 50 percent of the cases.[38] In many institutions, this uncertainty leads to an aggressive policy of immediate exploration.[39]

Diagnostic radiological modalities that are helpful in differentiating torsion from acute epididymitis include 99m scintigraphy, gray scale ultrasonography

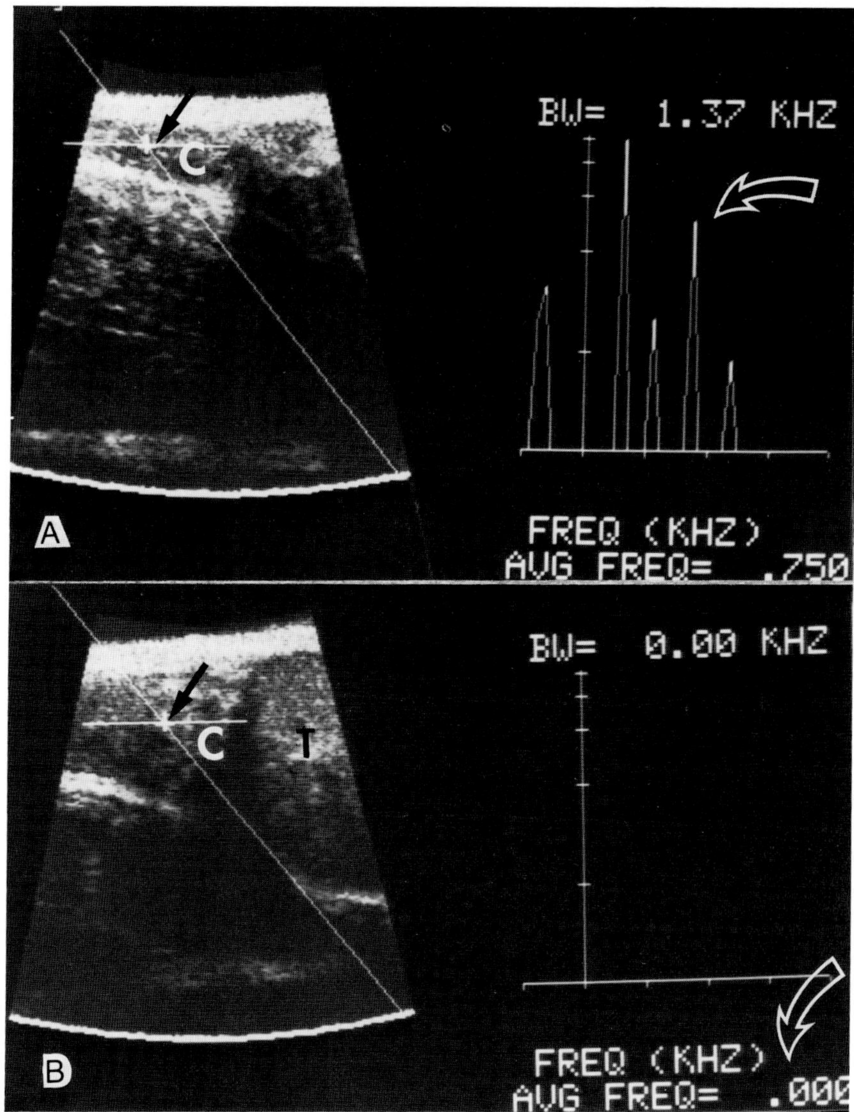

FIG. 11.17 (A) Pulsed Doppler from normal canine spermatic cord (C) shows normal blood flow (black arrow points to site of sampling in the cord). Graph on right documents flow (curved arrow). (B) Following spermatic cord torsion, pulsed Doppler shows markedly enlarged left spermatic cord (C). No flow through the spermatic artery or vein could be detected. Curved arrow points to average frequency of Doppler signal: O. T = testis.

and, more recently, Doppler ultrasonography.[40,41] While the results of nuclear medicine perfusion studies are encouraging, they have not been consistently successful.[44,45] The description of the sonographic findings, as well as predictive value of diagnostic ultrasonography, differs among the authors.[36,43,44] As a result of experimental studies,[36] it is seen that following acute spermatic cord torsion there is a spectrum of sonographic findings depending on duration of torsion. Unambiguous sonographic abnormalities can be seen within 1 hour of torsed testes. The spectrum of findings include testicular enlargement with an associated decrease in echogenicity of the testicular parenchyma, enlargement of the epididymal body, increase in spermatic cord size, scrotal thickening, and hydrocele. Unfortunately, similar sonographic changes can be seen in the case of acute epididymitis and, if doubt exists, a combination of gray scale sonographic findings and Doppler examination of the spermatic cord should achieve the correct diagnosis in a high proportion of cases. Early reports of Doppler techniques used a continuous-wave Doppler,[42] and the results of Doppler findings were sometimes misleading.[42-45] Greater accuracy is achieved using a duplex Doppler system, which allows precise monitoring of the site and sample volume of the vessels measured (Fig. 11.17).

We used a Diasonics 12 sector scanner with 10-MHz transducer. The unit is equipped with simultaneous Doppler system. Recently, we used Diasonics DRF 400, which allows even more precise measurements of the flow through the spermatic artery.

The flow through the spermatic artery is easily detected, and repeat measurements can be obtained. Also, there are reports that in the immediate posttorsion period, when venous stasis with preserved arterial flow can occur, the duplex Doppler system allows precise measurements of the flow within the spermatic artery which can be separated from flow measurements from the spermatic vein. A sample from the arterial and venous side can be obtained, minimizing the incidence of false-negative diagnosis.

In diagnosis of testicular torsion, we believe that combined sonographic and Doppler features are promising in the diagnosis of acute spermatic cord torsion and its distinction from acute epididymal orchitis.

DIAGNOSIS OF VASCULOGENIC IMPOTENCE

Impotence caused by either psychogenic or organic factors represents a serious problem, affecting nearly 50 percent of all men at sometime in their life. It is now believed that up to one-third of impotent men have some definable underlying organic pathology.[24-27] Among various organic causes (pharmacological, infectious, anatomical, vascular, neurological, and endocrine),[28] anatomical and vascular causes of impotence are potentially surgically curable. In the evaluation of anatomically caused impotence (phimosis, priapism, and Peyronie's disease), physical examination is usually diagnostic. Gray scale sonography can be utilized as an extension to the physical examination. In Peyronie's disease, it will accurately assess the extent of the fibrous plaque as well as its proximity to the deep arteries of the corpora cavernosa (Fig. 11.18).[29]

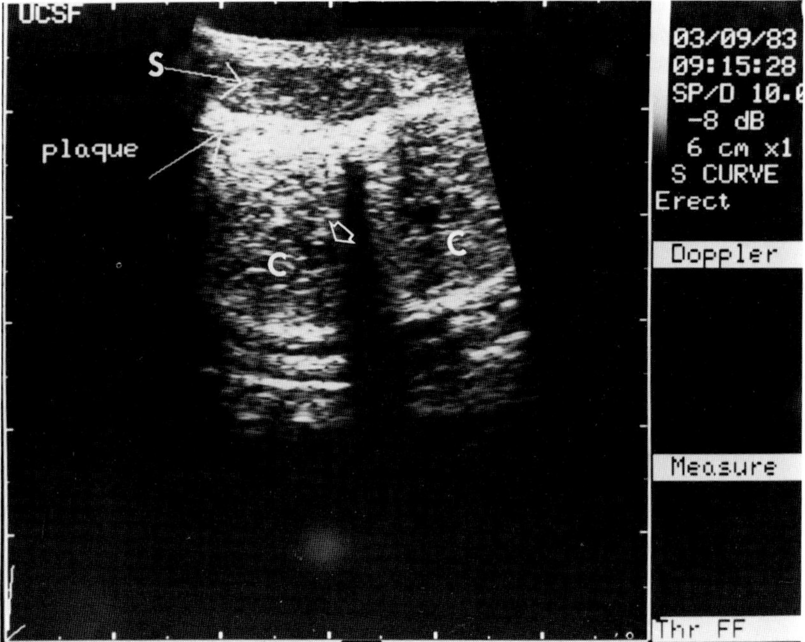

FIG. 11.18   Peyronie's disease. Transverse scan obtained following papaverine injection. The scan is performed from the ventral side of the penis. The corpus spongiosum (S) is seen anteriorly. Two corpora cavernosa (C) are visualized. Echogenic foci at the anterior part of the right corpus cavernosum indicate plaque. The proximity of the plaque to the dorsal artery (open arrow) is easily seen.

Penile erection is a neurovascular phenomenon resulting from arterial dilatation, venous outflow restriction, and sinusoidal relaxation.[18-21] Arterial compliance and adequate flow are essential to achieve erection, and venous outflow restriction is essential to maintain it.

In evaluating vasculogenic impotence caused by either arterial or venous insufficiency, radiological techniques are essential. Venous insufficiency can be caused by the deterioration of the tunica albuginea, leading to a venous leak. Repeated prolonged erection causes high pressure in the corpora cavernosa and speeds the deterioration of the tunica albuginea.[30] An erection cavernosogram can detect and assess the venous leak,[22,31] but the assessment of the arterial system is not possible.

Different methods have been proposed for the diagnosis of arteriogenic impotence. The penile-brachial index obtained by Doppler pressure studies of the dorsal and brachial arteries has been accepted as a valuable screening test.[32] Although its overall accuracy is good, a significant decrease in the dorsal penile artery/brachial artery pressure ratio can occur in the absence of detectable aortoiliac disease; conversely, patients with obvious aortoiliac disease may have normal penile hemodynamics.[33] The velocity/pulse rise time ratio of the penile vessels relative to the radial arteries appears more diagnostically promising, as acceleration may prove to be a more reliable factor in evaluating arterial insufficiency.[34] Blood flow into the corpora cavernosa in normal volunteers has been measured by xenon clearance studies.[35] In the flaccid state, the blood flow to the penis is 2.5 to 8.0 ml/min; in early erection, the considerable arterial influx to the penis results in average flow rates of approximately 90 ml/min; with full erection, the venous outflow restriction increases the pressure in the corpora cavernosa while the arterial and venous average flow rates are at their minimum, approximately 4 ml/min/100 g.

Arterial compliance and flow measurements can be accurately evaluated by a combination of static scan imaging and pulsed Doppler spectrum analysis. Sonographic techniques combined with papaverine-induced erection allows evaluation of penile vascular anatomy and physiology and is recommended as the initial radiological study in the evaluation of vasculogenic impotence.

Penile Sonography

Before diagnostic ultrasound, the patients should undergo routine evaluation consisting of a thorough history and physical examination, testosterone, chemistry panel (SMA 12), urinalysis, and snap-gauge (Dacomed) nocturnal tumescence monitoring. Patients are referred for sonography and pulsed Doppler studies if following all the above studies they are suspected of having vasculogenic impotence.

To perform penile sonography, we use Diasonics DRF 400V with an imaging frequency of 10 MHz (Fig. 2.7). The duplex probe contains two piezoelectric transducers positioned in a geometrical configuration that allows simultaneous imaging and Doppler analysis.[23] Blood flow studies are performed with the pulsed range-gated Doppler subsystem at a fundamental frequency of 4.5 MHz. The simultaneous display of the anatomical image during Doppler analysis provides visual guidance for the placement of the Doppler sample volume into the small vessel of the penis. The length of the sample volume can be varied from 0.6 to 10.0 mm; 1.3 mm was used in all penile studies. Blood flow was measured by the system's real-time gray scale spectrum analyzer with fast Fourier transform (FFT) analysis (50 FFTs/sec, with a frequency resolution of 50 Hz). The velocity data were automatically converted from frequency data, resulting in the display of peak and average velocities from any selected vessel. The flow volume was calculated by multiplying the time of the average velocity of several cardiac cycles by the cross-sectional area of the vessel of interest.[37] The measurements are always made at the base of the penis. Papaverine (60 mg in 20 ml of 0.9 percent normal saline solution) is injected into either corpus cavernosum. A rubber band is placed at the base of the penis for approximately 2 minutes to allow the action of papaverine to take effect and to prevent leakage into the systemic circulation. After the rubber band is removed, the patient is asked to stand for observation for 3 to 5 minutes to assess the erection and rigidity of the penis. The patient is then asked to

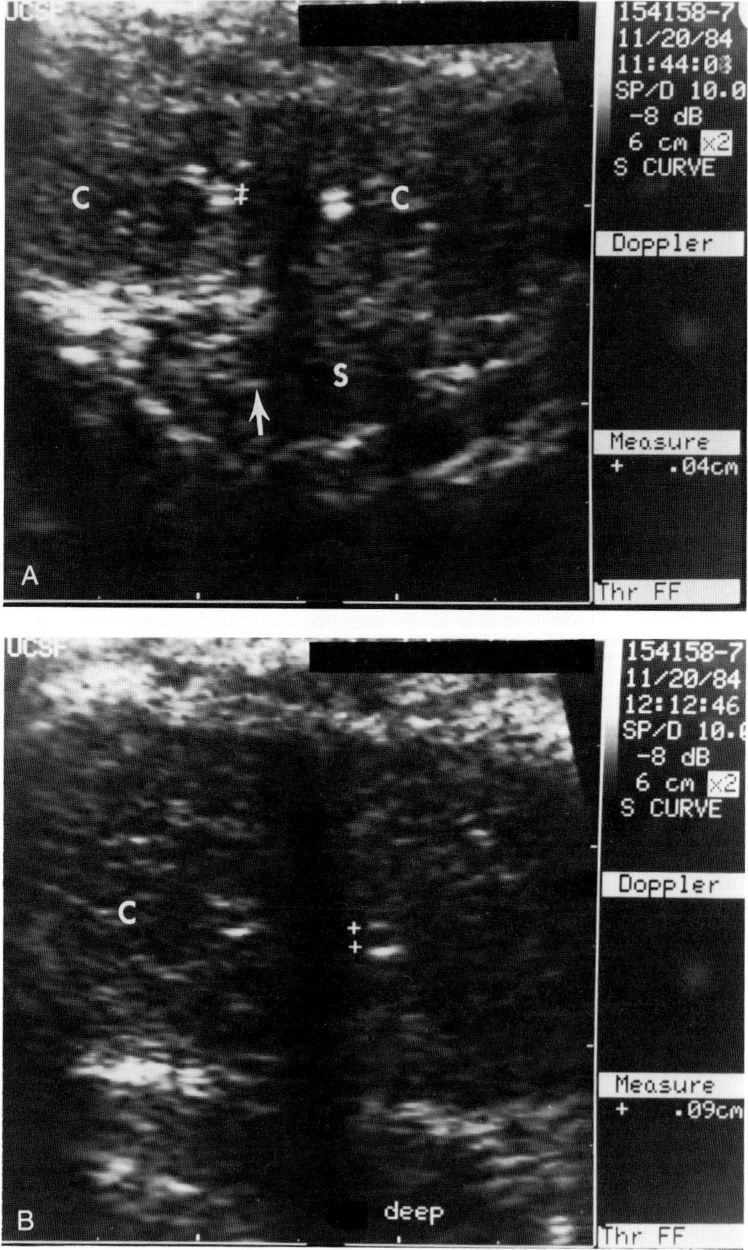

FIG. 11.19   (A) Flaccid penis; transverse scan. Both right and left corpora cavernosa (C) with dorsal artery (++) in the center are well imaged. Corpus spongiosum (S). Urethra (arrow). (B) Transverse scan obtained following papaverine injection shows dilatation of both deep arteries (++). The size of the artery changes from 0.04 cm in the flaccid state (Fig. 11.19A) to 0.09 cm in the erect state (Figure continues).

264

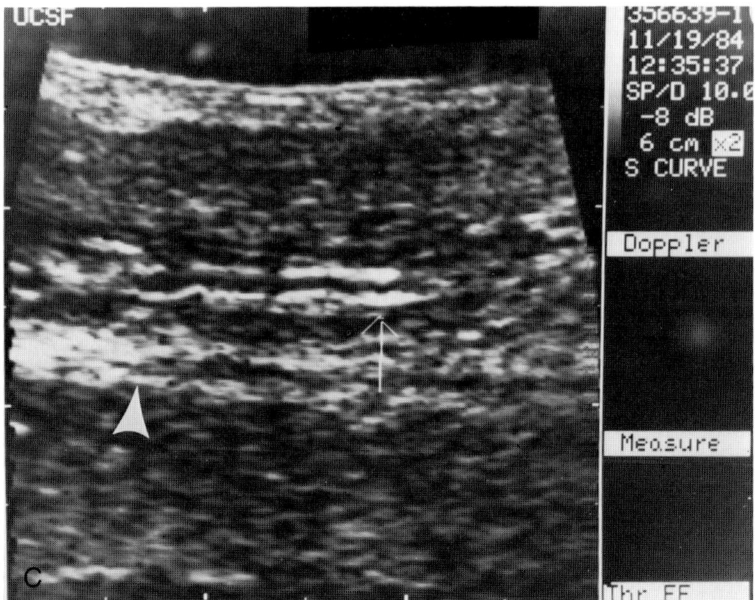

FIG. 11.19 Continued. (C) Longitudinal scan through the same section shows deep artery of the corpora cavernosa (arrow). Also, an asymmetrical position of the artery toward the septum (arrowhead) is seen.

resume the supine position, and high-resolution ultrasound and pulsed Doppler spectrum analysis repeated. This examination consists of measuring the inner diameter and blood flow of the deep arteries and blood flow only in the dorsal artery (Fig. 11.19). In some patients, intracorporeal pressure is measured with a 23-gauge butterfly needle.

The ultrasound study should be performed initially with the penis in the flaccid state to evaluate the size and shape of the corpora cavernosa, the corpus spongiosum, and the dorsal and deep arteries (Fig. 11.19). Electronic calipers can be used to measure the diameter of the dorsal and deep arteries (Fig. 11.19B).

The *complications* during penile sonography in our series of 90 were relatively minor. About one-fourth of the patients had a small-to-moderate hematoma at the site of injection; one patient experienced a slight drop in blood pressure; three experienced dizziness; and two complained of worsening erections.

The major concern is prolonged erection, which can occur in 15 percent of patients and lasts from 1 to 6 hours. Our policy is to aspirate the penis with a 21-gauge needle if the erection lasts for more than 1 hour. Two patients with Peyronie's disease required three aspirations in a 6-hour period. The others responded well to aspiration, with detumescence occurring within 1 hour.

CLINICAL RESULTS

Longitudinal, transverse, and coronal high-resolution gray scale images of the flaccid penis clearly showed the penile anatomy (Fig. 11.19). The sonographic appearance of the corpora cavernosa showed a homogeneous medium echogenic texture. Dense echogenic foci detected within the corpora cavernosa represented the parenchymal calcifications. The deep arteries of the corpora cavernosa on the transverse section were identified by their highly echogenic vascular walls and their location in the center of the corpora cavernosa; in the longitudinal section, the deep arteries were located asymmetrically within the corpora cavernosa and were seen close to the septum (Fig. 11.19C). The echogenic rim surrounding the corpora cavernosa is the tunica albuginea, and the medial highly echogenic line dividing the two corpora represents the septum (Fig. 11.19C). In the flaccid state, the echogenicity of the corpus spongiosum appeared similar to that of the corpora cavernosa. The urethra was seen as a focus of bright echoes within the corpus spongiosum.

After injection of papaverine, the erectile response varied from slight penile elongation to full erection and rigidity. Enlargement of the corpora cavernosa ranged from 99 to 263 percent; average area increased 165 percent. In addition, tissue echogenicity changed noticeably, showing an increased reflectivity at the periphery; furthermore, a hypoechoic area was seen in the periarterial region. The latter probably represents hyperemia within the periarterial sinusoids. The diameter of the deep arteries changed during erection.

The wide variation in penile size and length makes it difficult to establish a normal range for arterial flow. Before onset of full rigidity, the flow and diameter of the deep arteries increased in all patients. In those who achieved full erection, the diameter increased two- to threefold, and the flow rate increased markedly (Fig. 11.19); in those who experienced only a moderate or poor erectile response, the increase in diameter was small or minimal, and the flow increase was less marked.[37] More experience is needed to determine the normal values for this study.

Arteriogenic impotence can be recognized by lack of arterial dilatation and less-than-normal blood velocity after papaverine injection. As volume flow is the result of both vessel diameter and blood velocity, both parameters should be evaluated. It should be noted that patients with atherosclerotic disease, including penile vascular sclerosis and generalized atherosclerosis, have diminished erection capability caused by narrowing or occlusion of the iliac arteries. Because segmental stenosis in large vessels will increase the flow rate, an increase in velocity alone does not necessarily indicate an increased volume. We have noticed repeatedly that some patients may have arterial dilatation but still demonstrate a sluggish flow because of proximal narrowing, whereas others may have rapid flow but minimal arterial dilatation. Since the penile artery is close to its terminus, it should dilate to accommodate a free flow that will initiate and maintain erection. Tentatively, we now accept a diameter of less than 1.0 mm and a peak flow velocity of 30 cm/sec as our normal limit, providing a calculated flow of 3 ml/min (Figs. 11.20, 11.21). Arteriogenic

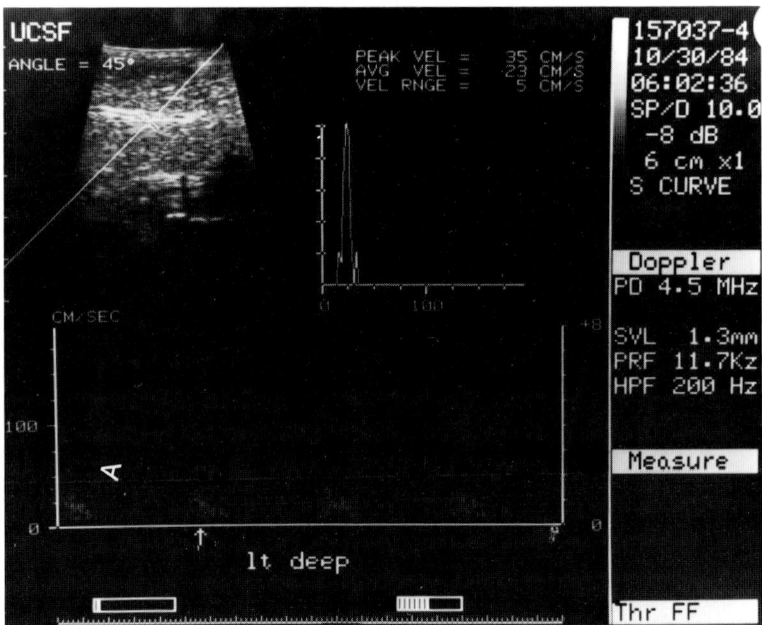

FIG. 11.20   Transverse scan in full erection. The flow throughout the left deep artery has a peak velocity of 35 cm/sec, and the arterial response to papaverine was within normal limits.

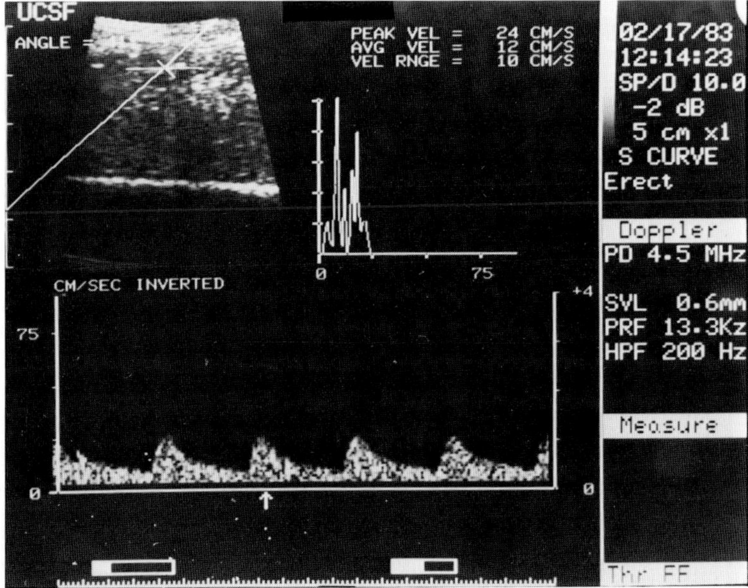

FIG. 11.21   Poor response to papaverine injection. The flow through the dorsal artery has a peak velocity of only 24 cm/sec. Also, arterial dilatation was minimal indicating that the vascular impotence was arteriogenic.

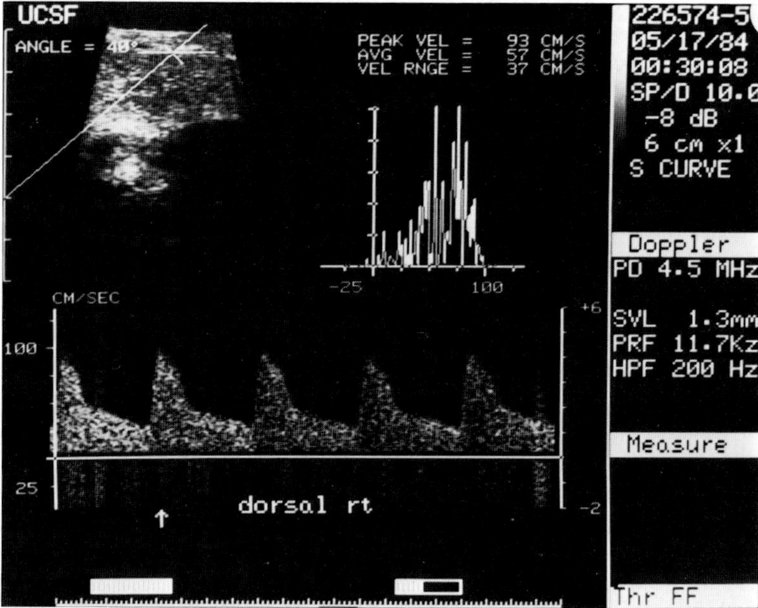

FIG. 11.22   Following papaverine injection, there was excellent flow through the dorsal artery with peak velocity of 93 cm/sec. Full erection was not achieved, and the vascular arterial response in the deep artery was poor.

impotence is a complex and dynamic process, encompassing a wide range of severity. Anticipating a wider range of normal variations, the data should be viewed in the context of the patient's habitus and the degree and duration of erection. If arterial vessels undergo dilatation and demonstrate increased flow during papaverine-induced erection, arteriogenic impotence is excluded. Should the degree and duration of erection be less than normal, venous leakage is suspected, and the patient should be referred for an erection cavernosogram.[31]

The initial size of the artery is not a good indicator for arterial disease; arterial compliance and the ability to dilate are more important functions. Also, evaluation of the dorsal artery seems less important (Fig. 11.22): good flow through the dorsal artery, but a very poor vascular response of the corpora, has been seen. Further studies are needed, but it appears that the evaluation of vasculogenic impotence with combined sonography and Doppler spectrum analysis has a valuable diagnostic potential.

REFERENCES

1. Satomura, S: Study of flow patterns in peripheral arteries by ultrasonics. J Acoust Sci Jap 15:151, 1959
2. Lunt, MJ: Accuracy and limitations of the ultrasonic Doppler blood velocimeter and zero crossing detector. Ultrasound Med Biol 2:1, 1975

3. Johnston KW, Maruzzo BC, Cobbold RSC: Inaccuracies of a zero-crossing detector for recording Doppler signals. Surg Forum 28:201, 1977

4. Johnston KW, Maruzzo BC, Cobbold RSC: Doppler methods for quantitative measurement and localization of peripheral arterial occlusive disease by analysis of the blood flow velocity vaveform. Ultrasound Med Biol 4:209, 1978

5. Light LH: A recording spectrograph for analyzing Doppler blood velocity signals in real time. J Physiol (London) 207:42, 1970

6. Coghlan BA, Taylor MG, King DH: On-line display of Doppler shift spectra by a zero line compression analyzer. p. 55. In Reneman RS (ed): Cardiovascular Applications of Ultrasound. Elsevier-North Holland, New York, 1974

7. Cooley JW, Tukey JW: An algorithm for the machine calculation of complex Fourier series. Math Comp 19:297, 1965

8. Kubak RJ, Nevrtal M, Tovarek L et al.: A method of analysis of the Doppler velocity-meter signal for determination of hemodynamic parameters. Scripta Medica 47:61, 1974

9. Nichols BT, Rittgers GE, Norris CS, Barnes RW: Non-invasive detection of renal artery stenosis. Bruit 8:26, 1984

10. Spies JB, Hricak H, Slemmer TM et al.: Sonographic evaluation of experimental acute renal arterial occlusion in dogs. Am J Roentgenol 142:341, 1984

11. Reid MH, MacKay RS, Lantz BMT: Noninvasive blood flow measurements by Doppler ultrasound with applications to renal artery flow determination. Invest Radiol 15:323, 1980

12. Taylor KJW, Burns PN, Woodcock JP, Wells PNT: Blood flow in deep abdominal and pelvic vessels: Ultrasonic pulsed-Doppler analysis. Radiology 154:487, 1985

13. Munda R, Alexander JW, Miller S et al.: Renal allograft artery stenosis. Am J Surg 134:400, 1977

14. Doyle TJ, McGregor WR, Fox PS et al.: Homotransplant renal artery stenosis. Surgery 77:53, 1975

15. Lindsey ES, Garbus SB, Golladay ES, McDonald JC: Hypertension due to renal artery stenosis in transplanted kidneys. Ann Surg 181:604, 1975

16. Berland LL, Lawson TL, Adams MB et al.: Evaluation of renal transplants with pulsed Doppler duplex sonography. J Ultrasound Med 1:215, 1982

17. Arima M, Takahara S, Ihara H et al.: Predictability of renal allograft prognosis during rejection crisis by ultrasonic Doppler flow technique. Urology 19:389, 1982

18. Lue TF, Takamura T, Schmidt RA et al.: Hemodynamics of erection in the monkey. J Urol 130:1237, 1983

19. Shirai M, Ishii N, Mitsukawa S et al.: Hemodynamic mechanism of erection in the human penis. Arch Androl 1:345, 1978

20. Lue TF, Zeineh SJ, Schmidt RA, Tanagho EA: Physiology of penile erection. World J Urol 1:194, 1983

21. Newman HF, Northrup JD, Devlin J: Mechanism of human penile erection. Invest Urol 1:350, 1964

22. Ebbelhoj J, Uhrenholdt A, Wagner G: Infusion cavernosography in the human in the unstimulated and stimulated situations and its diagnostic value. p. 41. In Zorgniotti A, Ross G (eds): Vasculogenic Impotence: Proceedings of the 1st International Conference on Corpus Cavernosum Revascularization. Charles C Thomas, Springfield, Ill. 1980

23. Wetzner SM, Tutunjian J, Marich, KW: Duplex scanning:A vascular diagnostic technology. Am Rev Diagnostics 1:31, 1983

24. Federman DD: Impotence: Etiology and management. Hosp Pract 17:155, 1982

25. Martin LM: Impotence in diabetes: An overview. Psychosomatics 22:318, 1981

26. Bohannan NJ, Zilbergeld B, Bullard DG, Stoklosa JM: Treatable impotence in diabetic patients. West J Med 136:6, 1982

27. Beutler LC, Gleason DM: Integrating the advances in diagnosis and treatment of male potency disorders. J Urol 128:338, 1981

28. Smith AD: Causes and classification of impotence. Urol Clin North Am 8:79, 1981

29. Gelbard M, Sarti D, Kaufman JJ: Ultrasound imaging of Peyronies plaques. J Urol 125:44, 1981

30. Tudoriu T, Bourmer H: Hemodynamics of erection at the levels of the penis and its local deterioration. J Urol 129:471, 1983

31. Lue T, Hricak H, Shinn-N L et al.: A new diagnostic approach for penile impotence. In Proceedings of the American Urological Association, 1984 (J Urol 131:231A, 1984)

32. Abelson D: Diagnostic value of the penile pulse and blood pressure: A Doppler study of impotence in diabetics. J Urol 113:636, 1975

33. Blaivas JG, O'Donnell TF, Gottlieb P, Labib KB: Comprehensive laboratory evaluation of impotent men. J Urol 124:201, 1980

34. Velcek D, Sniderman KW, Vaughn ED, Jr et al.: Penile flow index utilizing a Doppler pulse wave analysis to identify penile vascular insufficiency. J Urol 123:669, 1980

35. Wagner G, Uhrenholdt A: Blood flow by clearance in the human corpus cavernosum in the flaccid and erect states. p. 41. In Zorgniotti A, Ross G (eds): Vasculogenic Impotence: Proceedings of the 1st International Conference on Corpus Cavernosum Revascularization. Charles C Thomas, Springfield, Ill. 1980

36. Hricak H, Lue T, Filly RA, Alpers CE, Zeineh SJ, Tanagho, EA: Experimental study of the sonographic diagnosis of testicular torsion. J Ultrasound Med 2:349, 1983

37. Lue T, Hricak H, Marich KW et al.: Evaluation of vasculogenic impotence using high-resolution ultrasonography and pulsed Doppler spectrum analysis. Radiology 155:777, 1985

38. Bunce PL: Scrotal abnormalities. In Glenn (ed): Urologic Surgery. Harper and Row, Hagerstown, Md., 1975

39. Cass AS, Cass BP, Veeraraghavan K: Immediate exploration of the unilateral acute scrotum in young male subjects. J Urol 124:829, 1980

40. Holder LE, Melloul M, Chen D: Current status of radionuclide scrotal imaging. Semin Nucl Med 11:232, 1981

41. Holder LE, Martier JR, Holmes ER et al.: Testicular radionuclide angiography and static imaging. Anatomy, scintigraphic interpretations and clinical indications. Radiology 125:739, 1977

42. Pederson JR, Holm HH, Hald T: Torsion of the testes diagnosed by ultrasound. J Urol 113:66, 1975

43. Goodman JD, Haller JO: The scrotum. Diagnostic ultrasound in pediatrics. Clin Ultrasound (8) 264–275, 1981

44. Bird KL Jr: Emergency testicular scanning. Diagnostic ultrasound in emergency ultrasound. Clin Ultrasound (7) 55–70, 1981

45. Skoglund RW, McRoberts JW, Radge H: Torsion of the spermatic cord. A review of the literature and an analysis of 70 new cases. J Urol 104:604, 1970

CASE NO. 1   Sharon L. Abrams

Obstetrical Ultrasound for Fetal Age

A 17-year-old gravida 1, para 0 woman was referred for an obstetrical ultrasound for dating of her pregnancy. The examination demonstrated a single living fetus with a composite age of 19 menstrual weeks. Figure 1 is a coronal scan through the fetal abdomen and thorax. Figure 2 is a longitudinal oblique sonogram through the fetal abdomen with the fetal thorax on the left. Figure 3 is a longitudinal scan through the fetal pelvis.

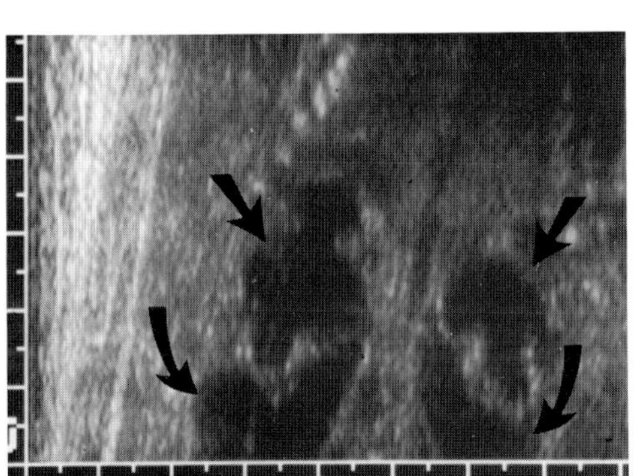

FIGURE 1

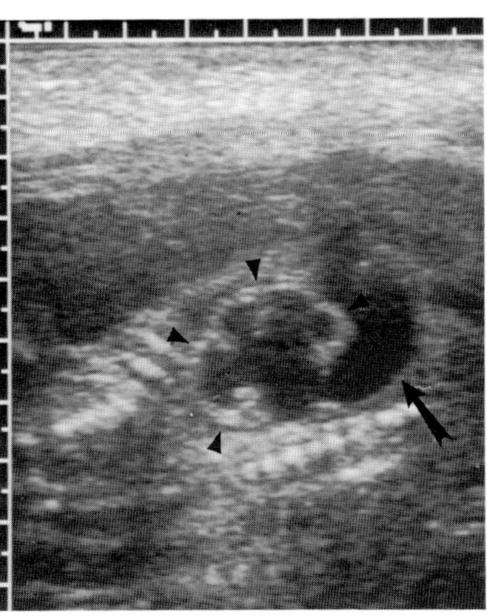

FIGURE 2

DISCUSSION

The ultrasound examination demonstrates bilateral hydronephrosis (straight arrows) and hydroureter (curved arrows) in Fig. 1, with a markedly dilated fetal bladder (arrowheads) and posterior urethra (arrow) in Fig. 3. A perirenal urinoma (arrow) formed from spontaneous decompression of the collecting system is seen in Fig. 2. The renal parenchyma is thinned with mildly increased echogenicity (arrowheads), but no parenchmal cysts. There is mild-to-moderate oligohydramnios. These findings are diagnostic of posterior urethral valves or urethral atresia in a male fetus.[1] Fetal ascites and abdominal wall distention may be present as well. In a female, the etiology is usually a caudal regression abnormality.[1]

The fetal outcome in this setting is determined by the degree of renal dysplasia caused by the obstruction. The kidneys are definitely dysplastic if macroscopic cysts are seen on the sonogram. However, if no cysts are visualized, increased echogenicity in the renal parenchyma is a less reliable indicator of dysplasia.[2] In this patient, urine from the fetal bladder was aspirated to evaluate renal function. Analysis of the urine electrolytes and osmolality indicated normal urine composition and, therefore, nondysplastic kidneys.[2] However, the patient elected to have a therapeutic abortion after extensive counseling. Chromosome analysis revealed a normal male fetus.

Diagnosis:

Posterior urethral valves.

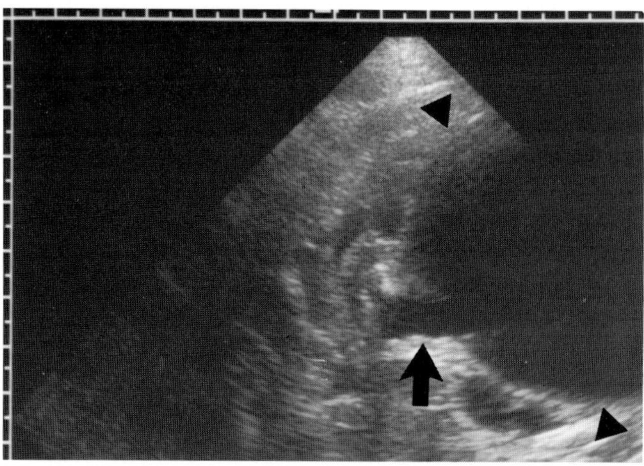

FIGURE 3

REFERENCES 1. Harrison MR, Golbus MS, Filly RA: The Unborn Patient: Prenatal Diagnosis and Treatment. Grune and Stratton, Orlando, Fla., 1984, p. 101

2. Glick PL, Harrison MR, Adzick NS et al.: J Pediatr Surg, in press

CASE NO. 2   Sharon L. Abrams

Seizures in an 11-Year-Old Girl

An 11-year-old girl was admitted for grand mal seizures. She had no history of urinary tract problems, and serum electrolytes, BUN, and urinanalysis were normal. Longitudinal sonograms through the right kidney are shown (Fig. 1 and 2). The left kidney had a similar sonographic appearance.

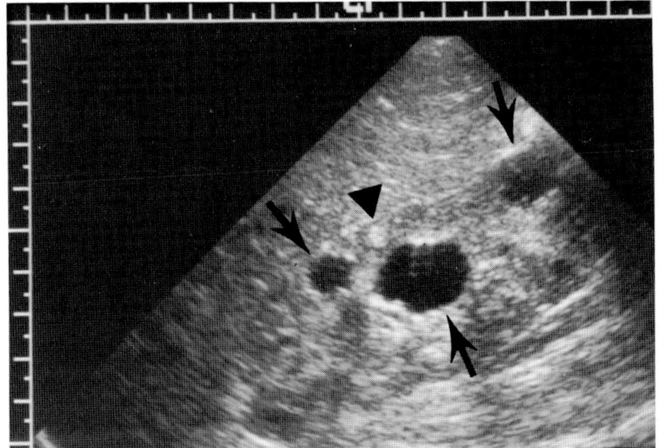

FIGURE 1

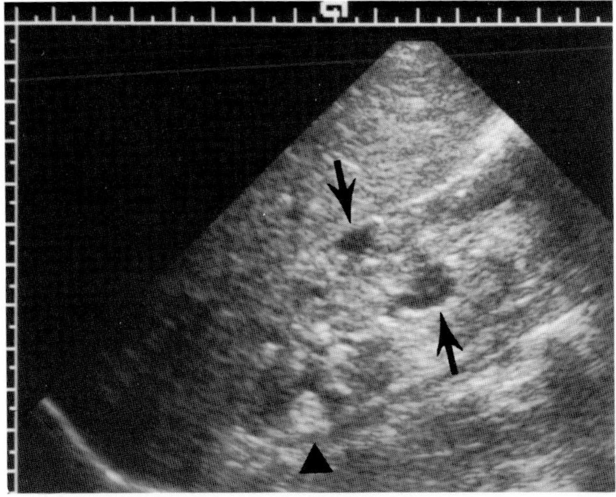

FIGURE 2

DISCUSSION

The ultrasound examination reveals multiple cysts (arrows) and hyperechoic masses (arrowheads) of varying size in the kidney, ranging from several millimeters to 3 cm. Echogenic renal masses may be due to angiomyolipomas, although this appearance is not diagnostic for this entity. The simultaneous occurrence of bilateral cysts[1] and hyperechoic masses[2] in the kidneys is highly suggestive of tuberous sclerosis. This patient had adenoma sebaceum, mental retardation, and epilepsy, the classic disease triad, as well as skin depigmentation.

Multiple, bilateral, small angiomyolipomas are seen in 40 to 80 percent of patients with tuberous sclerosis.[3] They are composed of blood vessels, smooth muscle, and fat, and the highly echogenic appearance on ultrasound is attributed to the fatty component of the tumor. Renal cysts are seen in 10 percent of patients with tuberous sclerosis.[3] There is no association between renal cysts and angiomyolipomas, and they can occur simultaneously in the same patient. These lesions are usually asymptomatic, but they can gradually increase in size and progress to renal failure due to loss of normal renal parenchyma. Hematuria is present in less than 25 percent of patients with angiomyolipomas.[3]

Diagnosis:

Tuberous scelerosis with multiple, bilateral renal cysts and angiomyolipomas.

REFERENCES   1. Mitnick JS, Bosniak MA, Hilton S et al.: Cystic renal disease in tuberous sclerosis. Radiology 147:85, 1983

2. Totty WG, McClennan BL, Melson GL et al.: Relative value of computed tomography and ultrasonography in the assessment of renal angiomyolipoma. J Comput Assist Tomogr 5:173, 1981

3. Elkin M: Radiology of the Urinary System. Little, Brown, Boston, 1980, p. 344

CASE NO. 3 Sharon L. Abrams

Chronic Active Hepatitis in an 11-Year-Old Girl

An 11-year-old girl underwent an ultrasound-guided liver biopsy for chronic active hepatitis. The longitudinal sonogram through the liver and right kidney (Fig. 1) was performed prior to the biopsy. The left kidney had a similar appearance.

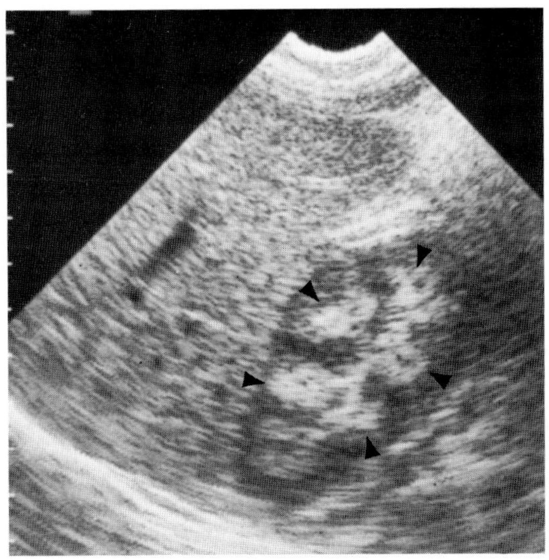

FIGURE 1

DISCUSSION

The renal sonogram shows increased echogenicity throughout the renal pyramids (arrowheads) without posterior acoustic shadowing. The echogenicity of the cortex is normal. These findings suggest medullary nephrocalcinosis.[1] This patient had primary hypoparathyroidism as part of her autoimmune polyendrocrinopathy-candidiasis syndrome. She received therapeutic doses of dihydrotachysterol and calcium supplements for treatment of her hypocalcemia, causing iatrogenic medullary nephrocalcinosis. Medullary nephrocalcinosis may also be caused by hyperparathyroidism, renal tubular acidosis, Cushing's syndrome, sarcoidosis, bone metastases, multiple myeloma, hyperthyroidism, milk-alkali syndrome, hyperoxaluria, and medullary sponge kidney. The major complications are infection, fibrosis, and renal failure.[2]

This patient's polyendocrine-deficiency syndrome included hypoparathyroidism, cutaneous candidiasis, pernicious anemia, glucomineral corticoid insufficiency, and chronic active hepatitis. The disease syndrome may also include thyroiditis, diabetes mellitus, hypogonadism, vitiligo, postnecrotic cirrhosis, alopecia totalis, steatorrhea, myasthenia gravis, and collagen vascular disease.[3,4]

Diagnosis:

Medullary nephrocalcinosis.

REFERENCES   1. Glazer GM, Callen PW, Filly RA: Medullary nephrocalcinosis: Sonographic evaluation. AJR 138:55, 1982

2. Elkin M: Radiology of the Urinary System. Little, Brown, Boston, 1980, p. 603

3. Dillon RS: Handbook of Endocrinology. 2nd Ed. Lea & Febiger, Philadelphia, 1980, p. 695

4. Rabin D, McKenna TJ: Clinical Endocrinology and Metabolism: Principles and Practice. Grune and Stratton, New York, 1982, p. 625

CASE NO. 4   Sharon L. Abrams

A 39-Year-Old Man with Acute Renal Failure

A 39-year-old Turkish man presented with acute renal failure 5 years prior to admission. Gallium scan demonstrated bilateral renal uptake at that time. With therapy, the patient's creatinine improved, and the patient did well for 5 years. He was readmitted in acute renal failure with BUN 119, creatinine 12, and 17 g proteinuria for 24 hours. Hypertension, pericarditis, and anemia were present as well. An emergency renal venogram was normal, excluding renal vein thrombosis as the cause. A longitudinal sonogram through the right kidney and liver is shown (Fig. 1). The sonographic appearance of the left kidney was similar.

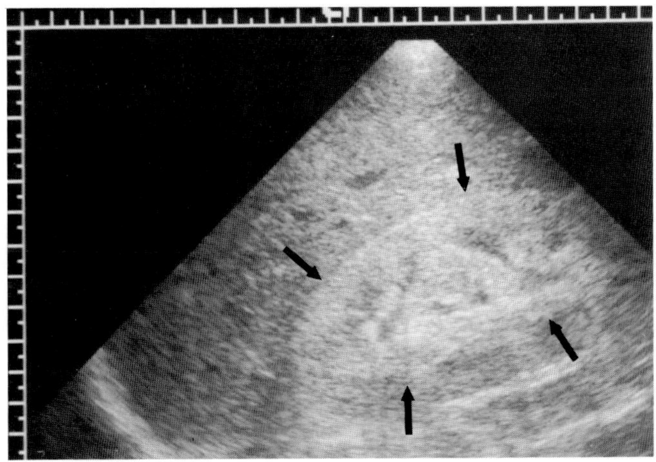

FIGURE 1

DISCUSSION

The renal ultrasound shows an enlarged echogenic kidney (arrows) without hydronephrosis. The renal echogenicity is greater than that of the liver and equal to the renal sinus fat. Renal biopsy revealed severe renal amyloidosis and acute interstitial nephritis. This patient also had familial Mediterranean fever, which is complicated by amyloid in 26 to 40 percent of individuals.[1] Amyloid is usually the cause of death in these patients.[2] Enlarged kidneys are seen in the acute stage of amyloidosis, and the kidneys decrease in size with advanced disease.[3] However, renal enlargement was present in 36 children with renal amyloidosis secondary to familial Mediterranean fever.[1]

The etiology of the interstitial nephritis in this patient was not known. Histologically, it was compatible with a drug hypersensitivity reaction. Both active interstitial disease and amyloid may cause increased cortical echogenicity on ultrasound.[4]

Diagnosis:

1. Renal amyloidosis secondary to familial Mediterranean fever.
2. Acute interstitial nephritis.

REFERENCES   1. Ekelund L: Radiologic findings in renal amyloidosis. Am J Roetgenol 129:851, 1977

2. Elkin M: Radiology of the Urinary System. Little, Brown, Boston, 1980, p. 1000

3. Subramanyam BR: Renal amyloidosis in juvenile rheumatoid arthritis: Sonographic features. AJR 136:411, 1981

4. Rosenfield AT, Siegel NJ:Renal parenchymal disease: Histopathologic-sonographic correlation. AJR 137:793, 1981

CASE NO. 5   Sharon L. Abrams

Possible Sepsis in a 7-Day-Old Infant

A 7-day-old girl presented with possible sepsis and dehydration. The initial urinalysis showed 10 to 25 WBC/HPF. All cultures were negative, but the urine specimen was obtained after the first dose of antibiotics. An abdominal ultrasound was performed. Longitudinal scans through the liver and right kidney (Fig. 1) and right lower abdomen and pelvis (Fig. 2) are shown.

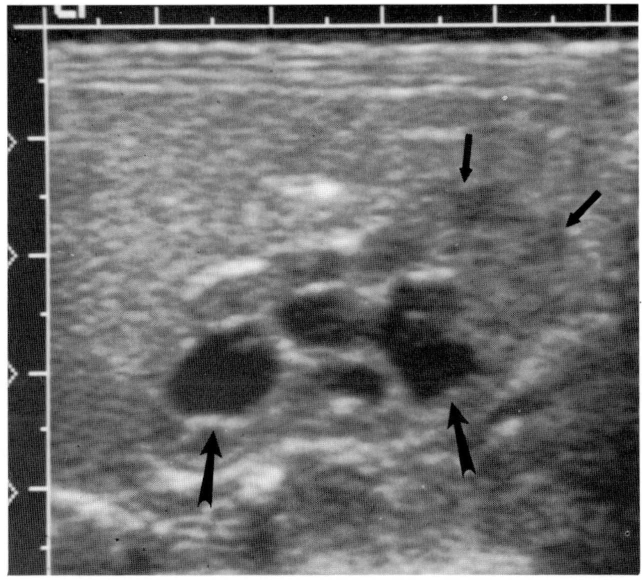

FIGURE 1

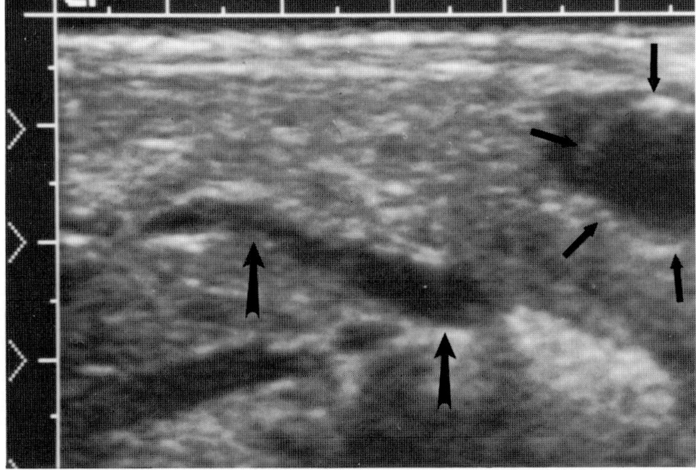

FIGURE 2

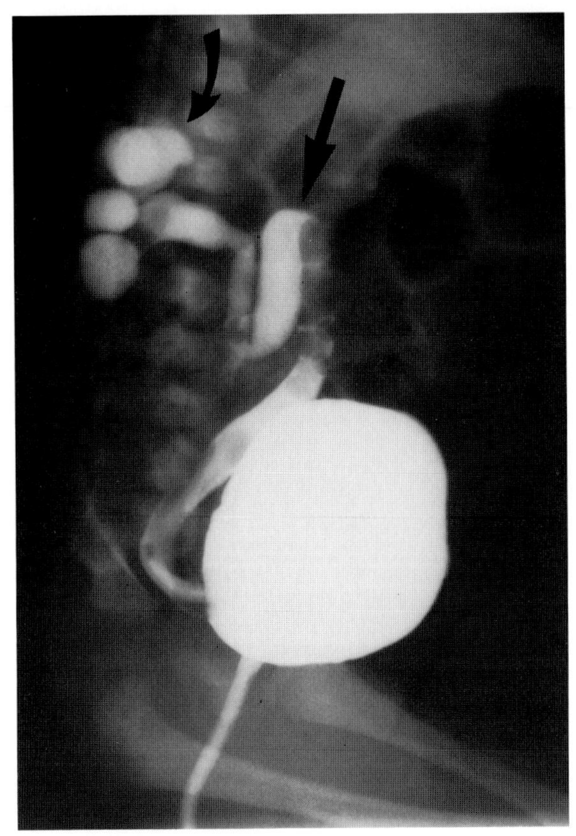

FIGURE 3

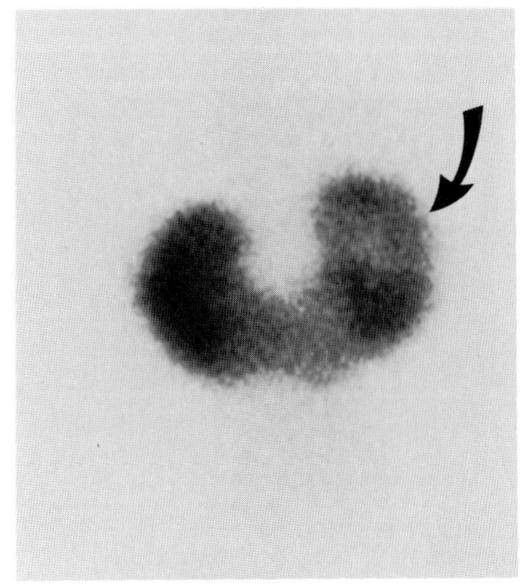

FIGURE 4

DISCUSSION

The abdominal ultrasound demonstrates hydronephrosis (Fig. 1, large arrows) of the upper pole moiety in a right duplex kidney. An ectopic ureterocele (Fig. 2, small arrows) with right hydroureter (large arrows) is well visualized. The voiding cystourethrogram (Fig. 3) shows the ectopic ureterocele with significant reflux into a dilated right ureter (straight arrow) and right intrarenal collecting system (curved arrow). A dimercaptosuccinic acid radionuclide scan was then obtained. The posterior view (Fig. 4) shows a horseshoe kidney with decreased activity in the upper pole of the right kidney (arrow) compatible with obstruction. In retrospect, the lower pole of the right kidney does extend toward the midline, forming the isthmus of the horseshoe kidney (Fig. 1, small arrows). Ultrasound is useful in identifying horseshoe kidneys,[1] collecting-system duplications,[2] ectopic ureters, and ureteroceles.[3]

Cystoscopy confirmed the presence of three ureteral orifices, one ectopic and two in their normal position. The patient expired at 6 weeks of age after readmission for *Escherichia coli* pyelonephritis and unsuccessful resuscitation after cardiac arrest.

Diagnosis:

1. Horseshoe kidney.
2. Right renal duplication with obstruction of upper pole moiety and ectopic ureter secondary to ectopic ureterocele.

REFERENCES 1. Gay Jr BB, Dawes RK, Atkinson Jr GO et al.: Wilms' tumor in horseshoe kidneys: Radiologic diagnosis. Radiology 146:693, 1983

2. Schaffer RM, Shih YH, Becker JA: Sonographic identification of collecting system duplications. J Clin Ultrasound 11:309, 1983

3. Mascatello VJ, Smith EH, Carrera GF et al.: Ultrasonic evaluation of the obstructed duplex kidney. Am J Roentgenol 129:113, 1977

CASE NO. 6   Sharon L. Abrams

Three-Year-Old Child with Persistent Hematuria

A 3-year-old Chinese boy was evaluated for a 2-month history of persistent hematuria. A cystoscopy and an intravenous urogram were performed. Ultrasound examination of the kidneys was normal. Longitudinal and transverse real-time sonograms through the pelvis are shown in Figs. 1 and 2, respectively.

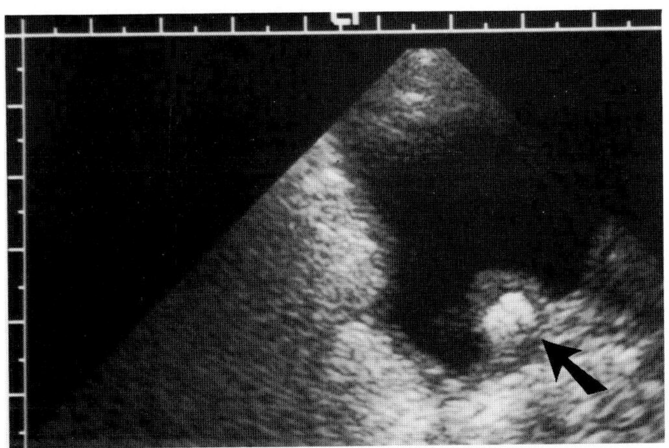

FIGURE 1

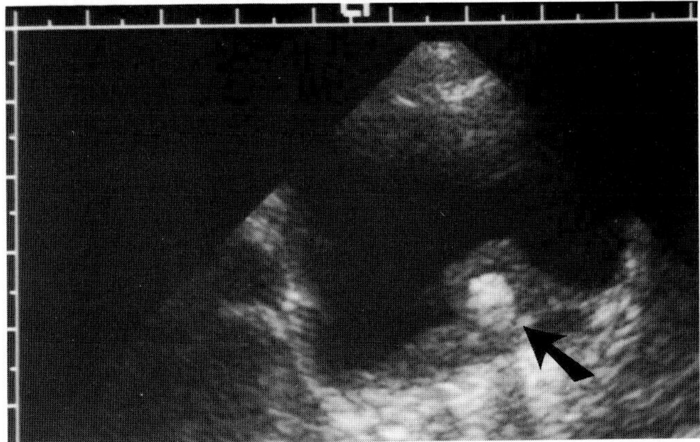

FIGURE 2

DISCUSSION

The ultrasound examination through the urinary bladder demonstrates two foci of high-amplitude echoes (arrows) with posterior shadowing compatible with stones. The calculi are within a ureterocele. The findings confirm those seen at cystoscopy and intravenous urography. At surgery, the ureterocele was incised, and two stones were removed.

Simple ureteroceles are usually associated with nonduplicated renal collecting systems, as in this case, and are due to congenital or acquired narrowing of the ureteral orifice. The typical cobra-head appearance on intravenous urography is caused by prolapse of the dilated distal ureter into the bladder lumen. The ureter usually enters the bladder in its normal position. Simple ureteroceles may be complicated by hydronephrosis, infection, and calculi. They are not usually associated with reflux.[1]

Diagnosis:

Simple ureterocele containing calculi.

REFERENCE 1. Ney C, Friedenberg RM: Radiographic Atlas of the Genitourinary system. 2nd Ed. Vol II. J.B. Lippincott, Philadelphia, 1981, p. 1134

CASE NO. 7   Sharon L. Abrams

Scrotal Swelling in a Middle-Aged Man

A 42-year-old man presented with headaches 6 weeks after a right pontine hemorrhage. He incidentally noted the acute onset of right scrotal swelling on the day of admission. On physical exam, the testis was enlarged, firm, nontender, and the scrotum transilluminated. A scrotal ultrasound was performed and right longitudinal (Fig. 1) and transverse (Fig. 2) sonograms are shown.

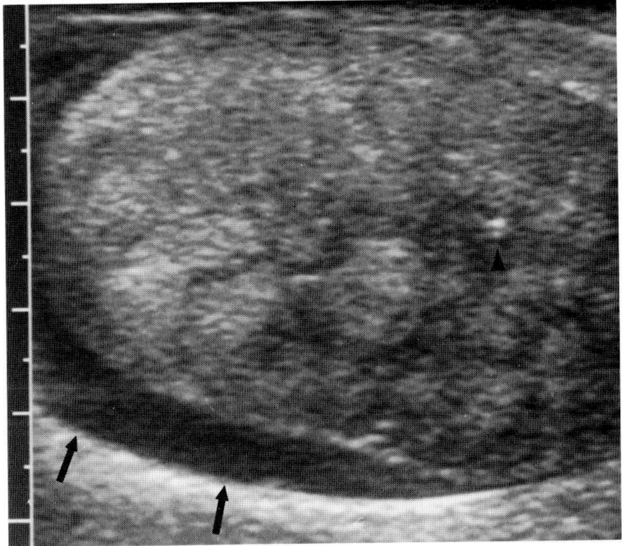

FIGURE 1

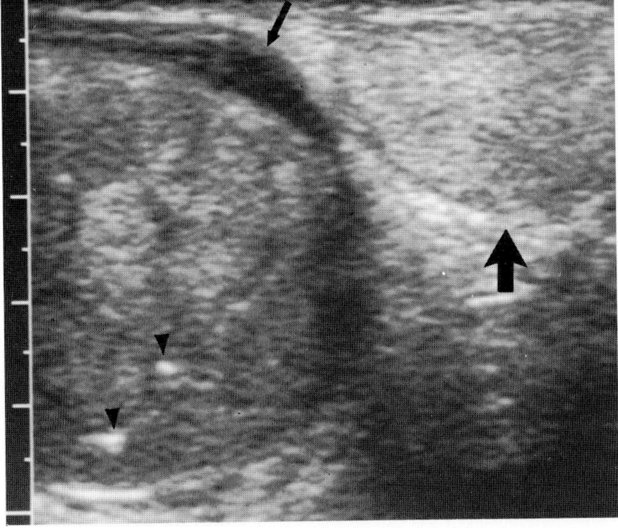

FIGURE 2

DISCUSSION

The ultrasound examination demonstrates an enlarged right testis with a diffusely inhomogeneous echo texture. Several punctate calcifications are present within the mass (arrowheads). There is an intrascrotal fluid collection representing a hydrocele (small arrows). The left testis is normal (Fig. 2, large arrow). A radical orchiectomy was performed. The surgical specimen revealed a seminoma without invasion through the tunica albuginea.

Most testicular neoplasms (97.6 percent) are malignant germinal cell tumors with four basic histological patterns: seminoma, embryonal carcinoma, teratomas, and choriocarcinoma.[1] Sonographically, testicular tumors demonstrate parenchyma inhomogeneity throughout the testis. Localized tumors usually appear as well-circumscribed, hypoechoic masses within an otherwise normal testis. Less commonly, hyperechoic or mixed echogenic masses may be seen. Ultrasound is sensitive (80 to 90 percent), but nonspecific, in detecting testicular neoplasms.[1] The sonographic appearance may be mimicked by orchitis, hemorrhage, infarction, abscess, or chronic torsion. Less than 10 percent of hydroceles are associated with testicular neoplasms.[1]

Diagnosis:

Seminoma.

REFERENCE   1. Hricak H, Filly RA: Sonography of the scrotum. Invest Radiol 18:112, 1983

Index

Page numbers followed by f denote figures; page numbers followed by t denote tables